D0646361

Memory, Amnesia, and the Hippocampal System

Memory, Amnesia, and the Hippocampal System

Neal J. Cohen and Howard Eichenbaum

A Bradford Book
The MIT Press
Cambridge, Massachusetts
London, England

This book was set in Trump by DEKR Corporation and was printed and
bound in the United States of America.

Library of Congress Cataloging-in-Publication Data

Cohen, Neal J.
    Memory, amnesia, and the hippocampal system / Neal J. Cohen and
Howard Eichenbaum.
        p.   cm.
    "A Bradford book."
    Includes bibliographical references and index.
    ISBN 0-262-03203-1
    1. Memory—Physiological aspects. 2. Animal memory—Physiological
aspects. 3. Amnesia—Physiological aspects. 4. Amnesia—Animal
models. 5. Hippocampus (Brain) 6. Recollection (Psychology)—
Physiological aspects. I. Eichenbaum, Howard. II. Title.
    QP406.C64   1993
    612.8'2—dc20   92-27982
                                                              CIP

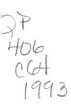

To Maureen, my wife and partner in crime for lo these many years; to my parents, Albert and Natalie Cohen; and to cousin Sheila, for her remarkable courage and amazingly good grace.
N.J.C.

To my parents Victor and Edith Eichenbaum for teaching me that there are at least two ways to look at absolutely anything (although I don't recollect them mentioning memory as one of those things), and to my family—Karen, Alex, and Adam—for my best declarative memories.
H.B.E.

Contents

12 Comparing the Theory to Other Accounts: Human Amnesia   271

13 On the Functional Role of the Hippocampal System in Memory   285

Preface

This book is for students of memory who are interested in cognitive, neuropsychological, or neuroscientific bases of memory, or, better yet, the convergence of all three. The book arose directly out of a challenge from H.B.E. to N.J.C. a little more than ten years ago. Well, actually, the beginnings of this project lie in the housing situation that got us together one day in Boston, but that sounds like another book. The nature of the challenge was that if the hippocampal system *really* played the role in memory that N.J.C. had just proposed in his thesis work with Larry Squire on human amnesia—mediating declarative memory, operating independently of procedural memory—then it should be the case that *rats* with hippocampal-system damage would show a parallel pattern of impairment and sparing of memory functions if tested with the kind of stimuli about which normal rats learn rapidly, namely odors. The point was that to really understand memory, amnesia, and the hippocampal system it would be very important to bring the cognitive and neuropsychological work on humans together with the behavioral, neuroanatomical, and neurophysiological work on animals.

We took on that challenge by putting the notion to a particularly tough test. We proposed to teach rats about some odors and then assess their retention on a test of reversal learning on which, given the claims of the theoretical view that N.J.C. had offered, hippocampal system damage should produce *better-than-normal performance*, in contrast to the literature on animal models of amnesia to that point. Indeed this was just the result observed.

This success convinced us to take on the larger challenge, that of seeking and taking advantage of convergences among the lines of evidence forthcoming from cognitive psychology, cognitive science, neuropsychology, cognitive neuroscience, and the neurosciences about memory, amnesia, and the hippocampal system. We embarked a systematic program of collaborative work on the idea of corresponding memory mechanisms in humans and rodents, supported by the National Science Foundation and, in the earlier stages, by the Sloan Foundation. What was required in order to really work simultaneously on humans and rodents was an articulation of the functional role of the hippocampal system in memory, and of the nature of the memory impairment in amnesia, that would permit experimental predictions for studies performed on any species and that would permit us to make contact with and contribute to work ranging from cognitive processes to neural mechanisms.

About two years ago we realized that the theoretical work we had to do to permit our own dialogue, and the dialogue among the different areas we were trying to synthesize, together with the results we had obtained in our collaborative work permitted us to offer a comprehensive accounting of memory systems in normal and amnesic performances across species. Taking advantage of a leave that N.J.C. was able to take at Wellesley College—resulting in the first and only time during our collaboration that we were actually able to physically work together for any extended period of time—we set out to put these ideas down in a review paper. As sometimes happens in such situations, the thing got out of control and became, with work over the past two years, the present book.

Each of us would like to thank a large number of colleagues with whom we have had multiple discussions over the years about issues of concern to this book, and whose ideas have influenced our own. To name all of them individually, however, would exceed the space we have been allotted. The best way we know to thank them is to endeavor to represent in the book as fairly as we are able their views and contributions to the field, although we cannot promise that they will agree with the final conclusions we offer.

Special thanks are owed to several people for guidance, encouragement, support, and other kind acts that have been extended to one or both of us, and for continued dialogue over the years with one or both of us: David Amaral, Sue Corkin, John Gabrieli, Michela Gallagher, Bill Greenough, Jim McGaugh, Richard Morris, David Olton, Tim Otto, Pat Goldman-Rakic, Jim Ranck, Matt Shapiro, and Larry Squire. There are some people, in addition to those above, with whom one or both of us has collaborated directly in studying

memory and amnesia, and who have contributed to our work: Jay
Buckingham, Anne Fagan, Carol Ann Paul, Harvey Sagar, Edie Sul-
livan, Cindy Wible, Sid Wiener, and Stuart Zola-Morgan.

N.J.C. would, in addition, like to express his deep gratitude to
Larry Squire and to Suzanne Corkin for providing him early in his
career with an opportunity to work on issues of memory and amnesia, and with an environment in which that work could thrive,
and for teaching him much; to John Gabrieli for his friendship and
his expertise in matters central to this book; to Manny Donchin,
Bill Greenough, and a remarkable collection of colleagues in the
Psychology Department and the Beckman Institute at the University of Illinois, who have collectively provided an ideal environment
in which to bring this work to fruition; to Jeff Corwin for support,
encouragement, and friendship at critical times in this project; and
to Ralph, Cary, and Chuck at Champagne Audio who, through the
wonders of high-end audio, have been instrumental in maintaining
the sanity of this author during the period in which the book was
being written.

H.B.E. would like to express his gratitude for the mentoring and
support of Charlie Butter, Bernie Agranoff, and Steve Chorover, and
Fote Macrides during his successive stages of training. Making time
for research behind the ideas presented here was not easy while at
Wellesley College, whose primary mission is first-class undergrad-
uate teaching. So a considerable debt is owed to those who made
that time possible, in particular, Mary Coyne, Carol Ann Paul, and
a whole lot of very bright young students. This author also wishes
to express gratitude particularly to Richard Morris, who created a
sabbatical environment in which many ideas expressed here came
together, and to Michela Gallagher for creating the productive environment of a combined laboratory in Chapel Hill; both are
thanked as well for listening endlessly to and challenging some of
the ideas expressed here.

In the end, each of us owes the other the greatest intellectual
debt for stimulating, challenging, and refining the ideas in this book.
This project has been a truly collaborative effort in its most productive and rewarding sense. And it has been great fun.

We would like to acknowledge the very able and (under the circumstances) remarkably cheerful assistance of Linda May for her
help with references and figures for the book. Amy Marks did a

great job of researching and summarizing literature relevant to this book, and of working on figures to use in the book. Thanks to Violet Pogorzelski for help with indexing. Matthew Shapiro, Brian Ross, Russ Poldrack, and Scott Selco offered helpful suggestions on various chapters. Fiona Stevens and Katherine Arnoldi, our editors at MIT Press, have been wonderful; we thank them for shepherding this book, and us, through this process.

Finally, we wish to thank our wives, Maureen and Karen, for refusing to allow the task of putting this book together to get in the way of our marriages and of our friendship. The usual difficulties of writing a collaborative book were magnified by the fact that the two authors have lived in two different parts of the country throughout the time they have been collaborating and have each moved to yet different parts of the country during the course of writing the book. But, it has been our great good fortune to have both a professional relationship and a friendship that has lasted all these years despite the distance, and that continues to bring our two families together. The writing of this book is in many ways a celebration of both.

Funding for our work together has come from several sources that we would like to acknowledge. Main support for direct collaboration came from the National Science Foundation for the project entitled "Corresponding memory mechanisms in humans and animals." Support for the early stages of the collaboration, during which we did much of the conceptual work in attempting to bring together the different relevant literatures and levels of analysis, came from a grant to N.J.C. from the Sloan Foundation. In addition, support from the U.S. Public Health Service and Office of Naval Research to H.B.E. for continued behavioral investigations on declarative memory in animals and for research described in the book involving single neuron recording in the hippocampal system of behaving animals has been very helpful. Finally, funds from Johns Hopkins University to N.J.C., and funds from Wellesley College and a British Council grant to R.G.M. Morris for H.B.E.'s sabbatical period made an additional contribution.

Memory, Amnesia, and the
Hippocampal System

1 Introduction

The question of how we learn, remember, and forget has long been the subject of much speculation. Considering how importantly the successes and failures of our memory abilities affect our lives, this interest seems eminently justified. We depend on our memories for so much of what we do, such as whenever we are engaged in identifying, appreciating, and responding appropriately to the objects and persons we encounter in our environment and to the events in which we participate; in speaking, reading, writing, or otherwise communicating; in thinking, reasoning, and problem solving; and in reminiscing about our experiences. It is our memory that holds, and permits us to use, the knowledge we have acquired about ourselves and the world and that captures the ways in which we have adapted to the world so as to better cope with it. So much do we depend on our memory that we have become mostly unaware of its constant contributions, other than to appreciate the pleasant memories that are sometimes triggered by an idle thought or some outside prompt, or to curse the occasional inability to retrieve some particular name or word on demand.

Within the scientific arena, too, memory has aroused very considerable interest and is the subject of an enormous, and ever rapidly increasing, body of research. The research has addressed questions about the structure and organization of memory and about memory's neural substrates—What is the nature of memory? How does it work? How is it instantiated in the brain? This has been the goal of work in several different scientific disciplines, including neuroscience, neuropsychology, psychology, and cognitive science. Although these disciplines share common overall goals, and there are any number of scientists who move across disciplinary boundaries, the disciplines differ from one another substantially in regard to the specific questions about memory that they take to be interesting, and, given the research techniques available to them, that they take to be amenable to empirical inquiry.

In neuroscience, for example, research on learning and memory has been conducted largely within the context of plasticity. The goal of this work has been to characterize the way in which the brain is itself modified by—and thereby supports a lasting representation of—experience. This research aims to identify the plastic changes that occur in brain physiology and anatomy during behavioral learning and memory; it seeks to characterize the nature of the plasticity exhibited at each of several different levels of organization of the nervous system. The questions posed by this work span at least the following levels: Which brain systems are capable of plasticity and are involved in the expression of plasticity? What are the synaptic events that constitute plasticity within the participating brain systems, i.e., that code experience and mediate the storage of memory in those systems? What are the physiological mechanisms of plastic change that give rise to the observed synaptic events?

Research efforts in the cognitive sciences, by contrast, have been concerned with understanding the nature of memory representation and of the cognitive processes that act on them in mediating learning and memory performance. Among the questions posed by such work are the following two: How do we characterize the distinct stages of processing involved in the initial encoding and acquisition of memories, the storage and maintenance of memories, and the subsequent retrieval and expression of memories? Are there functionally distinct types or forms of learning and memory, reflecting functionally separable component processes or systems?

The fact that memory research is proceeding in so many different scientific disciplines, across various levels of analysis, is very encouraging to those who, like us, feel that gaining insight into how experiences can modify our brains and thereby shape our behaviors is critical for a fuller understanding of the human condition. However, there is another, much less salutary, result of this state of affairs: Work on learning and memory is divided among the different disciplines in such a way as to make it difficult for the ideas and theories within a given discipline and at a given level of analysis to be enriched and *tested* by work in other disciplines or at other levels. As a consequence, all too often theories are offered about the nature of memory representation and the cognitive processes operating on them without any regard paid to the question of whether such representations and processes could plausibly or even conceivably be instantiated by the hardware of the brain. Likewise, all too often neurobiological mechanisms are "identified" as candidate brain substrates of memory without any evidence about their actual functional significance.

The ideas described in the present book are guided by the principle that *if we want to understand the nature of memory as actually instantiated in human brains, we must take into account—and provide an account of—both behavioral performance data and facts about the constraints imposed by the hardware of the brain.* We believe, and endeavor to show in this book, that the time is ripe for bringing together the developments and insights forthcoming from various disciplines involved in memory research. It is our intention to demonstrate that a convergence of findings and ideas from various disciplines provides the critical clues and constraints for the development of a more comprehensive *cognitive neuroscience* understanding of memory.

Perhaps a few words are in order here about the notion of convergence and constraints, in advance of formally making our case. Of the ways in which a memory device could be organized to exhibit the functionalities of human memory, that is, of the ways in which memory could, in principle, be structured to solve the problem of producing the range of human memory performances, only the solution that is actually instantiated in human brains is of interest to us. Surely the brain hardware that as a result of the evolutionary process has come to mediate human memory performances is constrained in the functionalities it can now conceivably support. And, just as surely, to the extent that an understanding of this hardware offers any insights at all about constraints on the functionalities it can and cannot support, theories of memory would profit by taking such constraints into account.

Let us consider a brief example here. There are any number of ways in which a visual processing system *could* be organized; and, indeed, several very different plans have appeared in nature. Insects have compound or mosaic eyes made up of many ommatidia, each with its own lens and light-sensitive cells. Eyes of this design cannot form a simple, single image, but instead produce a mosaic image in which there is represented the contribution from each of the separate ommatidia simultaneously. Vertebrates, by contrast, have a camera-like eye in which a lens system produces a sharp, *single* image on a light-sensitive retina, and a set of muscles that move the eye and that regulate the size and shape of the lens and pupil to permit the focusing of images under an enormous range of different viewing distances and lighting conditions. The radical differences in design of these two types of eye give rise to differences in the specific functionalities each can now support. The compound eyes of insects are particularly well suited for detecting motion, because any moving object will be seen to move across the many ommatidia comprising the mosaic image. The type of eye that we possess, given its overall design, is particularly suited for clarity, sensitivity, and acuity of vision.

A further comparison between different visual systems, this time between that of the frog and that of primates, is likewise instructive. The brain of the frog has no neocortex with which to accomplish higher-order visual processing. Its highest visual processor is in the midbrain and corresponds to the human superior colliculus, a structure that is critical for localizing objects in space. In the absence of any higher brain systems for accomplishing sophisticated visual processing, the functionalities of the frog's visual system are closely tied to the spatial localization properties of the midbrain processor, and also on certain parallel specializations of the frog's retina, which performs considerably more sophisticated analyses than does the retina of humans. The result is a visual system that is superbly suited for detecting and guiding the tongue to potential prey—"bug detection." But the hardware of the frog's visual system, no matter how successful at its specialty, just cannot accomplish the various computations that can be performed upon visual input by the human neocortex. As a result of the development in humans (and mammals in general) of multiple highly specialized visual processors implemented in neocortical neural networks, each capable of integrating and performing transformations on multiple inputs, we have developed various visual capacities that go beyond the capabilities of the frog, including far greater visual acuity, depth perception, and visual memory.

The point is that the particular hardware configuration that has evolved for supporting visual processing in a particular species determines the range of functionalities it can support. The computations and algorithms that can now be performed by the human visual system is determined by the currently existing hardware configuration. It seems evident that knowing more about that hardware and its functional constraints would be helpful in developing a full account of the *functional architecture* of human vision. So, too, is it the case for memory.

But what about moving across levels or disciplines in the other direction? Neuroscientists who, on the basis of their research on the neural substrates of memory (e.g., the brain systems mediating memory), have drawn inferences about the *functional architecture* of memory (e.g., the functional role played by particular brain systems) would certainly benefit from knowledge of the functional properties of human memory. It stands to reason that knowledge about the functionalities actually exhibited by human memory would be useful for efforts to ascribe particular memory functions to specific brain systems or neural mechanisms. Much of our knowledge about the functionalities exhibited by human memory necessarily comes from cognitive-level analyses of behavioral performances.

This idea about constraints and convergence may be controversial to some cognitive scientists and some neuroscientists alike, or at least to that subset whose commitment to the independence of their own level of analysis might cause them to deny the potential relevance to their own work of investigations framed at other levels. What we are asserting here, by contrast, is that findings and ideas from different disciplines can inform, enrich, and provide constraints on work conducted in other related disciplines. This is certainly the trend of *cognitive neuroscience*, an emerging discipline that holds the promise of providing a more complete understanding of learning and memory (or perception, attention, etc.) and that is capable of bridging the different levels of analysis without in any way rejecting the contributions to be made from any of the individual disciplines. Indeed, the point is precisely that each of the separate disciplines, or different levels of analysis, has much to offer the others. We see the trend of making use of the contributions of the different levels in articulating more comprehensive accounts as both eminently reasonable and thoroughly inevitable.

Daniel Dennett's (1984) notion of "cognitive wheels" seems particularly germane at this juncture. Hopefully he will forgive us for whatever liberties we take in the treatment of that idea we offer here. Dennett noted that engineers charged with solving the problem of land locomotion are drawn inexorably to the wheel. That is, they would undoubtedly design vehicles with various combinations of wheels. The wheel provides such an elegant solution to the problem of land locomotion, in fact, that those unschooled in biology might assume that wheels must no doubt be found in nature, too. Surely, if wheels truly provide such an elegant solution, then one would expect that nature, in her infinite wisdom, would have bestowed wheels on any number of the creatures whose habitat requires land locomotion; or, more scientifically, having wheel-like adaptations for land locomotion would provide such a strong advantage that they would be selected for and hence emerge in the course of evolution.

But, of course, as soon as one actually turns to biology, it becomes apparent that wheels do not exist anywhere in nature. Because of various hardware and competing-function constraints, and the fact that nature does not have the engineer's luxury of designing from scratch (nature, unlike the typical engineer, must build new structure on top of preexisting structure), wheel-based solutions to land locomotion have never developed in the course of evolution. A purely functional analysis of design considerations, by itself, would seem to provide rather little insight into biological solutions to real-world locomotion demands, in this case at least.

Dennett worries that the same may be true of at least some of the purely functional accounts offered in cognitive science. That is, for at least some of the accounts, the specific cognitive processes or systems proposed to support particular types of performance may constitute the same sort of elegant engineering solution that is as unknown (or unavailable) to nature—hence, cognitive wheels.

Accordingly, it seems prudent to begin to look carefully at the brain, to ascertain whether or not brain systems exist that actually possess the machinery and the anatomical connections needed to perform the computations and support the functionalities proposed. To the extent that a particular functional/cognitive account both provides an elegant solution to the behavioral phenomena of interest and also conforms with neuroscientific facts about particular brain regions, the concern about cognitive wheels is considerably mitigated, and the goal of mapping the functional architecture of cognition onto the neural architecture of the brain comes closer to being realized.

All of this, so far, is just a promissory note. The rest of the present book can be construed as our effort to cash it in. We endeavor to demonstrate that a more complete understanding of learning and memory is now possible by appreciating *and providing an account of* the convergence of findings from across different disciplines. The scope of the findings to be incorporated here includes issues about the nature of memory impairments exhibited in amnesia, about the functional role played by the hippocampal system (the hippocampus and related structures in the medial temporal-lobe region of the brain, as shown in figures 1.1 and 1.2, below), and about the componential structure of normal memory. (Readers interested in getting to know the anatomy may want to jump ahead to chapter 4.) It is this set of issues about memory, amnesia, and the hippocampal system—issues that lie at the intersection of the neuropsychological, neuroscientific, and cognitive levels of analysis of memory—that constitutes the subject of the present book. We offer here an explication of a theory of memory capable of accounting for a large set of seemingly unrelated findings taken from these different disciplines, a theory that emerges from the mutual constraints provided by the different findings.

SCOPE OF THE PRESENT ACCOUNT

The major findings that constitute the scope of the account offered here can be summarized by the following six points:

1. Damage to the hippocampal system in humans can cause an impairment of long-term memory called *amnesia* that, despite resulting in a severe, pervasive deficit in storing and/or using the "data" ordinarily acquired as the outcome of one's learning experiences, leaves intact the capacity for acquisition and expression of skilled performance. Somehow such patients can learn new skills normally and show other experience-dependent modifications of skilled performance without being able to explicitly remember their training experiences, and without any sense of familiarity for the materials they have encountered.

This finding is the starting point for this book, and much space is devoted to seeking an understanding of the phenomenon and of its implications about the organization of normal memory. But, in seeking an explanation, the following five other findings are discussed and incorporated into our comprehensive theory.

2. In normal subjects, too, there is a dissociation between explicit remembering of new facts or events and the acquisition and expression of skilled performance. Learning and expressing skilled performance with a given set of stimulus materials can proceed independently of explicit remembering of the materials: Different variables influence skilled performance and explicit remembering; and there are circumstances in which skilled performance is no more or less likely to be exhibited for materials that a subject can recognize as having previously occurred than for materials that the subject fails to recognize, even when his or her recognition memory ability is excellent.

3. Damage to the hippocampal system in rodents and nonhuman primates also produces an amnesia that exhibits selectivity in the aspects of memory that are impaired. Such animals show impairments in learning and remembering of spatial relations among environmental cues, configurations of multiple perceptually independent cues, contextual or conditional relations, and comparisons among temporally discontinuous events. They are impaired when information learned in a given context must be expressed in or related to novel contexts. Yet the same animals can show normal learning and remembering of a large variety of conditioning, discrimination, and skill tasks.

4. The hippocampal system receives inputs from, and in return projects to, the neocortical brain regions that serve as the highest-order processors of the various categories and modalities of information handled by the brain. Thus, the anatomical connections of the hippocampal system place it in a privileged position to receive the outcomes of processing of the brain's various processing modules, and to relate them.

5. The activity of neurons in the hippocampus of awake, behaving animals is responsive to relationships among significant cues or objects in the environment. In rats who are actively exploring their environment, many hippocampal neurons are found to have "place fields"—each of these neurons fires preferentially when the animal

is in one or another specific "place" in the environment, providing a physiological parallel to the spatial learning deficit seen in rats with damage to the hippocampal system. When the same rats are engaged in olfactory discrimination learning, however, the same neurons are sensitive to other relationships, such as the conjunction of particular odors and particular odor-delivery ports, or particular temporal orders of the olfactory stimuli. Thus, just as damage to the hippocampal system produces a deficit in learning of both spatial and various nonspatial relations, so activity of hippocampal neurons reflects the coding of both spatial and nonspatial relations.

6. The hippocampal system supports a particularly robust form of synaptic plasticity called long-term potentiation (LTP), in which brief patterned activation of particular pathways, especially by converging inputs arriving in close temporal contiguity, produces a stable increase in synaptic efficacy lasting for hours to weeks. The conditions for invoking this mechanism of plasticity, and its characteristics, suggest a mechanism for handling memory for conjunctions.

Each of these major findings will be elaborated and discussed in the ensuing chapters, emphasizing particularly the behavioral phenomena indicated in (1), (2), and (3). All six of these major findings will be explained by and used to support a theory of memory and amnesia that assigns to the hippocampal system a critical role in one particular kind of memory called *declarative memory*. The theory gives a descriptive account of the nature and characteristics of declarative memory, and the way in which the representations it supports give rise to a particular class of memory performances.

OUTLINE OF THE BOOK

We begin with the amnesia findings. The remainder of this chapter provides a brief introduction to amnesia and considers why studying disorders of memory offers illumination about the organization of *normal* memory. In chapter 2, we discuss the phenomena suggesting the selective nature of amnesia and introduce the idea behind, and the initial difficulties encountered in, trying to develop animal models of amnesia in rodents and nonhuman primates. We argue strongly that a theory of memory, amnesia, and the hippocampal system will have to account for data from both the human and animal literatures; starting in chapter 3, we offer just such a comprehensive account.

Anatomical and physiological considerations about the hippocampal system, of which findings (4), (5), and (6) considered above are illustrative, are discussed in chapters 4 and 5. The way in which these findings converge with the behavioral data and are accommodated by our comprehensive theory of memory and amnesia is discussed.

In an effort to present the theory itself as clearly and completely as possible, we have taken the tack of presenting it in several ways: First, we present the theory formally in chapter 3, defining and describing the characteristics of the proposed *declarative* and *procedural* memory systems. Second, to communicate how the theory works, we then apply it to and show how it accounts for and is supported by the major behavioral, anatomical, and physiological data (chapters 4 to 9). Particular emphasis is placed, in chapters 6 to 9, on evaluating the fit of the theory to the behavioral outcome of hippocampal system damage for each of the major paradigms in both the human amnesia and animal models literatures. Another way to present a theory is to articulate how it might be tested; accordingly, chapter 10 considers exactly what kinds of experiments and data would provide critical tests of the theory. The last way in which the theory is presented, in chapters 11 and 12, is by comparing it to and distinguishing it from other treatments of memory and amnesia in the literature.

The book concludes with a final chapter (chapter 13) that speculates more generally about the functional role of the hippocampal system in memory. Here we attempt to move beyond our theory of the type of memory or representation that the hippocampal system supports to consider the place it occupies (functionally speaking) in the overall machinery of memory processing. We do so by offering a tentative description of how the hippocampal system is engaged by a single learning event, and how it interacts with other brain systems in supporting declarative-memory–based remembering.

STUDYING AMNESIA AS A WAY OF UNDERSTANDING NORMAL MEMORY

Center stage is given in this book to findings from studies of amnesia. But what exactly *is* amnesia? And what exactly can study of the memory impairments seen in amnesic patients, or in animals with damage to the brain regions, tell us about the nature and organization of *normal* memory? The remainder of this chapter attempts to provide an answer to these two questions.

Memory impairment occurs in a variety of individuals in the context of certain neurological and psychiatric conditions. It is typically associated with other motor, perceptual, or cognitive deficits, as occurs in the dementias (most notably in Alzheimer's disease, Parkinson's disease, and Huntington's disease), in many examples of severe brain trauma, in depressive illness, and in drug-altered stages. Occasionally, however, memory impairment occurs in striking isolation from other deficits. When circumscribed memory impairment occurs following some instance of brain insult, it offers the opportunity to study the role ordinarily played in memory by the affected brain structures. To see how this is possible, we begin by introducing the patient known as H.M.

An Example of Amnesia: Patient H.M.

The case most often cited as exemplifying amnesia is the patient H.M. (e.g., Corkin, 1984; Milner, Corkin, & Teuber, 1968; Scoville & Milner, 1957). In 1953, at the age of 27, this man underwent resection of hippocampal-system structures bilaterally (figures 1.1, 1.2), in an experimental surgical procedure designed to relieve what was an otherwise medically intractable seizure disorder. He had been suffering both major and minor epileptic seizures since the age of 16, and by the age of 27 it was clear that even massive doses of anticonvulsant medications were ineffective in controlling his seizure disorder. The surgery succeeded in reducing the severity of his seizure disorder; it became, and has to this day remained, relatively well controlled by medication. However, the surgery also produced a severe and pervasive disorder of learning and memory, which has also remained to the present day. He has an impairment both in the ability to acquire and retain new material across a delay (anterograde amnesia [AA]) and in the ability to make use of some premorbid material acquired normally before the onset of amnesia (retrograde amnesia [RA]).

To the researchers who have studied H.M., including ourselves, it appears that his amnesia has resulted in what Scoville and Milner (1957) described as "forgetting of the events of daily life as quickly

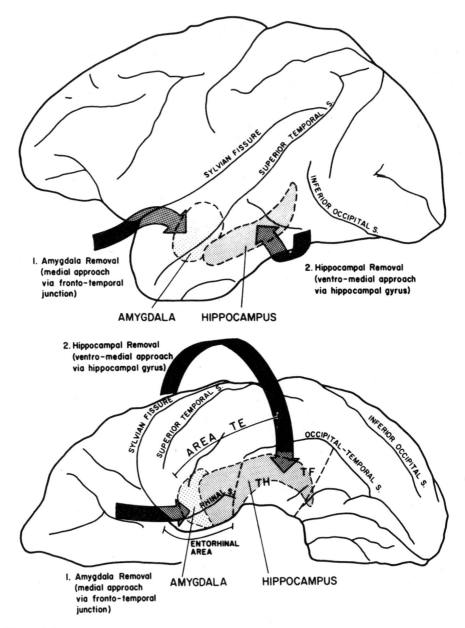

Figure 1.1
Schematic lateral (*top*) and ventral (*bottom*) views of the left hemisphere of the monkey brain illustrating the anatomical location of hippocampal system structures. The figure indicates an anatomical approach to these structures used in work by Squire and Zola-Morgan to produce amnesia in monkeys. (From Squire & Zola-Morgan, 1983.)

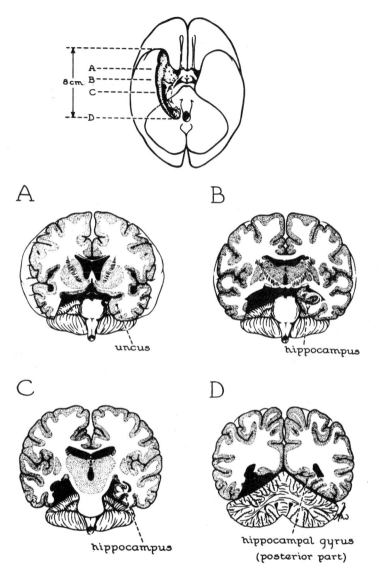

A

B

uncus

hippocampus

C

D

hippocampus

hippocampal gyrus
(posterior part)

Figure 1.2
Schematic of surgeon's estimate of the extent of hippocampal system removal in the patient H.M. Illustrated is the extent of removal on one side
of the brain at four cross-sectional levels (A, B, C, and D) along the anterior-
posterior extent of the brain shown at the top. Although the surgical
removal was bilateral, one side of the brain is shown intact for illustrative
purposes. (From Scoville and Milner, 1957.)

as they occur." Now, nearly 40 years after his surgery, H.M. does not know his age or the current date; does not know where he is living; does not know the current status of his parents (who are long deceased); and does not know his own history since his high school years, many years prior to the surgery in 1953. The sheer severity of his deficit cannot be minimized. He has consistently scored at literally chance levels on nearly every, even very sensitive, test of recognition memory ever administered to him when there was a significant delay interposed between study and test. The only real exception to this is on the test of recognition memory for colorful scenic slides administered by Freed, Corkin, and Cohen (1987), on which H.M.'s performance was at well above chance levels despite considerable delay intervals. But, this performance was the consequence of a special procedure in which he received 20 *times* the normal study time for each slide to compensate for his deficit; when given the normal amount of study time, he performs at chance levels on this task as well.

Despite the severity and pervasiveness of H.M.'s impairment, however, many other abilities were left intact. The surgery produced no known deficits in (non-mnemonic) cognitive, perceptual, or motor capacities.[1] Neuropsychological testing has repeatedly shown that his deficit was limited to the domain of memory. An unsuspecting person (without neuropsychological training) meeting H.M. for the first time would be hard pressed to note anything wrong. He or she might notice that H.M.'s conversation was devoid of any information about current events, or might be struck by the repetition of certain topics and stories in H.M.'s discourse. More likely, the impairment would become apparent to the observer only if his or her interaction with H.M. were interrupted for a period—upon subsequent continuation of the interaction it would become clear that H.M. can neither remember the earlier interaction nor, more than likely, even remember having ever met the person.

H.M.'s deficit is thus seen as being specific to the domain of memory. More interesting for the issues of concern in the present book, however, is its specificity to particular domains *within* memory. The anterograde deficit affects long-term memory but not working (or short-term) memory; thus, H.M. can keep track of a conversation, of his train of thought, and of whatever material he is currently "working on," as long as he keeps it active. His retrograde deficit is also restricted, affecting his memories for as many as 11 years prior to the surgery, but not for more remote memories; thus H.M. can remember his childhood experiences and the world knowledge he acquired early in his life (e.g., Corkin 1984; Sagar, Cohen, Corkin, & Growdon, 1985).

But the real surprise regarding the specificity of H.M.'s amnesia is the discovery that the anterograde deficit, while preventing him from storing and/or using the data usually acquired as the outcome of one's learning experiences, nonetheless leaves *intact* the ability to acquire and express skilled performance based on these same experiences. It is this aspect of selectivity that is most central to the issues of concern in the present book.

It must be understood that the specificity of amnesia described above is by no means limited to H.M. A like pattern of sparing and loss of memory is observed in any number of other patients who have sustained insult to the hippocampal system. Some introduction to these other examples of amnesia following hippocampal-system damage, as well as the amnesias associated with damage to different brain systems, is provided in chapter 2.

Understanding Normal Memory

But what does all this have to do with *normal* memory? Until fairly recently, many researchers interested in the organization of human memory felt that normal memory was hard enough to understand without having to also figure out how memory breaks down after brain damage. It turns out, however, that the study of amnesia can, and indeed has, contributed significantly to our current understanding of normal memory. By studying the specific patterns of memory impairment that occur after damage to critical brain regions—that is, by characterizing the *systematic* dissociations between the categories of impaired versus spared performances—we may draw inferences about the component cognitive processes that mediate these categories of performance in patients and normal subjects alike. Thus, observing the dissociations noted above we pose the question, *How must normal memory be organized in order for these particular patterns of behavioral performance to ever occur?*

What we want to know in the present context is just what the structure of memory must be in order for it to be possible to acquire skills across training sessions without being able to actually remember those experiences explicitly. The answer that seems most compelling, and that is at the heart of the cognitive neuropsychological approach in general, is that this behavioral dissociation reflects a selective disruption of particular component systems of memory, or memory subsystems, leaving other component memory systems or memory subsystems unaffected. The claim, then, is that hippocampal system damage (like certain other instances of brain insult) produces a fractionation of memory into its (impaired versus spared) component systems, thereby revealing the functionally distinct contributions each of these subsystems make to normal memory.

This approach has been applied particularly successfully in recent years to the study of such other cognitive domains as language, attention, and visual perception, as nicely documented by Coltheart (1985), Caramazza (1986), Shallice (1988), McCarthy and Warrington (1990), Posner et al (1987), and Farah (1990), to name just a few. Reports of neuropsychological studies of specific cognitive impairments now regularly grace the pages of many of the standard cognitive journals and, because of how such work informs theories of normal cognition, even those cognitive journals that were until very recently the exclusive province of work on normal subjects.

Two fundamental lessons about normal memory come from studying amnesia, it seems to us. First is that memory is a big word, encompassing a host of different capacities mediated by functionally distinct components or subsystems that collectively produce the performances we call memory. Second is that amnesia provides a particularly effective tool for studying the subsystems of memory. Ordinarily, the various component systems operate in concert seamlessly in producing memory performance. But damage to brain regions such as the hippocampal system permits aspects of the componential or modular structure of memory to be revealed.

The major thesis articulated in the present book is that the hippocampal system is responsible for mediating one of the brain's component memory systems, the declarative memory system, that supports a particular class of memory performances. When this system is damaged in amnesia, that class of memory performances dependent on its special contribution are profoundly compromised. Other memory systems of the brain, including the procedural memory system, operate independently of the hippocampal system, support different classes of memory performances, and are unaffected in hippocampal amnesia.

Bringing Together Studies of Normal Subjects with Studies of Amnesic Patients

If the inferences we draw about the organization of normal memory from study of amnesia are correct, then it should—at least in principle—be possible to design tests that would reveal the operation of functionally dissociable components or modules in normal subjects as well. Happily, there is now abundant evidence that this is indeed the case. Some of this evidence, and its implications for the multiple memory system theory we offer here, will be discussed at length in chapters 8 and 12.

Memory and Brain

Investigations of amnesia permit study of the relationship between brain and cognitive processes. To the extent that damage to particular brain regions is systematically related to disruption of specific component memory systems, then the neuropsychological study of amnesia permits the mapping of the functional organization of memory onto the neuroanatomical architecture of the brain. The fact that damage to the hippocampal system reliably produces impairment of the declarative memory system ties this brain system to a particular set of memory processes. Evidence for this linkage converges with the anatomical and physiological data about the hippocampal system that we bring to bear on our characterization of its role in declarative-memory–based remembering in chapters 4, 5, and 13.

WHAT THIS BOOK IS *NOT* ABOUT

Having given some idea of the ground to be covered in this book, it seems important to be clear about what is *not* going to be included in our exposition. The discussion of memory, amnesia, and the hippocampal system will focus on the areas where several different research strategies overlap and converge. Accordingly, much superb research being done within each of the individual strategies, which was not squarely in the area of overlap, had to be left out. For example, many of the questions guiding research in the cognitive literature on learning and memory is just not amenable at this time to either neuropsychological or neuroscientific analysis, and hence plays little role in the synthesis we offer here. Likewise much work on molecular mechanisms of plasticity has no convergent agenda in the cognitive or neuropsychological arena as of yet, and thus receives scant attention here.

Our treatment of the literature on the anatomy and physiology of memory and the hippocampal system will be highly selective. Considerable progress has been made in outlining the details of connectional pathways and topographical organizations of the relevant circuits, as well as the fundamental physiological properties of the participating neurons. However, many of the specific findings go beyond the level of detail that can be incorporated usefully into an account of the functional role of the hippocampal system in memory. Thus we have abstracted only the general principles and functional implications of the anatomical and physiological data that intersect with and speak directly to the hypotheses we offer about memory function. In these sections of the book we cite several excellent reviews that provide more comprehensive accounts of anatomical and physiological detail.

Within the area of the neuropsychology of memory, we have had to be selective, too. First, we have limited our scope to the particular types of memory impairment that are called amnesia. Other types of memory impairment occur in neuropsychological populations currently being studied intensively and productively by various investigators that have no bearing on the particular issues of concern here. Thus, for example, work on impairments of either the brain's knowledge systems (such as those supporting language, object recognition and other perceptual abilities, or motor programming) or the brain's working memory systems (supporting the on-line comprehension of the world and selection of appropriate responses)—both of which are quite intact in H.M. and similar amnesic patients of interest here—is necessarily outside the scope of this book. The reader interested in these neuropsychological issues is encouraged to look at the volumes by McCarthy and Warrington (1990), Shallice (1988), Farah (1990), Vallar and Shallice (1990), Humphreys and Riddoch (1987a, b), and Ellis and Young (1988), among others.

Second, even for the examples of memory impairment on which we focus here, there is much neuropsychological work whose research agendas are outside the current scope of concern. For example, there are excellent studies of amnesia that deal with the agenda of clinical classification, concerned with describing the precise nature of memory impairment associated with particular etiologies of amnesia, such as that exhibited by patients with Korsakoff's disease compared to various dementing illnesses (e.g., Butters & Miliotis, 1985; Corkin, 1982; Gabrieli, 1991; Heindel et al., 1989). Other work has focused on issues concerned with the neuroanatomy of amnesia, inquiring about the relative contributions made by damage to different structures within the hippocampal system in producing amnesia, or about the contributions to amnesia made by additional damage to various cortical areas or subcortical nuclei (e.g., Damasio et al, 1985; Moscovitch, 1984; Squire, 1987). As much as these research agendas contribute to our understanding of memory and the brain, they are not central to the issue of the specific role that the hippocampal system plays in normal memory and amnesia, and hence they receive scant attention here.[2]

Finally, this book will not offer a quantitative, computational model of hippocampal function. That is, it does not attempt to model *how* the hippocampal system performs its functional role in terms of specific mechanisms. For example, although we shall discuss notions about the possible contribution of the hippocampal system to memory consolidation processes in chapter 13, it will offer neither a detailed account of the mechanisms by which consolidation might be achieved nor a comprehensive review of the supporting evidence. Rather, the book offers a high-level theory of the *nature* of the hippocampal system's functional role, expressed in terms of the type of representations it mediates, of the characteristics of hippocampal-mediated representations, and of the nature of the memory performances that are supported by them. Such a high-level description would seem a necessary component of, if not actually a prerequisite for, attempts to produce quantitative, computational models of "hippocampal function." Any attempt to produce such a model must have some clear answer to the question "In service of what specific functionality do the hippocampal-system mechanisms that are being modeled actually operate?" The present book offers the most detailed description to date of that functionality.

2 Toward an Account of Amnesia in Human Patients and Animal Models: Taking Care of the Preliminaries

The goal we have articulated for the present book is to offer a comprehensive theory of the relationship between memory, amnesia, and the hippocampal system, that, while starting with the remarkable findings from human amnesic patients, goes well beyond human neuropsychology to incorporate converging findings from animal models of amnesia, from anatomical and physiological studies of the hippocampal system, and from studies of normal memory. Each of these areas of research has provided findings of importance to the theory we will develop here. Research on the neuropsychology of memory, at least as much as any other field in neuroscience or cognitive neuroscience, is filled with seeming contradictions in the findings, both within and across species, and with controversies in the interpretations of these findings. What follows, then, is an outline of the sets of findings and theoretical controversies for which an accounting must be offered before we can move on, as well as some indication of those that will not bear importantly on our agenda. This chapter starts it off with discussion of animal models of amnesia.

ANIMAL MODELS: WHY AND HOW?

The initial report of H.M.'s amnesia following resection of hippocampal-system structures (Scoville & Milner, 1957) had an enormous impact not only on neuropsychologists but also on neuroscientists, a number of whom were stimulated to try to produce animal models of this disorder by placing experimental lesions in lab animals in the same brain regions damaged in H.M. By the end of the 1960s there were already numerous reported attempts to approximate amnesia in nonhuman primates with lesions to the hippocampal system, including several papers by the two authors of the original report of H.M. (Orbach, Milner, & Rasmussen, 1960; Correll & Scoville, 1965a, b, 1967, 1970). Other investigators have taken up this agenda in more recent years, with several different research aims in view.

The first aim is neuropsychological. Work with animal models can address the same issues about the nature of memory impairment characterizing amnesia and the brain structures whose damage actually cause amnesia as does work with humans. Working with animal models rather than with patients is attractive when addressing this aim because it permits the investigator to maintain very strong control of the learning experiences of the subjects, and it permits systematic studies to be performed to delineate precisely which structures within the hippocampal system are the critical ones. A second aim is comparative. By looking at the effects of damage to the same hippocampal system structures in a variety of species, it becomes possible to search for fundamental cross-species commonalities and differences in the functional role of this very important region of the brain. It also permits inquiries about the kinds of mechanisms that have evolved to support memory in species with different environmental challenges and behavioral demands. A third aim is concerned with discovering underlying neurobiological mechanisms. Work with animal models, if successful in delineating the brain structures that contribute critically to memory, provides the opportunity to conduct systematic exploration of these structures' physiological properties and functional organization with methods not amenable for use with humans. Thus, recording of the activity of single neurons during the performance of memory tasks as well as neuroanatomical and neurochemical studies of the connections and local circuit interactions of the relevant brain structures is now possible with animal studies, and contributes much to our knowledge of the organization of memory and the functional role played in memory by the hippocampal system.

INITIAL LACK OF CORRESPONDENCE

From the very beginning of this effort to develop animal models of amnesia, however, researchers were struck by the great discrepancy in the apparent scope of the learning impairment between human amnesic patients and animals receiving damage to the very same brain regions. H.M.'s amnesia, *as described at the time*, was quite obviously a *global* disorder (Corkin, 1984; Milner, Corkin, & Teuber, 1968; Scoville & Milner, 1957), apparently extending to *all* kinds of new information, regardless of sensory modality or mode of response. His impairment in new learning included such materials as "words, digits, paragraphs, faces, names, maze routes, spatial layouts, geometric shapes, nonsense patterns, nonsense syllables, clicks, tunes, tones, public and personal events, and more" (Cohen, 1984). The only limitation of his deficit seemed to be along temporal dimensions, with intact immediate or short-term retention, but impaired performance when significant (especially interference-filled) delays must be bridged.

Yet, animal subjects whose brain damage was designed to match H.M.'s could learn a wide range of the most common conditioning, maze learning, and discrimination tasks studied by experimentalists, and could learn them as rapidly as could intact control animals. These animals did show clear impairments of learning on some tasks, but these tasks did not seem obviously different in the extent to which they depended on memory compared to those tasks on which performance was spared. This difficulty in demonstrating a consistently profound memory impairment in hippocampal-damaged animals was so much in contrast with the success of neuropsychologists in demonstrating amnesia on a wide range of tasks in patients such as H.M. that it was taken by many as a failure to model amnesia in animals. As a consequence, much of the animal model work turned away from the view of hippocampal system being involved in memory per se. Some authors argued that the deficits in learning that were observed in animals with hippocampal system damage could be attributed to impairments in certain non-memory psychological dimensions, such as response inhibition (Douglas, 1967), attention (Kimble, 1968) or cognitive processing in a particular cue-modality (i.e., spatial processing: O'Keefe & Nadel, 1978). These ideas still persist today, in that at least some current computational approaches are based in attention theory (e.g., Schmajuk & Moore 1988) or spatial computations (e.g., O'Keefe, 1989).

Considering how strongly the findings from H.M. and the other human amnesia data tied the hippocampal system to memory, the movement of the animal model work toward nonmemory accounts constituted an enormous divergence, and explains why these two literatures had so little to say to one another for so long.

WHY ANIMAL MODELS MIGHT FAIL: THREE POSSIBLE EXPLANATIONS

How can we understand the discrepancy between the phenomena of human amnesia and the phenomena of animal amnesia? What can we make of this apparent failure to model amnesia in animals? At least three classes of reasons can be cited as to why discrepancies might emerge in comparisons of the effects of hippocampal-system damage in humans versus other animal species.

1. Evolutionary changes may have produced differences between humans and other animal species in the functional role played by hippocampal system structures.

2. Investigators may have misunderstood which particular hippocampal system structures are the critical ones whose damage produces human amnesia, and thus have chosen the wrong lesions to produce in their animal model work.

3. There may be important differences among species in the behavioral tests that have been or must be used to reveal amnesia. One version of this idea is that the impairment in human amnesia was mischaracterized and, consequently, that the wrong behavioral tests have been used in animal model work. An alternative version of this idea is that there might be important differences between humans and other animal species in the way in which memory can be assessed experimentally and in which memory impairment is expressed, obscuring basic commonalities in hippocampal system function.

Faced with this state of affairs, most investigators have chosen to work with a single species, with a single or limited set of lesion loci, and with a restricted set of behavioral paradigms. That is, various investigators have adopted the strategy of assessing the effects of relatively limited variations in behavioral demands or in locus of brain injury on a species-by-species basis. To the extent that each of the investigators can capture at least some aspect of human amnesia in their animal models, then at least progress can be made in understanding the role of hippocampal system structures in memory for rats or for rabbits or for monkeys. The hope is that the data and theoretical accounts that emerge from work on different species will share enough commonalities that they will eventually converge on a single account; or that the differences that emerge will be systematic enough to permit an understanding of the evolutionary trend that has led to the memory systems and mechanisms instantiated in human brains.

Such an approach is not without certain risks, however. In particular, it runs the risk of encouraging what we shall call *limited-domain* theories, namely, accounts that are capable of accommodating the data for a particular domain, such as for rats tested with a particular set of paradigms, but prove to be less capable for other domains, such as for monkeys tested with a different set of paradigms or, ultimately, for human amnesia. This has in fact proved to be a serious problem in the field, hampering progress toward a comprehensive account of memory, amnesia, and the hippocampal system. Nonetheless, to the extent that the limited-domain accounts have captured some important regularities about the memory-dependent performance impairments caused by damage to the hippocampal system in different species, they have helped to guide the way to and will be incorporated in the comprehensive theory we offer here.

DIRECTLY ADDRESSING THE DISCREPANCY

In contrast to the limited-domain strategy, however, we and several other investigators have attempted to address the apparent discrepancy between the human amnesia and animal model literatures directly. We turn now to the three explanations for the failure of animal models noted above and consider their relative merits.

Evolutionary Changes in Functional Role

The first approach focuses on possible evolutionary differences in the functional role played by the hippocampal system. There are both anatomical and physiological grounds on which the hippocampus does appear to differ among species. In addition to the gross morphological differences in the size and location of hippocampus in the brain of rodents versus primates, there are a number of cytoarchitectural differences in the organization of hippocampal subdivisions (Rosene & Van Hoesen, 1988), as illustrated in figures 2.1 and 2.2. Also, major species differences have been observed in the gross physiological activity of hippocampus as reflected in the behavioral correlates of hippocampal EEG. In rats, the theta rhythm (a large, regular 4 to 12 Hz activity) predominates in the hippocampal EEG during exploratory activity as is common when performing in learning tasks, but it is nearly absent whenever the rat is not moving or is engaged in "automatic" behaviors such as drinking or grooming. In rabbits, however, the theta rhythm is usually evoked by sensory stimulation even when the animal is immobile. In primates, there has been little indication of theta rhythm even during active learning performance (Crowne & Radcliff, 1975; Winson, 1972). More recently, however, a clear pattern of 7 to 9 Hz rhythmic activity in the monkey hippocampus has been reported; this EEG pattern has the same laminar profile, sensitivity to pharmacological manipulation, and correlation with movement as theta activity described in nonprimates (reviewed in Stewart & Fox, 1990).

But do these anatomical and physiological species differences translate into *functional* differences above and beyond whatever variations exist among species in behavioral repertoires and predispositions? One way that this question can be addressed is through analyses of the behavioral correlates of single unit activity. Although most of the electrophysiological studies have been limited solely to rats, the available cross-species data suggest that the firing correlates of hippocampal neurons across a large range of experiences are similar in the fundamental aspects of experience encoded, as illustrated in figure 2.3. Hippocampal neurons in both rats and rabbits can be found to fire selectively as the animal is sampling significant visual, auditory, or olfactory cues or is engaged in exploration within large open fields. In these circumstances neuronal firing can be related to specific spatially and nonspatially defined combinations of stimuli and behavioral responses (e.g., Eichenbaum et al., 1986; O'Keefe, 1979; Wiener, Paul, & Eichenbaum, 1989; discussed in greater length in Eichenbaum, Otto, & Cohen, 1992; see chapter 5). It is now clear that in monkeys and humans, as well, many hippocampal neurons fire in relation to specific meaningful stimuli or during the execution of meaningful behavioral responses, including in various spatially and nonspatially directed behaviors

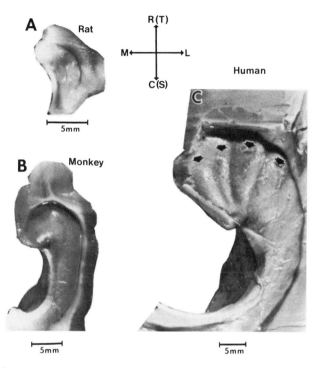

Figure 2.1
Comparative hippocampal gross anatomy: grossly dissected hippocampal formation as it appears from the ventricular side in the rat (*A*), monkey (*B*), and human (*C*). Note that the caudal (C) end of the primate hippocampal formation corresponds to the septal (S) end of the rat hippocampal formation. However, in the rat, the septal end of the hippocampal formation is located rostrally rather than caudally. In the primate the temporal (T) end of the hippocampal formation is located at the rostral end of the inferior horn of the lateral ventricle. In *C*, the arrows mark the convolutions of the human hippocampus. (From Rosene & Van Hoesen, 1987).

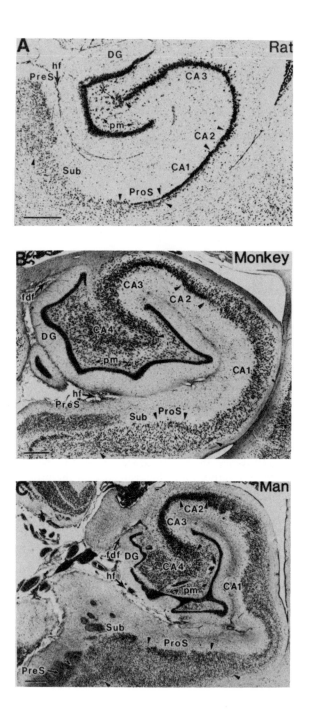

(Heit, Smith, & Halgren, 1988; Rolls, 1987; Rolls et al., 1989; Watanabe & Niki, 1985; Wilson, Brown, & Riches, 1987).

While hardly conclusive, these data point to the functional constancy of hippocampal processing across species. At this time, there are no compelling data for attributing cross-species differences in the behavioral outcome of amnesia to cross-species differences in the functional role of the hippocampal system. Accordingly, we have proceeded on the assumption that there are *no* fundamental functional differences. The appropriateness of this assumption will of course be tested by our effort to offer a comprehensive cross-species account of memory, amnesia, and the hippocampal system; the merits of the assumption will be demonstrated only to the extent that the account offered here succeeds in accommodating the data obtained from different species.

Differences in Locus of Lesion

The second possibility is that the particular hippocampal system structures whose damage produces human amnesia may not be the same ones that have been experimentally lesioned in the animal model work. The hippocampal system has many anatomical components, as will be discussed in chapter 4; readers interested in such anatomical matters are encouraged to jump ahead to that discussion. All of these components were removed in whole or part in H.M.'s surgical resection. A number of investigators are currently

◄───

Figure 2.2
Comparative hippocampal cytoarchitecture: Nissl-stained coronal sections through the hippocampal formation of the rat (A), monkey (B), and human (C) with the approximate boundaries of the corresponding cytoarchitectonic subdivisions marked by arrowheads. The asterisk in A marks the small cluster of hilar neurons that may correspond to the CA4 subfields of monkey and man. Note that while there is striking similarity in the overall arrangement of the hippocampal formation in all three species, this similarity decreases as one proceeds from the dentate gyrus (DG) through the CA subfields toward the subiculum. Furthermore, it is also clear that the CA1 and subicular subfields occupy a proportionally larger part of the hippocampal formation as one proceeds from rat to monkey to human. DG, dentate gyrus; Sub, subiculum; PreS, presubiculum; ProS, prosubiculum; CA1, CA2, CA3, CA4, subdivisions or fields of Ammon's horn; hf, hippocampal fissure; pm, polymorph layer of the dentate gyrus; fdf, fimbrio-dentate fissure. (From Rosene & Van Hoesen, 1987.)

studying in various animal models the effects of damage to different anatomical components of the hippocampal system and of disconnection of its input-output pathways (Aggleton, Blindt, & Rawlins, 1989; Aggleton, Hunt, & Rawlins, 1986; Bachevalier, Parkinson, & Mishkin, 1985; Gaffan, 1974; Horel & Pytko, 1982; Jarrard, 1986; Jarrard, Okaichi, Steward, & Goldschmidt, 1984; Mahut, Zola-Morgan, & Moss, 1982; Mishkin, 1978; Murray & Mishkin, 1986; Zola-Morgan, Squire, & Amaral, 1989a, b; Zola-Morgan, Squire, & Mishkin, 1982; Zola-Morgan, Squire, Amaral, & Suzuki, 1989). Such research has proven quite productive and indicates that damage to different structures within the hippocampal system may indeed cause different components of the amnesia seen in H.M., and also suggests that differences across experiments in the locus of lesion within the hippocampal system may well contribute to apparent cross-species discrepancies.

Yet we include in our consideration of the literature all lesions producing significant interruption of hippocampal system function. It is our contention that all subjects with significant hippocampal system dysfunction, regardless of the precise localization of their damage within the system, have impairment of the same *domain* of memory. That is, while there may well be differences in the exact phenomenology of their behavioral impairments, and almost certainly in the severity of their amnesia, so far it seems that they all are impaired on the same type of memory tests and spared on the

---→

Figure 2.3
Behavioral correlates of hippocampal firing across species. (A) Activity of a hippocampal neuron in a monkey performing a visual recognition task where pattern stimuli are presented repeatedly at four different locations on a video screen. The monkey had to respond differentially to a pattern repeated at the same location as its original presentation. Firing rate for each pattern is given for first (novel) and second (familiar) presentations of stimuli (numbers given) at each of the four locations. Compare responses to the spontaneous firing rate of the cell (spont). This cell fires differentially in association with stimulus locus and familiarity. (From Rolls et al., 1989.) (B) Activity of a hippocampal neuron in a monkey (M) shown various stimuli at different orientations of view. A and C show responses to the sound of a human walking at different loci, with the monkey at two different orientations. B shows responses to a human walking and other stimuli. This cell fires in association with the allocentric location of a particular stimulus. (From Ono et al., 1991.)

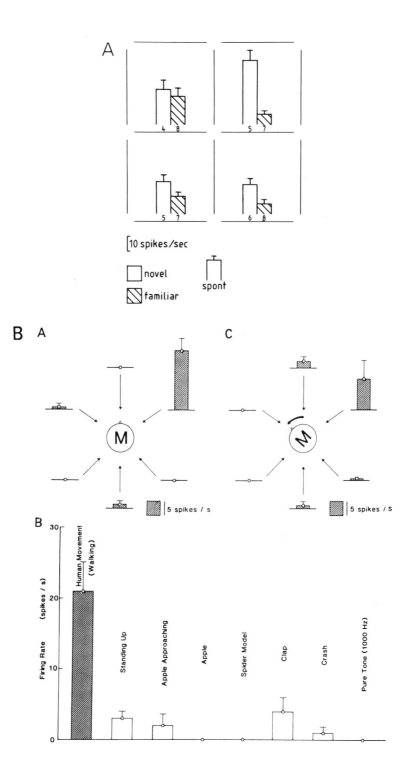

A

10 spikes/sec

novel

familiar

spont

B   A

M

5 spikes / s

C

M

5 spikes / S

B   30

Human Movement (Walking)

Firing Rate   (spikes / s)

Standing Up

Apple Approaching

Apple

Spider Model

Clap

Crash

Pure Tone (1000 Hz)

20

10

0

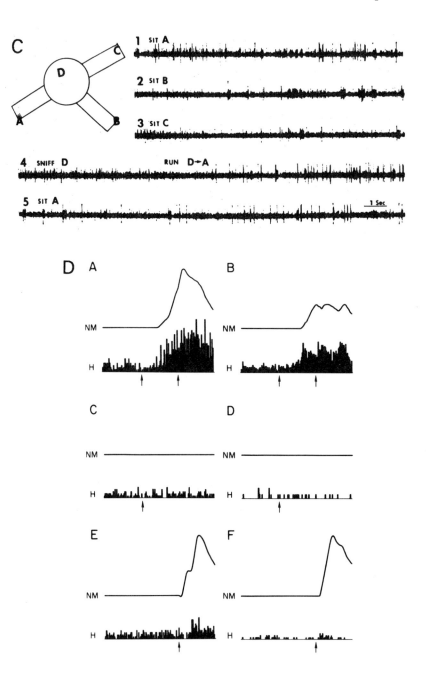

same types of other memory tests.[1,2] The legitimacy of this contention and, therefore, the appropriateness of taking as fair game all instances of significant hippocampal system damage, is empirically testable; its merits will be demonstrated by the extent to which performances resulting from the different types of hippocampal system lesions conform sufficiently to permit inferences to be drawn about the nature of the tasks impaired versus spared in amnesias. If an account of impaired versus spared memory capacities in amnesia can be formulated for humans and other animal species despite our inclusiveness, then our decision will have been vindicated.

It should be said that the position we have taken forces us to bear a significant cost. In treating all hippocampal system lesions as fair game for our analyses, we are faced with incorporating performance data from animals or patients with *partial* lesions of the hippocampal system along with data from subjects with complete ones. Among investigators working with animal models, the specific lesions administered in order to interfere with hippocampal system function differ considerably, sometimes involving only one of the hippocampal system structures or a particular input-output pathway, and sometimes involving the entire set of hippocampal system structures that were resected in the patient H.M. Likewise, different etiologies of human hippocampal amnesia vary markedly in the extent of damage to various hippocampal system structures. By considering together all subjects with significant interruption of

◄───

Figure 2.3 (continued)
(C) Activity of hippocampal neurons in a rat performing a foraging task on a three-arm maze. The raw recordings show firing of the large cell (long vertical lines) when the rate is running (RUN) or sitting (SIT) in each arm. This cell fires preferentially when the rat is running or sitting in arm A. (From O'Keefe, 1976). (D) Activity of hippocampal neurons in a restrained rabbit performing an eyeblink conditioning task. In each panel NM represents the eyeblink movement (up is eye closure) and H represents the activity of a single hippocampal pyramidal cell over a 750-msec period. A and B show activity of two different cells recorded after conditioning involving pairing of a tone CS and airpuff UCS. The arrows represent onset of the CS and UCS. Other panels show control tests. C and D show activity of two different cells around presentations of an unpaired tone (arrow). E and F show activity of two different cells around presentations of an unpaired airpuff (arrow). These cells fire only preceding and during conditioned eyeblink responses. (From Berger et al., 1983).

hippocampal system function, permitting variance in the completeness of the hippocampal system damage, we will surely be faced with instances of false negatives—that is, observations of no deficit (intact performance) that will turn out to be due *not* to the preservation of that type of performance in amnesia, but rather due to failure to cause sufficiently complete interruption of hippocampal system function.

However, this cost is mitigated in two ways. First, when other data from subjects performing on the same test but with more inclusive lesions reveal behavioral impairments, we can identify partial lesion effects (i.e., the instances of intact performance due to incomplete interruption of hippocampal system function) and dismiss them from our analyses. Second, we place particular emphasis on data from tasks that produce systematic results across different laboratories using somewhat different lesions of the hippocampal system. A good example comes from work on delayed nonmatch-to-sample (DNMS), a task used in numerous studies of the effects of hippocampal system damage in monkeys (Gaffan, 1974, 1977; Gaffan & Saunders, 1985; Mishkin, 1978, 1982; Zola-Morgan & Squire, 1985) and rats (Aggleton et al., 1986, 1989; Raffaele & Olton, 1988) (see chapter 7). Studies by Mishkin and colleagues in monkeys and Aggleton and colleagues in rats failed to show the profound impairment usually reported on this task (discussed at length in chapter 7). But these studies differed from the others in that they used partial lesions, restricted to particular components of the hippocampal system. When the same authors tested performance following more complete hippocampal system damage, the usual full-blown impairments were observed. Moreover, other studies of DNMS in monkeys (Gaffan, 1974; Zola-Morgan & Squire, 1986b) or rats (Raffaele & Olton, 1988) found that even partial lesions *can* be sufficient to produce serious impairment. Thus, there is no doubt that significant hippocampal system damage disrupts performance on DNMS.

Having contended that the hippocampal system as a whole supports a particular domain of memory functioning, with damage to any component of that system producing deficits for the same domain of memory, it seems likely to us that different brain structures within the hippocampal system support memory for one or another subset of that domain. On this view, particular structures of the hippocampal system would have a smaller scope in its domain of memory functioning than does the hippocampal system as a whole. Accordingly, damage to different components of the hippocampal system could well produce deficits on different tasks—different subsets of the full range of deficits—and there will be tasks for which deficits will appear only after damage to a large enough portion of the whole hippocampal system (for further detail on this issue see Eichenbaum, Otto, and Cohen, 1992). It is the latter class of deficits with which we concern ourselves here.

Differences in Behavioral Tasks

The third approach follows from observations about the differences between the tasks typically administered to human amnesics and those administered to subjects in animal model work (see Iversen, 1977; Squire & Zola-Morgan, 1988; Weiskrantz, 1978). One obvious difference concerns the absence of an animal counterpart to verbal testing (cf. Iverson, 1976). Accordingly, some investigators developed nonverbal tasks for humans paralleling more closely those used for animals, such as maze learning and discrimination learning (Aggleton, Nicol, Huston, & Fairbairn, 1988; Milner et al., 1968; Squire & Zola-Morgan, 1988). Given that H.M. and other amnesic patients have now been shown to perform as poorly on those tasks as on more conventional verbal learning tasks, however, an explanation of the discrepancy in terms of administering verbal versus nonverbal tests has not proven viable.

More recent work has succeeded in demonstrating significant differences in the tasks administered to humans versus other animal species when considered in terms of the demands they place on memory processing. These differences take on importance with the discovery that human amnesia is not as global a disorder as was previously thought. We now understand that amnesia is a selective memory impairment whose detection depends critically on choice of memory task—that is, on the demands placed on memory by different tests. As the field's characterization of human amnesia has undergone significant change, we have come to understand that the kinds of memory task used to probe amnesia in animal models have traditionally *not* paralleled those used with human patients. For example, human memory is often tested by having subjects *use* their previous experiences to answer some question or solve some problem, whereas animals' memory is typically tested by having them *repeat* some training experience and assessing whether their performance has been facilitated. Thus, tests of humans often entail asking questions that can be answered with knowledge gleaned from one or more previous learning experiences, such as in tests of memory for lists of items, public events, famous faces, former television programs, and so forth. Tests of animals, for which the verbal question-and-answer format is obviously inappropriate, usually entails repeated assessments of performance during repetitions of a set of experimental circumstances.

It turns out, as we shall see, that this difference between the way memory is tested has a significant impact on the demands that are placed on the systems that store, maintain, and permit access to memories. In fact, they encourage or require the use of different memory systems. What we shall show in the following chapters is that, by contrast, when we aim for *memory-processing equivalence or representational equivalence* rather than a surface-level task equivalence the cross-species discrepancy in behavioral outcome of hippocampal system damage disappears.

TOWARD A CORRESPONDENCE: MODELING AMNESIA AS A SELECTIVE MEMORY DEFICIT

Making choices about what would constitute an appropriate test of amnesia in animals, and an adequate animal model of amnesia, is critically dependent on the description of the impairment in human amnesia. A description of human amnesia as a truly global memory impairment is incompatible with the selectivity of the memory deficits seen following hippocampal system damage in animals. But a description of human amnesia that emphasizes *not* its inclusiveness but rather its restricted or selective nature makes it possible to bring the animal models into correspondence. We turn now to some of the evidence that indicates that human amnesia is indeed a selective memory impairment.

It was first shown in the 1960s that the profoundly amnesic patient H.M. could demonstrate impressive learning of motor skills across days of testing (Corkin, 1965, 1968; Milner, 1962). An example of this, involving mirror tracing, is illustrated in figure 2.4. H.M. was asked to trace the outline of a five-pointed star that can

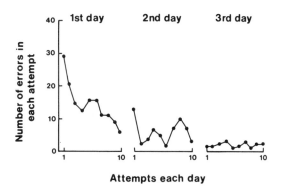

Figure 2.4
Performance by the patient H.M. on three successive days of testing on mirror drawing. (From Milner, 1965.)

be glimpsed only through a mirror; the only visual information about the position of the hand and pen with respect to the star is through mirror reflection. Challenged with this task several times on each of several successive days, H.M. was able to demonstrate robust improvement across trials (Milner, 1962). Subsequent work confirmed and extended this finding with other amnesic patients, including postencephalitic patients with damage to hippocampal system structures and patients receiving bilateral electroconvulsive therapy (ECT) with presumed (transient) dysfunction of hippocampal system structures. It has also been extended to patients with Korsakoff's disease and the noted patient N.A., with damage to midline diencephalic brain structures, which have connections to but are not part of the hippocampal system. All of this work has shown that the learning of perceptual-motor skills, such as those required in continuous manual tracking tasks (e.g., rotary pursuit), can be fully preserved despite amnesia (Brooks & Baddeley, 1976; Cermak, Lewis, Butters, & Goodglass, 1973; Cohen, 1981).

Further work of ours and of others documented that the domain of preserved learning extended beyond motor skills to include perceptual and cognitive skills as well. For example, normal learning could be observed in amnesia for reading of mirror-reversed text (Cohen & Squire, 1980; Martone, Butters, Payne, Becker, & Sax, 1984; Moscovitch, Winocur, & McLachlan, 1986), as illustrated in figure 2.5. In the study by Cohen and Squire (1980), subjects saw words presented as unrelated word triplets in mirror-reversed form, with the task of reading each word aloud as quickly as possible. Several blocks of triplets were presented in each of several sessions. Amnesic patients of various etiologies showed a normal reduction across blocks in the average time required to read each triplet.

Normal performance could also be observed for solving the Tower of Hanoi puzzle (Cohen, Eichenbaum, DeAcedo, & Corkin, 1985; Saint-Cyr, Taylor, & Lang, 1988), although it has not been universally the case (an issue taken up in chapter 8). There are also reports of amnesic patients learning to use simple numerical algorithms, specifically the Fibonacci rule (Wood, 1974) and a rule for mental squaring of two-digit numbers (Charness, Milberg, & Alexander, 1988; Milberg, Alexander, Charness, McGlichey-Berrot, & Barrett, 1988), although the learning here may not be fully normal (see chapter 8).

What is particularly intriguing about these skill-learning phenomena is that they occur despite the patients' *profoundly impaired recall and recognition of the specific materials* used to train and test skilled performance, despite *poor recollection of the learning experiences* during which skilled performance was developed, and despite *poor insight into the nature of the knowledge* underlying the skilled performance (see Cohen, 1984). Thus, for example,

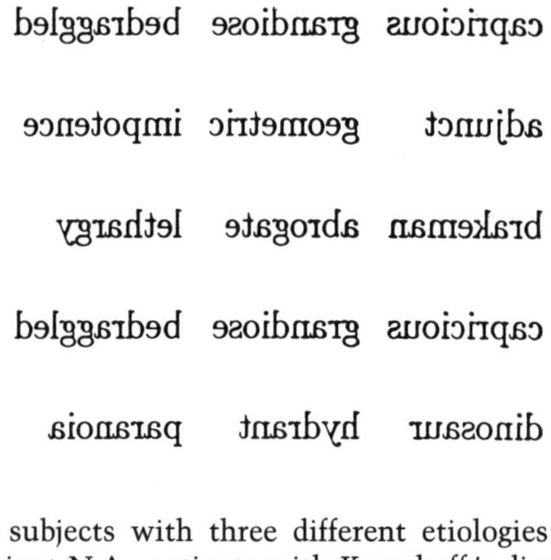

beldggeibed esoibnsig suoioiiqso

adjunct geometric impotence

brakeman abrogate lethargy

capricious grandiose bedraggled

dinosaur hydrant paranoia

Figure 2.5
Performance of subjects with three different etiologies of amnesia (the diencephalic patient N.A., patients with Korsakoff's disease, and patients who received a course of bilateral ECT for relief of endogenous depression)

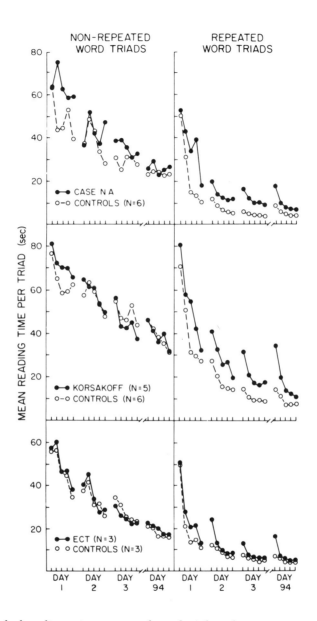

on speed of reading mirror-reversed word triplets that were seen only once (*left*) or were repeated in each block of trials (*right*). Performance was assessed on a series of blocks of trials on each of three successive days and then a fourth day 3 months later. (From Cohen, 1981.)

H.M.'s success on the Tower of Hanoi puzzle was accompanied by verbal reports in which he made clear that he had no recollection of his training experiences with the puzzle, could not remember having ever seen the puzzle previously, and claimed that he could not solve it.

There is another, parallel, body of work demonstrating the selectivity of the memory impairment in amnesia, which has of late received considerably more attention than the examples of skill learning. Beginning in the late 1960s with the seminal work of Warrington and Weiskrantz (1968, 1970), studies of amnesia have shown that exposure to stimuli influences the later processing of those stimuli, even when the prior occurrence of those stimuli cannot be explicitly remembered. Thus, having been exposed to some words or line drawings during an initial study phase, amnesic patients—like normal control subjects—will show a facilitation, biasing, or *priming* of those specific items when the subsequent test requires identification, naming, fragment completion, or categorization of stimulus materials including the previously presented ones (for excellent reviews see Schacter, 1987b; Shimamura, 1986; Tulving & Schacter, 1990; further discussion of these phenomena can be found in chapter 8).

An example of this phenomenon, based on Warrington and Weiskrantz's (1968) and Milner, Corkin, and Teuber's (1968) work with the Gollin incomplete figures test, is shown in figure 2.6. A series of visually degraded or incomplete line drawings of objects was presented, one drawing at a time, with the task of trying to identify the object depicted. The amount of visual degrading or incompleteness of each drawing was varied systematically, so that the drawings became progressively more complete and hence more identifiable. Increasingly more complete drawings of each object were presented until the subject could identify all of them. Then, after a delay, the entire procedure was repeated. To the extent that there was priming of the objects based on the earlier learning experience, subjects would be expected to identify the objects earlier in the sequence, that is, with more degraded or incomplete drawings as the stimuli. This is exactly what was observed in several amnesic patients, including H.M. Such priming effects occur despite the patients' impaired recall or recognition of the repeated test materials and

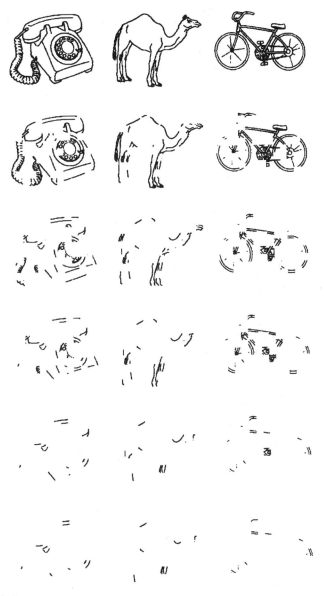

Figure 2.6
Examples of incomplete or fragmented pictures used to test for object priming. Line drawings of three objects are shown here in various degrees of completeness or fragmentation, ranging from undiscriminable (bottom-most) to fully complete (topmost). (From Snodgrass & Feenan, 1990.)

impaired (if any) recollection of the experiences responsible for the priming.

A rapidly growing and increasingly influential body of work on priming effects in normal subjects has demonstrated that the separation between priming and explicit remembering (e.g., recall and recognition) does not require the presence of amnesia or of hippocampal system damage. Even in normal subjects, with intact ability to recall and recognize the test materials, priming effects can occur independently of—that is, can occur in a way that is not predicted by—explicit remembering of the materials. Such findings and their implications for our understanding of the amnesia data are discussed in chapter 8.

These demonstrations of the influence exerted by previous experience on the performance of amnesic patients (discussed at length in subsequent chapters), together with other examples from studies of eyeblink conditioning (Weiskrantz & Warrington, 1979) and long-lasting perceptual aftereffects (Benzing & Squire, 1989; Savoy & Gabrieli, 1988; Weiskrantz, 1978) in amnesic patients, suggest that the label "global amnesia" is misleading and that the memory loss in amnesia is rather more selective than was previously appreciated.

Hippocampal and Nonhippocampal Amnesias

Our discussion thus far has noted that preserved skill learning and/ or repetition priming effects can be observed in patients with amnesias of diverse etiologies. Findings from the literature discussed above include some that come from patients with hippocampal system damage as well as some from those whose amnesias are due to damage outside of the hippocampal system. What we need to do here is first provide some information about the etiologies of amnesia that are most frequently encountered, and then explain why we should consider *non*hippocampal amnesias in a book on memory, amnesia, and the hippocampal system.

For each of the following etiologies of hippocampal system damage, the dissociation between amnesia on tests of explicit remembering and the spared acquisition of skilled performance has been documented: *herpes simplex encephalitis*, an often deadly virus with a predilection for the medial temporal lobes (Drachman & Adams, 1962; Rose & Simonds, 1960); *vascular accident*, such as occlusion of the posterior cerebral artery, feeding the medial temporal lobes (Benson, Marsden, & Meadows, 1974); *hypoxic ischemia* (Victor & Agamanolis, 1990; Volpe & Hirst, 1983); certain instances of *closed head injury* (Levin, Papanicolaou, & Eisenberg, 1984; Russell & Nathan, 1946; Schacter & Crovitz, 1977); and *bilateral electroconvulsive therapy*, a series of treatments with seizure-producing electric shocks for the relief of severe depressive illness (Squire, 1982a).

Amnesias caused not by damage to the hippocampal system but rather by damage to brain structures along the midline of the diencephalon (including the dorsomedial nucleus of the thalamus and the mammillary nuclei of the hypothalamus) have received much attention in the literature. Such amnesias occur in the following circumstances: *Korsakoff's disease*, resulting from many years of chronic alcohol abuse (Butters & Cermak, 1980; Talland, 1965; Victor, Adams, & Collins, 1971); *vascular accident*, such as infarction of the paramedial artery, feeding midline thalamic structures (Winocur, Oxbory, Roberts, Agnetti, & Davis, 1984); and *tumors* of the third ventricle region (Williams & Pennybacker, 1954). While not all of these examples of amnesia have been tested with regard to the pattern of sparing and loss of memory that has been the subject of our discussion, the amnesia associated with Korsakoff's disease has received intensive scrutiny—more so than any other etiology of amnesia—and has been found to exhibit this type of selectivity.

Given that Korsakoff's disease is a *non*hippocampal etiology of amnesia, why should data from such patients play any role in our discussion of the nature of the hippocampal system's role in memory? The answer is that there is a critical correspondence between Korsakoff amnesia and that resulting from hippocampal system damage in terms of the pattern of sparing and loss of memory abilities: They both show intact acquisition and expression of skilled performance despite impaired explicit remembering. Although there has been some work and much discussion about possible differences in the nature of the amnesias associated with Korsakoff's disease versus the hippocampal amnesias (see discussion in Squire & Cohen, 1984; Weiskrantz, 1985; Zola-Morgan & Squire, 1985), the available evidence suggests that they both result in impairment of the same *domain* of memory. That is, while it is undoubtedly the case that hippocampal system structures have different specific processing functions than do midline diencephalic structures, such functions seem all to be in service of one particular memory system: *declarative memory*. Based on our current understanding, any differences likely to emerge between Korsakoff amnesia and hippocampal amnesia would be in the processing locus of impairment within declarative memory. Accordingly, data from patients with Korsakoff's disease can be considered together with data from patients with hippocampal amnesia in exploring the difference between the acquisition and expression of skilled performance and the explicit remembering of learning experiences and their content, with certain caveats discussed below.

However, one aspect of Korsakoff's disease is problematic in trying to understand memory, amnesia, and the hippocampal system. Korsakoff's disease is often accompanied by certain problem-solving or other cognitive deficits not seen in patients with hippocampal system damage. Such accompanying deficits may well cause impairments on skilled performance tasks that would otherwise be spared in amnesia; for a given finding of impaired learning performance in Korsakoff's amnesia, if not also confirmed in hippocampal amnesia, it might be difficult to determine whether to attribute impairment to a deficit in *learning and memory* abilities or in problem-solving and other cognitive abilities. (Of course, on the other hand, a finding of *intact* performance on some test of skill learning or repetition priming in patients with Korsakoff's disease is all the more impressive, occurring in the face of both their amnesia and their additional cognitive deficits.) Possible interpretive difficulties arising in work with Korsakoff's amnesia will be illustrated in chapter 8. As a result of this problem, we shall endeavor to make use of reports of impaired performance in Korsakoff amnesia only if also confirmed in hippocampal amnesia.

There is one other set of *non*hippocampal amnesias germane to the issues of concern in this book, namely the amnesias associated with Alzheimer's disease, Huntington's disease, and Parkinson's disease, in which the damage sustained may include cortical brain areas and basal ganglia structures or basal forebrain nuclei. These patients will be considered briefly near the end of this chapter and in chapter 10 because they have memory problems that compromise at least some of the memory abilities that are *spared* in hippocampal amnesia (e.g., see Gabrieli, 1991; Heindel et al., 1989).

MULTIPLE MEMORY SYSTEM THEORIES OF HUMAN AND ANIMAL AMNESIAS

The selectivity of the impairment in amnesia raises a pair of connected questions: If amnesia is not a global loss of memory functions, then just what kind of memory loss is it? and What aspects or dimensions of memory are required for performance on the tasks on which amnesics are impaired but are not required for performance on the tasks on which amnesics succeed? Three general answers to our pair of questions have been offered.

1. The tasks on which amnesic patients demonstrate preserved capacity are more sensitive to whatever is stored in memory than are those tasks on which the patients show impaired performance. Amnesia produces an impoverished memory, resulting in a quantitative relationship between sensitivity of a memory test and its ability to detect evidence of memory in amnesic patients: Tasks that are most sensitive to the presence of memory might be able to evoke robust performance despite degraded memory (Meudell & Mayes, 1981).

2. The tasks on which amnesic patients demonstrate success differ from those on which they fail by virtue of the nature of the retrieval cues they offer or that they require for revealing memory. On this view, the tasks preserved in amnesia are those providing the types of cues necessary to overcome the patients' deficit, for example, by aiding impaired retrieval processes that would otherwise be insufficient for accessing an intact store of memory; or else they are tasks that do not require certain attributional processes unavailable to amnesic patients (Jacoby, 1984; Warrington & Weiskrantz, 1974, 1978; Weiskrantz, 1978 [although later writings by the latter two authors offer a different interpretation; see chapter 12]). These first two answers assume a *unitary* memory system, and assign the selectivity of amnesia to differences among tasks in their ability to provide access to the contents of that single memory store.

3. The difference between tasks spared and impaired in amnesia rests on the *representational demands* they place on memory, that

is, on what kind of memory they require for successful performance. The notion here is that the hippocampal system supports only one type of memory—only one of the memory systems in the brain. The selectivity of amnesia comes from the deficit being restricted to a particular type of memory or domain of representation. The tasks on which amnesic patients show preserved performance are those whose representational demands can be fully met by the hippocampal-independent memory system. This answer, then, is a *multiple memory system account.*

It is the third answer, involving the multiple memory system view, that we have offered in our work (Cohen, 1981, 1984, 1985; Cohen & Squire, 1980; Cohen et al., 1985; Eichenbaum, Fagan, & Cohen, 1986; Eichenbaum, Fagan, Mathews, & Cohen, 1988; Eichenbaum, Mathews, & Cohen, 1989; Eichenbaum et al., 1990, 1991, 1992) and that will be elaborated and extended here. This answer is to be preferred for three reasons: independence between the categories of performance that are spared versus impaired in amnesia, double dissociation between the two categories of performance, and different characteristics of the memory representations necessary for the two categories of performance.

Independence

Performances on tasks for which amnesic patients show impairment and performances on tasks for which amnesic patients show sparing can be fully independent of one another; they do not show the correlations that would be expected if they were based on a common unitary representation of experience. That is, if the reason for skill learning and repetition priming performances remaining preserved in amnesic patients is that these performances are more sensitive tests of memory than are recall and recognition, then a certain correlation would have to be predicted: Whenever memory storage for a given set of stimulus materials or a given learning experience is sufficient to mediate performance on the less sensitive tests (recall and recognition), it must also be sufficient to mediate performance on the more sensitive tests (skill learning and repetition priming) as well. In other words, such a unitary-memory-system explanation of these performances requires that successful recall and recognition *predict* successful skill learning or recognition memory. However, this is just *not* the case. Repetition priming for a given set of materials can be shown to be no better or worse (no more or less likely) for items that the subject successfully remembers having previously encountered than for items that the subject fails to remember having previously encountered. This is evident both for amnesic patients, whose ability to explicitly remember the items is profoundly impaired, and for control subjects, with good explicit remembering. Hence, performance on the repetition priming measure cannot be predicted by performance on the recall or recognition measure. This independence, or lack of correlation, is logically equivalent to that between two successive flips of a coin: Because the outcome of a coin flip (heads versus tails) on any given occasion is uninfluenced by the outcome of a subsequent coin flip, the two outcomes will be uncorrelated and therefore independent.

Double Dissociation

The notion that skill learning and repetition priming performances survive in amnesia because they are sampled by tests that are more sensitive to residual memory than are the tests of recall or recognition, and are therefore easier for memory-impaired amnesic patients to perform, is also contradicted by findings of other types of memory-impaired patients who have the opposite pattern of sparing and loss. Patients with Huntington's disease or Parkinson's disease have been reported to have a disproportionate deficit in skill learning and repetition priming (Heindel et al; 1989; Gabrieli, 1991; see figure 2.7). The general finding that some patients (here, amnesic patients such as H.M.) are impaired on performance of test category A (here, recall and recognition) but not on performance of test category B (here, skill learning and repetition priming), and other patients (here, Parkinson's and Huntington's patients) are impaired on test category B but not test category A is what neuropsychologists call a double dissociation; such a finding is taken to provide particularly strong evidence for claiming a distinction between the cognitive processes or systems mediating the dissociated categories of performance. This is because the tests that one group of patients find more "difficult" are the same tests that other patients find "easy." A double dissociation that parallels this one has been demonstrated in animals (Packard, Hirsh, & White, 1989).

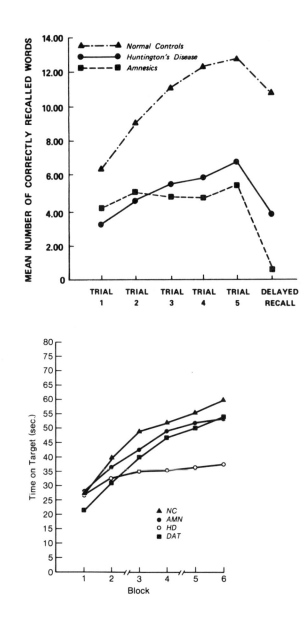

Different Representations

Last, and perhaps most central to the account we offer in this book, the memory representations mediating performance on tasks impaired in amnesic subjects seem to be fundamentally different from and cannot be used in the same ways as the memory representations mediating performance on tasks spared in amnesic subjects. This will become clearer when we articulate our theory in the next chapter, but, to anticipate, we shall argue that the hippocampal-dependent *declarative memory* system supports a relational form of representation exhibiting the critical property of *flexibility*, capable of being accessed and expressed in novel contexts; whereas *procedural memory*, operating independently of the hippocampal system, supports a fundamentally *in*flexible form of representation that can be expressed only in virtual repetitions of the initial learning situation. Evidence for this claim, and a full description of the nature of the representations mediated by hippocampal-dependent and hippocampal-independent memory systems, will be provided in the subsequent chapters. The point here is that such a state of affairs has no place in a unitary memory system view.

DISTINGUISHING AMONG MEMORY SYSTEMS ACCORDING TO QUALITATIVE AND QUANTITATIVE PROPERTIES

While our focus here will be on the above stated differences in the *nature of representation* between hippocampal-dependent and hippocampal-independent systems, there is also the possibility that such anatomically and functionally distinct systems also differ quantitatively in operating characteristics that affect *learning and forgetting rates* and thus might distinguish amnesia from normal memory performance. Indeed, there is ample evidence that declar-

◀──────────────────────────────────────

Figure 2.7
Disproportionate deficit in procedural memory in Huntington's disease. (*Top*) The performance of patients with Korsakoff's amnesia and patients with Huntington's disease is shown to be comparably impaired compared to controls on a test of free recall of words. (From Butters et al., 1985). (*Bottom*) The performance of patients with Huntington's disease (HD) is shown to be selectively impaired compared to patients with Korsakoff's amnesia (AMN), patients with Alzheimer's disease (DAT), and controls (NC) on motor learning for rotary pursuit. (From Heindel et al., 1988).

ative and procedural systems do differ, at least sometimes, in terms of the incremental strength of memories resulting from single experiences and in the persistence, or decay rate, of such "traces."

The declarative system is apparently capable of supporting memories at full strength after but a single exposure to new material, and such memories typically persist for durations (minutes to hours or more) longer than the short-term (seconds) retention subserved by immediate memory. Furthermore, the persistence of such memories can be significantly increased to durations of days, months, or longer with a few repetitions of the experience. By contrast, the most common examples of procedural learning (described in detail below) are characterized by the acquisition of representations as relatively small, incremental tunings, biasings, or primings of various processors. The persistence of each individual change is long lasting and accumulates additively, assuming that subsequent processing events involve tuning, biasing, or priming of the processor consistently in a similar direction. These strength and persistence differences, rather than distinctions in the qualitative nature of memory representation, sometimes may be the primary basis for observed dissociations in memory performance between amnesic and normal subjects.

We will argue that these properties are major factors in, for example, experiments on object discrimination and recognition memory (see chapter 7). Not surprisingly, this has given rise to some confusion and misunderstanding of the data, especially when comparing results across different types of learning materials and across species, since each of these factors may also be associated with differences in learning and forgeting rates. Furthermore, consistent with the view we will offer that procedural memory is itself a nonunitary system, learning and forgetting rates among the hippocampal-*independent* systems are quite variable; in addition to the common examples of slow incremental learning there are a range of demonstrations involving significant one-trial learning that is unaffected in amnesia, such as the phenomenon of priming in humans, and flavor aversion learning and conditioned emotional responses in animals. Thus, it turns out that learning and forgetting rates do not provide reliable markers for declarative versus procedural memory systems. Instead, we must rely on explorations of the qualitative nature of memory representations to understand how these systems function differently.

BUT SHOULDN'T WE ASPIRE TO UNITARY VIEWS OF MEMORY?

Some investigators have avoided a multiple memory system account, arguing that it is unitary theories of memory to which we should aspire because they are fundamentally more parsimonious accounts. That is, there has been an attempt to wield Occam's razor here: Any account capable of explaining memory performances in amnesia by postulating a unitary memory system is seen to be preferred over any account that postulates multiple memory systems. But this only reflects confusion about how parsimony is to be understood and used as a criterion for judging competing theories. One cannot invoke claims of parsimony about components of a theory; rather, parsimony and elegance of theories can only be judged for the theory as a whole. Let us be more concrete. If, in order to make a unitary memory system account work for amnesia, it becomes necessary to postulate additional memory processes and multiple loci of deficits in amnesia, then such an account is *not* more parsimonious than the multiple memory system theory that accounts for the data with fewer memory processes and just a single locus of deficit in amnesia. This issue is discussed in chapter 12, in which we show that current unitary theories suffer from just this problem of having to postulate additional processes and multiple deficits.

There is another reason to be skeptical about aspiring to unitary theories of memory. One of the clearest lessons from modern neuroscience and from cognitive neuroscience more particularly is that the brain is fundamentally modular, with various evolutionary additions and modifications of brain systems that have increased and varied our functional repertoires. It is clear that there are multiple brain mechanisms and brain systems supporting perceptual processing, attention, motor performance, and—yes—memory. Modularity and multiple mechanisms seem to be the rule in the brain, with the various mechanisms and systems each contributing particular functionalities to the total package. In this context, unitary theories of memory (or perception, or attention, or motor performance) seem unlikely.

THEORETICAL COMMITMENTS OF A MULTIPLE MEMORY SYSTEM VIEW

There is one last piece of business to which we should attend before finally offering a specific proposal. We need to be clear about what theoretical commitments are entailed by a multiple memory system view. Four points should be addressed, presented here as admonitions about views to which a multiple memory system account does *not* entail a commitment. First, by rejecting the unitary memory system view, in which tasks that are impaired differ from tasks that are spared by virtue of—*and only by virtue of*—the types of retrieval cues they offer for revealing memory, we need *not* deny the possible importance of retrieval-cue differences. What we are committed to is rejection of the view that it is *only* the difference in retrieval cues offered by the different tasks that is critical. The multiple memory system view assumes that the different tasks rely crucially on different memory systems that can be distinguished by the type of representations they support as well as the (retrieval and encoding) processes that permit those representations to be built, stored, and accessed.

Second, and closely related to the first, the multiple memory system view does *not* commit us to rejection of the idea that amnesia is a retrieval deficit. There is no commitment at all about the stage of information processing that might be impaired in amnesic patients. The multiple memory system view is theoretically neutral on the question of whether amnesia reflects a deficit in processes that permit the encoding of memory, the storage, consolidation, and maintenance of memory, or the retrieval of memory. Its commitment is solely to the idea that it is a particular type of memory or domain of representation in which impairment of one or more processes will be manifested. Likewise, while we shall have much to say about the representations supported by the hippocampal system, we are *not* committed to the view that the hippocampal system is the device that physically creates or actually stores declarative representations. We shall return to this point in chapters 3 and 13.

Third, the multiple memory system view does *not* commit us to the idea that all amnesias are the same. It does commit us to the idea that all amnesias, of the sort we are considering, have damage to the same memory system. The patients may differ greatly in the nature of the damage to that system, for example, reflecting impairment of encoding or retrieval processes versus storage or consolidation processes. Indeed, we think it likely that such differences do exist (see Squire & Cohen, 1984; and discussion earlier in the present chapter).[3] What is important for the present purposes, however, is that any heterogeneity among patients is orthogonal to the type of memory or domain of representation affected.

Fourth and last, viewing the difference between tasks spared and tasks impaired in amnesia as reflecting a distinction between two different memory systems does *not* commit us to the idea that there are *two and only two* memory systems or types of memory. That is, although our inquiry organizes the data dichotomously, and although we shall advocate a particular dichotomy between memory systems or types of memory, we do *not* suggest that the two types of memory under discussion exhaust the set of possible types. It is for this reason that we call this approach a multiple memory system account. Adopting a truly dichotomous view runs a risk that we freely acknowledge of distorting the differences and correspondences among complex phenomena. As Stephen Jay Gould (1984) has pointed out:

Since the world is so full of things . . . we must try to catalogue and simplify in order to comprehend. But the reduction of complexity entails a great danger, since the line between enlightened epitome and vulgarized distortion is so fine. Dichotomy is the usual pathway to vulgarization.

We offer a dichotomous view here to point out the inadequacy of unitary models and to express the necessity of multiple memory system models. It reflects our conviction that analysis of the differences between tasks that are preserved versus impaired in amnesia helps to illuminate—indeed, may be the best available way to reveal—the workings of two of the brain's (however many) distinct memory systems.

3 The Hippocampal System and the Procedural-Declarative Memory Distinction: A Comprehensive Proposal

The relationship among memory, amnesia, and the hippocampal system revolves around the claim that the hippocampal system supports a particular type of memory or memory system that is selectively compromised in amnesic patients such as H.M. The critical data from amnesia concern the difference between memory tasks or performances that are spared and those that are impaired. In the account proposed here, this difference is understood in terms of the memory representations that are available and not available, respectively, after hippocampal system damage. Accordingly, we offer a description of two forms of memory representation that we claim are supported by hippocampal-*in*dependent versus hippocampal-dependent memory systems. The present account draws on the procedural-declarative distinction originally applied to amnesia by Cohen and Squire (Cohen, 1981, 1984, 1985; Cohen & Squire, 1980; Cohen et al., 1985; Squire & Cohen, 1984), but in a newly extended and elaborated form that provides for the first time a detailed explication of how the properties of declarative versus procedural memory (1) actually explain impaired versus preserved memory performances in hippocampal amnesia in humans and animals, and (2) conform with and follow from the anatomical and physiological characteristics of the relevant brain systems.

MEMORY REPRESENTATION AND TASK PERFORMANCE

In framing our theory at a level of analysis involving the underlying memory representations supported by hippocampal-dependent and hippocampal-independent memory systems, we are insisting on translating observable performances into details of the representational demands of those performances. Thus, throughout our presentation, the focus will be on what sorts of memory representations

and which performance strategies *must have been used* in performing any given task and how they influence the subject's success,
rather than on which sensory cues were available in the stimulus
array, or on which strategies might have been sufficient for solution.
It turns out that relatively simple variations in parameters of a task,
using exactly the same cues or stimulus materials, can result in
striking differences in the effects of hippocampal system damage
on learning and memory performances.

A particularly clear example of this parameter sensitivity comes
from one of our studies of olfactory learning, in which rats were
trained on a series of two-odor discrimination problems (Eichenbaum et al., 1988). In each problem, animals had to learn that one
of a pair of odors was rewarded (S+) and the other was unrewarded
(S−). When the discrimination trials for each problem involved
simultaneous presentation of the two odors from a pair of odor ports
and rats had to indicate their choice by going to the left port or the
right port (figure 3.1, top panel), hippocampal system damage produced a deficit in learning. But when discrimination trials involved
successive presentation of the two odors from a single port and rats
had to indicate their choice by completing or discontinuing response to the common port (figure 3.1, bottom panel), hippocampal
system damage did *not* interfere at all with learning: "amnesic"
rats learned as well as did normal animals.

Similarly, work by O'Keefe and Conway (1980) showed that impairment in learning a spatial discrimination task depended completely on how the same environmental cues were configured. Rats
were trained to find a food reward located at the end of one goal
arm, starting the trial from any of the other three arms, in a plus-
shaped elevated maze. The maze was surrounded by a plain curtain,
with a small set of stimulus cues visible to help guide performance
(figure 3.2). When rats were trained with the spatial cues dispersed
in the testing environment, hippocampal system damage impaired
performance; but when rats were trained with the same cues concentrated at the goal arm, hippocampal system damage had no
effect.

At first blush, this seems to suggest that the amnesia produced
in animal models is a rather *fragile* phenomenon compared to the
severe and pervasive amnesia seen in patients such as H.M.; or,
perhaps, that we just do not know enough about the representa-

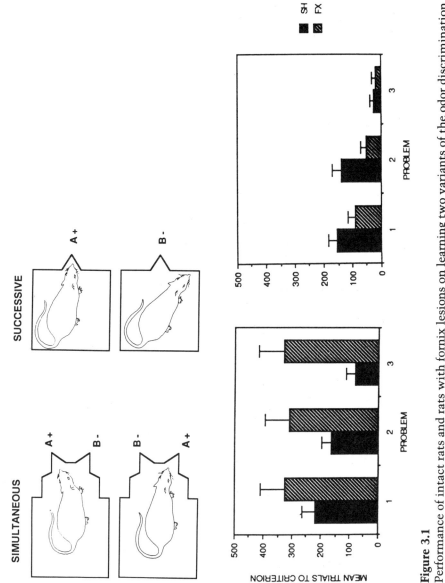

Figure 3.1
Performance of intact rats and rats with fornix lesions on learning two variants of the odor discrimination paradigm. (*Top*) Schematic diagrams and trial examples showing both configurations of odor presentation used in each task variant and a rat executing the appropriate response. (*Bottom*) Performance on these tasks (± S.E.) by sham-operated rats (SH) and rats with hippocampal system damage produced by bilateral fimbria-fornix transection (FX). (From Eichenbaum et al., 1988.)

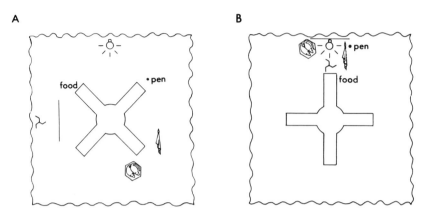

Figure 3.2
Two arrangements of the same cues for guiding spatial performance in the
O'Keefe and Conway study. In both situations a four-arm maze is surrounded by a plain curtain and the locations of six different cues predict
which arm is baited with food. (A) The cues are distributed around the
room and none is contiguous with the baited arm. (B) The cues are clustered
and their location is contiguous with the view down the baited arm. (From
O'Keefe & Conway, 1980.)

tional demands of tasks administered to animals. Yet, in human
amnesics, too, the parameters of the memory test can determine
whether or not impairment is seen for a given set of to-be-studied
materials. This is demonstrated especially clearly in a study by
Graf, Squire, and Mandler (1984), involving different measures of
retention of words whose initial three letters also formed the initial
stem of several different words in the language (e.g., the to-be-
presented words could include *mot*el and *cyc*lone, words whose
initial three letters also form the initial stems of *mot*her and *cyc*le,
not included on the study list). Subjects were presented with a list
of such words to study and were then tested for memory with the
three-letter stems (e.g., *mot* and *cyc*). When subjects were tested in
a cued recall condition—when their instructions were to use the
word stems as cues to help them recall items that had been on the
list—amnesic patients' retention was markedly impaired; but when
subjects receiving the same list items and the same stems were
tested in a word completion condition—when their instructions
were to report "the first word that comes to mind" that completes

each stem—the patients performed as well as control subjects, as shown in figure 3.3.

In each of the examples we have considered, the same to-be-learned materials led to either successful or unsuccessful performance depending on the precise details of testing. The point is that across different experimental conditions, the presence of the same stimulus materials does *not* guarantee that the same information will have been learned or that the same information must be represented in memory. Rather, different arrangements of the same cues and, for human subjects, different instructions, produce differences in how the subjects perceive the task and in what strategies they then choose to employ. These factors then determine what is stored, what is represented, and what is available at testing. Even simple experimental manipulations can change the representational requirements of the task and thereby change the kind of information that must be represented in memory and accessible at the time of retrieval in order to mediate successful task performance.

What ultimately determines the behavioral outcome of a given test, then, is the match between what subjects actually represent

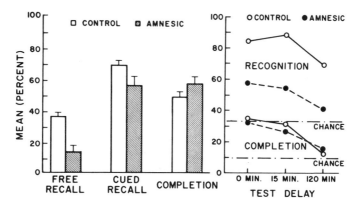

Figure 3.3
Performance of amnesic patients compared to controls on word-stem completion and on various measures of explicit remembering (free recall, cued recall, and recognition) for the same previously studied words. The amnesic patients were biased in their completion performance by the previous studied words to the same extent as were controls (*left*) and this priming effect lasted for the same duration as it did in controls (*right*). (From Graf et al., 1984.)

in memory and the representational requirements of the task. If, as we posit, memory performance is mediated by the cooperative action of a number of different memory systems that support different types of representation, and the hippocampal system plays a critical role in mediating one particular memory system—the declarative system—the "parameter sensitivity" of amnesia just illustrated begins to become clear. Manipulating experimental conditions (or instructions) can change the representational demands of the task, that is, change the relative importance of the different memory systems to that particular performance. Such changes can range from not needing at all the representations supported by declarative memory to being absolutely dependent on declarative representations; likewise, manipulating experimental conditions (or instructions) can change from *dis*couraging to encouraging subjects from relying on or using declarative representations. Either of these would result in the performance of amnesic patients—without the ability to support declarative memory—changing from being intact to being impaired relative to control subjects. If the task requires declarative memory or is at least structured to encourage its use, then the performance of amnesic patients will necessarily differ from that of normal individuals.

These points are a bit abstract at this juncture, in advance of our description of declarative memory and the representations it supports. So, let us turn now to the theory.

DECLARATIVE VERSUS PROCEDURAL MEMORY SYSTEMS

The view we propose here is that the hippocampal system plays a critical role in mediating declarative memory, one of the memory systems of the brain. Although ordinarily operating in concert with other memory systems to guide most behavioral performances, this system is rendered dysfunctional in hippocampal amnesia. Like all of the brain's memory systems, declarative memory has certain identifying properties that provide a signature of its use in particular performances. Other brain systems play a critical role in supporting procedural memory, which remains intact in patients with hippocampal amnesia. Procedural memory exhibits properties quite different from those of declarative memory, and hence leaves a very different signature of its use in behavioral performances. The nature and properties that we propose for procedural and declarative memory are outlined in the following theory, together with a description of their unique signatures.

DECLARATIVE MEMORY

Declarative memory is concerned with the accumulation of facts and data derived from learning experiences. This system represents the *outcomes* of processing by various (neocortical sensory, motor, and limbic) "modules," "processing systems," or "areas" that feed the hippocampal system.[1] That is, input to the hippocampal system consists of highly processed data from many higher-order cortical processing areas, each representing *functional descriptors* of the perceptually distinct objects and events encountered during learning, plus information about the affective and behavioral responses elicited. To understand, let us take visual processing as an example. The visual processing area that projects to, and receives return projections from, the hippocampal system is not striate or prestriate cortex, but rather the inferotemporal cortex (area TE). This area is thought to constitute the brain substrate for processes that permit identification of the functions or meanings of visual objects or scenes, irrespective of (i.e., maintaining constancy across) differences in visual size, location, and viewing perspective (Mishkin, 1982; see chapter 4). Accordingly, the type of visual information to which the hippocampal system has access, and is critical for representing in memory, reflects the outcome of processing for object identification. Analogously, the hippocampal system receives direct connections from the other higher-order sensory processing regions, providing it with the outcomes of sensory processing in the other modalities; and it is the recipient of similarly abstract movement representations from cortical areas receiving input from motor systems, affective representations from limbic system processors, and input from cortical association areas that provide it the outcomes of multimodal and other more integrative processing. Finally, a major output route for hippocampal system processing involves return (reciprocal) connections with these same sources of higher-order cortical input, providing for complex linkages among the areas via hippocampal processing.

These outcomes of processing are, due to the participation of the hippocampal system, represented in highly interconnected networks, with connections among informational elements forming multidimensional "spaces" that capture various possible relations. Thus, the form or nature of declarative representation is fundamentally *relational*. The relational dimensions captured by or represented in declarative networks are at all levels of abstraction: They include strictly sensory relationships, such as relative size, color, texture, shape, etc.; more integrative perceptual relationships such as relative positions of objects in space and time; and higher-order relationships based on the temporal contiguity of objects and events with other objects and events. These latter involve both noncausal coincidences, that is, the accidental conjunctions of objects or events, and causal contiguities, including the learned consequences of particular stimuli or events.

Activation of any given declarative memory (i.e., activation of any given element or set of elements in declarative networks) automatically gives rise to activation of other related memories (of other connected elements), revealing or producing all manner of relations among the stored items. This is a consequence of the relational nature we propose for declarative memory; it, in turn, gives rise to *representational flexibility and promiscuity*. That is, the full interconnectedness of such a representational system produces the ability of information to be activated regardless of the current context, by all manner of external sensory or even purely internal inputs. As a consequence, the representations are promiscuously accessible to—can be activated by—all manner of processes and processing modules; and they can be manipulated and flexibly expressed in any number of novel situations, independent of the circumstances in which the information was initially acquired.

Perhaps we can offer a feel for the relational quality of declarative memory by turning to a notion of representation that has had much currency in cognitive theory. Semantic knowledge, namely, the representation in human memory of meaning or of knowledge about the world, has been conceptualized by many cognitive scientists as being in the form of propositional or semantic networks. This form of representation involves networks of interconnected or associated facts. The networks are thought of as comprising a set of *nodes* embodying constituent pieces of the knowledge base, connected to other nodes by *links* that capture various relations among the bits of knowledge (figure 3.4). The act of perceiving some object in the environment or of thinking of some idea serves to activate nodes corresponding to (i.e., representing) that object or idea; that activation spreads along the links to many related or connected objects or ideas, thereby capturing and permitting the expression of the relationships stored in the networks. The conjunction of objects that constitutes a scene or event, as well as the association among separate bits of knowledge that constitutes a complex idea, make such information available to us by co-activating multiple nodes within such networks.

One aspect of representation in propositional or semantic networks that might be suggested by the above description, and that

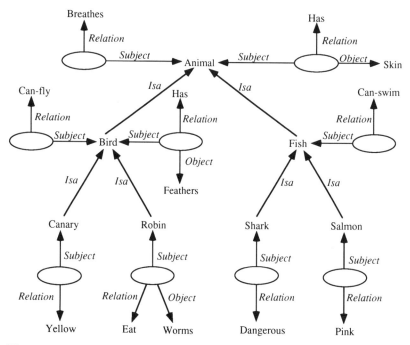

Figure 3.4
A cartoon of a small portion of a semantic network representing knowledge about animals. The key feature is the interrelatedness of the knowledge, depicted by a set of links among the knowledge nodes. Activation of nodes in the network automatically activate other connected nodes (From Norman & Rumelhart, 1975).

is a crucial feature of the relational representation we propose for declarative memory, is the property of *compositionality:* The representation of some scene or event, and the thinking or grasping of some complex idea, entails simultaneous representation both of the separate constituent pieces of knowledge and the larger structure they serve. Thus, for example, representation of an office entails both its office-ness (as opposed to, say, a bedroom or closet or auditorium), and its being composed of desk, chairs, windows, phone, books, and stacks of papers. Likewise, representation of an event such as a ball game involves simultaneously representing the event as distinct from other possible events, and also representing its constituent events and objects, such as parking the car, buying a hotdog, finding the seats, the players being introduced, and so forth. The important point is that a relational representation of scenes, events, and complex ideas in our proposed declarative memory system is *not* as blends, or configurals (see chapter 11), and does *not* involve conjoining of the multiple individual stimuli or constituent pieces of knowledge into unified knowledge structures. Rather, a relational representation preserves the status of the constituents of the larger structure while still permitting the larger structure to be appreciated.

This property of compositionality is critical to the generativity of language and, presumably, of thinking. This is because language and thought depend on the fact that the same constituent pieces of knowledge can be used to construct any number of larger structures (complex ideas, sentences, and even books), while still maintaining their own identity, an identity that must remain systematic across the different larger structures they help to form (see Fodor & Pylyshyn, 1988).[2] It is the compositionality of relational representations that contributes so much to the ability of declarative memory to be *manipulated* in our heads and thereby contributes to (at least one aspect of) its characteristic feature of representational flexibility (see the example just below).

An Extended Example of Declarative Memory in Action

The set of properties of declarative memory described to this point can be best understood by illustrating how declarative memory would come into play in a given processing situation. Consider, for example, what declarative memory might contribute to one's remembering of what is in this book. In the course of reading this book, the reader would engage the processing modules involved in visual pattern analysis, word identification, and text comprehension, among others. The outcomes of these various processing modules, outputted to and stored with the participation of the hippocampal-dependent declarative memory system, might well include the following: specific words or particularly felicitous phrases (if any) that were noted; ideas and issues that were grasped, impressions that were formed, or reactions that were elicited while reading; citations that were noticed (or citations whose absence was noticed); associations with and discrepancies from other work or other ideas that came to mind while reading; figures or illustrations that were particularly informative or compelling (or confusing); aspects or features of the layout of the book that were striking; and, perhaps, details about the context in which the book was read (where, when, what else was going on at the time, etc.).

Such information would be stored relationally and, as a result, would exhibit representational flexibility and promiscuity. Accordingly, this information would have the potential for being accessed and expressed in any number of ways, and in various—even completely novel—contexts. It would support three categories of performances that we would like to emphasize here.

First, declarative memory would support recall and recognition of the book and its contents. That is, words, phrases, figures, citations, and, hopefully, the substantive ideas in this book could be recognized if re-presented to the reader, and could be recalled if the reader were asked about the book. It would also support explicit remembering of the experience of reading the book, or first hearing about the book, or perhaps actually purchasing it. That memory might well include information about location or other activities ongoing in the background (e.g., music playing on the stereo while reading it at home, or people walking by the MIT Press booth while purchasing it at a convention), and so forth—that is, it would support representation of the conjunctions of objects and spatiotemporal context that characterize events.

Second, declarative memory would support the ability to access stored information about the book in a variety of circumstances, in response to various kinds of prompts. Thus, remembered details about the contents of the book could be reported whether the reader were asked explicitly to provide a report of the book; or asked to talk about whatever interesting things he or she had read recently; or queried about what Cohen and Eichenbaum are up to these days; or probed about new developments in the amnesia field; or asked about the books published recently by the MIT Press; and so forth.

Third, declarative memory would support the ability to *manipulate* in one's head information that was stored about the book. Declarative memory can be used by various processing modules to support the making of comparisons, judgments, abstractions, and generalizations across stored elements, and between stored elements and new inputs. Thus, declarative memory for the contents of the book could be used to: judge the plausibility and merit of the account proposed in this book and of the data offered support it, as compared to other theories in the literature; consider how the proposed account might deal with empirical data not discussed in the book; generate new experiments that might test the proposed account; and, perhaps, contemplate the possible consequences of making various additions or modifications to the theory.

An admonition to be noted, however: Of course, we can only talk about the potential offered by the hippocampal-dependent declarative memory system, namely, the performances this system can potentially support. Whether or not a particular item is actually recalled or recognized, and whether or not a particular item can actually be manipulated and used flexibly in novel contexts, depends on how well it was encoded and stored and how much forgetting may have occurred prior to testing.[3] Provided that the declarative memory is robust, however, it will be capable of supporting the performances described above. Furthermore, provided that it is retrieved, it can be used flexibly. Only declarative memory has the properties that would permit mediation of such performances.

Some of the means by which we commonly assess memory necessarily combine two or all three of these characteristics or potentialities of declarative memory (explicit remembering of the items, promiscuous access to the memories, and the ability to manipulate the information or otherwise use it flexibly), although their contributions to performance may not be readily apparent. The presence and contribution to performance of these three characteristics is more common in the recollection of everyday autobiographical memories than probably meets the eye. Consider the question "What did you have for breakfast yesterday morning?" Generating an answer typically involves conscious reflection on that morning's events (or memory search includes the generation of various events that can be used in a cognitively mediated way to cue other events in an attempt to get to yesterday's breakfast) leading to the identification of the particular representations of the food that was eaten, and ultimately producing an explicit oral description of those foods. Such a memory search engages all three of the categories of performance described above, including (1) simple reinstantiation (and recognition) of perceptual "images" associated with the food eaten, plus (2) the ability to gain access to these representations through linguistic queries in an entirely different context than the one in which the information was originally acquired (i.e., accessing neural processing devices distinctly different from those visual, olfactory, gustatory, and motor processors engaged during the breakfast event), and (3) the representational flexibility necessary to manipulate the various representations of the experience to extract just the context-appropriate information the questioner seeks, such as limiting the description to the class of food and not including specific details about the precise sensory features of the food items or of the various objects present in the same visual arrays (and, presumably, memory representations) as the food (for more discussion see chapters 7, 8, 11, and 12).

A similar conclusion can be drawn from the animal literature on place learning. Contrary to the view that learning the place of a reward (say, in a radial arm maze) or of some reward-related object (e.g., the escape platform in the Morris water maze) is formally identical to learning the reward association of some object or sensory cue—the two tasks putatively differing only in the cue "modality" (spatial versus visual or auditory)—place learning is much more complex *and more declarative* than that. The neural processes involved in approaching the learned place necessarily involve not only recognizing the place from familiar views, but also navigating different and perhaps novel views of the environment encountered along a variety of approach paths. This requirement arises from the fact that these tasks employ multiple starting locations that involve overlapping perspectives of the same, fixed perceptual stimuli within the environment being explored by the animals. Such overlapping perspectives of the same stimuli require that the memory representations be of a form that permits understanding that a given object or sensory cue is to the right of a particular cue under certain circumstances and to the left under others. Expression of the acquired knowledge must permit flexible responses guided by spatial relations among the cues and the position of the subject (for more discussion see chapter 7).

Viewed from this perspective it is difficult to imagine how memory for the events of daily life in humans and place learning in animals can be accomplished without declarative memory. And, indeed, except under unusual circumstances, amnesics are virtually always impaired in these kinds of learning.

A Second Example of Declarative Memory

Rather than emphasizing the representational flexibility and promiscuity of declarative memory, as was done in the previous example, this example stresses the unique capacity of declarative memory to support learning of relations among perceptually distinct objects. Consider the kind of memory representation necessary to learn and remember (in the sense of adding new knowledge to which one can gain access on demand) the specific names that go with particular people's faces, or the addresses and phone numbers that go with them. These relations are (nearly always) entirely arbitrary. Thus, whatever reasons there were for the respective parents of the current authors to name us Neal and Howard, it was *not* because there was something about our appearance that suggested those names. Hence someone trying now to learn our names (i.e., learn which name goes with which face) could not derive it from our appearance; rather, they would have to create specific representations of these relationships. Likewise, our phone numbers and addresses were certainly not suggested by nor are in any way meaningfully related to our names or appearance; hence, someone trying to learn them could not derive them from our name or appearance, and would instead have to create specific representations of these relationships. These representations would have to be robust and flexible, permitting the stored information about the faces, names, phone numbers, and addresses of people whom we know well to be accessible when queried in any number of ways and in any number of modalities: We can generate an image of persons whose names are mentioned orally or are printed in the phone book, or whenever we just happen to be thinking of them; generate the names of persons we see; remember the addresses of persons who invite us (orally or in writing) over; and so forth. Declarative memory is uniquely suited to mediate this form of memory representation.

In line with this attribution, H.M. is profoundly impaired at forming and using these kinds of relational representations. He cannot learn (in the sense described above) the names of his health care providers or the researchers with whom he has come into repeated contact, nor information about *his own* address or living arrangements for the place where he has lived for many years. More generally, the ability to learn arbitrarily paired items such as what is typically tested in "paired-associate learning" (e.g., being presented with a list of word pairings such as *crush-dark, obey-inch, school-grocery*, etc., and then being asked to remember the word that went with *crush* or with *obey* or with *school*), is notoriously impaired in hippocampal amnesia. Paired-associate learning provides a test that is most revealing of human amnesia.

Finally, let us complete our presentation concerning the nature and characteristics of declarative memory by moving to a description at the level of brain systems. As is captured in the cartoon (figure 3.5) borrowed from Halgren (1984), the hippocampal system is located in a position to receive and to "bind" or "chunk" together information represented as activity in multiple cortical areas. In the course of experiencing some event, various cortical networks are activated, each processing an aspect of the total event. By virtue of the connections of these various cortical networks to the hippocampal system, the co-activations representing the outcomes of the different analyses converge on hippocampal system networks. The hippocampal system is thereby in a position for mediating the representation of these conjunctions or co-activations. The hippocampal system is not to be seen as the repository for permanent storage of such information, however. Rather, the convergence of the projections from the various cortical processing areas onto the hippocampal system may permit the system to "maintain the coherence" of the cortical co-activations that represent the original event, as proposed by Squire, Cohen, and Nadel (1984); that is, it is

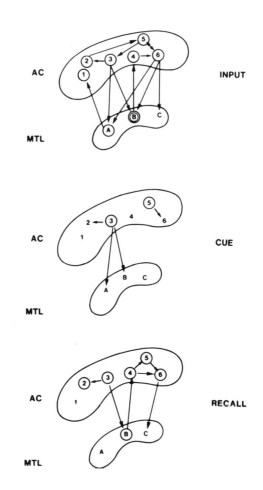

Figure 3.5
Halgren's scheme by which reciprocal interactions between the association
cortex (AC) and medial temporal lobe (MTL) mediate recall through mechanisms of long-term synaptic enhancement (LTE) [LTP in the text] and
pattern completion (*Input*) At the initial experience of an event, five association cortex neurons are activated (labeled 2 through 6). These AC
neurons excite MTL neurons A, B, and C, but only the synapses from 3 to
6 onto B are enhanced (A did not reach LTE threshold because it does not
participate in an active AC ↔ MTL positive feedback loop; C did not reach
LTE threshold because it received too little input from excited AC neurons).
(*Cue*) Aspects 3 and 5 of the previous event are presented as recall cues.
(*Recall*) Because the synapse from 3 to B is enhanced, excitation of 3 excites
B, which excites 4. Other aspects of the original experience (2, 4, 5, and 6)
are excited as a result of the interactions within the AC. Together these
processes lead to reconstruction of the AC neural activity pattern present

the cortical networks that actually store the memories. Then, if at some later time a portion or aspect of the original event is re-presented, activating a subset of the cortical networks originally activated, the reciprocal connections between cortex and the hippocampal system may serve to permit the original pattern of co-activations to be completed or recovered. We will have more to say in chapter 13 about the binding or chunking function we attribute to the hippocampal system. The physiological and anatomical support for several of the claims made above are presented in chapters 4 and 5.

Importantly, in providing a means for various subsets of the original input to gain access to the representation of the original event, that is, for completion or recovery of the original pattern of co-activations to be possible from a variety of different test-time cues, this scheme supports precisely the representational flexibility that is uniquely characteristic of declarative memory. It also provides for the compositionality of declarative memory, because the individual components or attributes are stored separately in the different cortical networks and then also form part of the larger relational representation when the hippocampal system participates in the circuit.

The reciprocal interconnections of the hippocampal system with various cortical networks, and the resulting convergence onto the hippocampal network of these cortical co-activations, gives rise to a very special functionality, namely the ability to represent in a single memory space the converging outcomes of processors that could not otherwise communicate. It is (only) in the hippocampal network that various combinations of objects can come together as a contemporaneous event or scene, and can be combined with affective information and information about behavioral responses and even information from previous events or other learning experiences to permit relational representations that go beyond what would be possible in any single cortical processor. That is, by bring-

---

at the original experience. (From Halgren, 1984.) This type of mechanism is envisaged in our account to extend to the hippocampal mediation of reciprocal interactions among neocortical processing networks or cell ensembles (and not just single cells) and to support the same type of completion phenomena on the network scale.

ing together and maintaining the coherence of the cortical co-activations, the hippocampal system provides the ability to construct
representations of new higher-order objects that are the conjunctions of the objects that can be represented in one or another of the
cortical networks that feed the hippocampus. These cortical networks are still essential in providing the outcomes that undergo
binding or chunking through the participation of the hippocampal
system, and are the necessary storage sites of the (distributed attributes of the) memories that are thus formed. But it is the hippocampal system that provides the relational memory space in which
the binding and chunking of the cortical outputs leads to the construction of declarative memory representations.

Two quick and final things to note about this: One is that the
co-activated elements in the hippocampal memory space, when
forming new relational memories, span across any number of different cortical networks, giving a very different feel than the semantic or propositional networks we considered earlier in the
chapter in discussing the relational properties of declarative memory. We offered semantic or propositional networks as an analogy
at the cognitive level for understanding the automatic spread of
activation we envision in declarative memory (as, for example, is
proposed by John Anderson [1983] and others). By contrast, our
discussion of cortical co-activations converging onto the hippocampal network, and the idea of the hippocampal system as a memory
space in which the construction of relational memories can occur,
is meant to be a proposal about the neurobiology of declarative
memory.

Second, among the processing outcomes that could converge onto
the hippocampal system and be chunked into relational representations are some potentially lower-level sensory inputs, *if they are
seen by the subject, or defined by the task, as being the outcomes
of processing.* That is, if the task makes discriminating among lines
presented at subtly different orientations the desired outcome of
visual processing, or if the task makes discriminating among the
particular sonic characteristics of the same piece of music through
different audio speakers the desired outcome of auditory processing,
then these will become part of the relational representations captured by declarative memory. The differences in sonic characteristics of the Thiel model 3.6 speakers versus the Duntech Sovereign

speakers are part of N.J.C.'s declarative memory of his visit to the summer 1992 Consumer Electronics Show in Chicago, together with other memories involving people he met and dinners he ate. In this case, as in the other cases we considered above, what enters into hippocampal-mediated declarative memories are the outcomes of processing.

To summarize, the declarative memory system receives, and plays a mediating role in the storage of, the outcomes of processing events. Declarative memory is a fundamentally relational representation system. The relational nature of declarative memory gives rise to two properties that give it its signature: representational flexibility and promiscuity. Thus, declarative memory is promiscuously accessible to, or can be activated by, various processing modules, regardless of which processing modules were engaged in the processing of the original learning event; and, once accessed, it can be manipulated and flexibility expressed in various test contexts, regardless of how much those contexts differ from the circumstances in which the information was initially acquired.

Features and characteristics of declarative *memory:*

• represents the outcomes of processing operations
• binds or chunks the outputs of various processors converging on the hippocampal system
• representation system is fundamentally relational (with compositionality)
• stored memory is promiscuously accessible to various processing systems
• memory can be expressed flexibly, capable of being used in even completely novel contexts

Features and characteristics of procedural *memory:*

• involves the tuning and modifying of the particular processors engaged during training
• representations are dedicated to the modified processors, unavailable to other processors
• representations are fundamentally individual
• memory can be expressed only *inflexibly,* only in a repetition of the original processing situation

PROCEDURAL MEMORY

By contrast, procedural representations, supported by memory systems that operate independently of the hippocampal system, are inflexible and dedicated. Their storage resides within and remains inextricably tied to the processing modules that were engaged during initial learning. This type of memory involves *not* the storage of outcomes of processing operations, but rather tuning of and changes in the way those operations actually run—that is, modification of the processing elements themselves. This type of representation is therefore *in*flexible; it is only accessible to those processing modules that were engaged during the original learning experiences, and only when they are again engaged. The representations therefore can only be expressed or otherwise exert their influence under testing conditions that so closely mirror the circumstances of original learning—from the perspective of the processors engaged by the task—as to constitute a repetition of the original learning situation.

Examples of Procedural Memory in Action

Let us consider the contributions that would be made by procedural memory in the example used earlier concerning memory for reading this book. The pattern analysis, word recognition, and text comprehension systems engaged during reading would be *tuned* by the action of procedural memory in accordance with the particular regularities of this text. These systems would be *biased* for a time such that there would be (a temporary) facilitation in reading of the particular words, phrases, and larger word-combinations read in this book if portions of this text were to be re-presented on a subsequent occasion particularly if re-presented in the same type font used originally. Facilitation in reading speed is another example of the repetition priming effects introduced in chapter 2 and discussed in more detail in chapter 8; it has been shown to occur in normal subjects and amnesic patients alike. The processors engaged in reading, having been organized by past experience, continue to be shaped and molded by new experiences, making and keeping them maximally tuned to the inputs they actually receive most frequently and recently. This tuning results in the often observed frequency effects in word identification and reading speed: Performance is fastest and most accurate for the words in the language that occur in text most often.

This contribution of the procedural system would be discerned *only* when the subject is presented with a repetition of the original learning event, in the sense of a test context that serves to again engage the pattern analysis, word recognition, and/or text comprehension processors engaged in originally reading the text. This would occur in the course of reading the text again or in the course of similar processing (e.g., in word identification, word-stem completion, or word-fragment completion tasks administered in the laboratory, such as the Graf, Squire, and Mandler [1984] word-stem completion work discussed earlier; for a fuller description, see chapters 8 and 12). That is, the modifications of these processors can be revealed or expressed only when they are again engaged, because of the inflexibility of procedural representations, *but by any task that does so.* Hence, a repetition of the original learning event in this case would be any task in which words are presented to be read, regardless of what the subject is supposed to do with the words. As long as the task includes reading the words, there will be the reengagement of the tuned processors, and some measure of procedural memory phenomena will be revealed. (Note that what constitutes a repetition of the original learning event as opposed to a novel context must be conceived from the perspective of the processing system or module that is being tuned procedurally, not from the perspective of the task. Any task that entails identifying and generating word forms would provide an opportunity to see the priming effects induced during reading.)

Let us consider another example, this time concerning evidence of changes in brain circuitry. Emerging findings on the plasticity of primary cortical areas suggests that there are procedural-like "shaping" or "tuning" mechanisms that operate throughout the lifetime of an animal to change the receptivity of the individual processing units within the basic processors of the brain. For example, Merzenich and colleagues (Merzenich et al., 1990; Recanzone et al., 1992) have shown rearrangements of the somatotopic representation in primary somatosensory cortex of monkeys following a variety of traumatic and more natural interventions in somatosensory input. Following digit removal, the cortical representation of neighboring digits invades the cortical zone whose afferents have been removed. In parallel studies, it has been found that surgical joining of the digits results in the establishment of a continuous somatic representation of formerly discontinuous zones for each digit.

Rearrangement of cortical representations can occur naturally during conventional behavioral training. For example, Merzenich and colleagues (Merzenich et al., 1991) have recently shown that tactile discrimination training results in altered sensory receptive fields in the somatosensory cortex—again, changes in the processing units themselves. When the training stimuli involve punctuate stimulation of small skin loci, receptive fields representing that area grow in size; conversely, when moving stimuli are employed, the receptive fields shrink. In addition, the responsiveness of these neurons to other formerly effective inputs is reduced. These changes are accompanied by decreases in response latencies and increases in the temporal synchronization of the local neuronal circuitry. Indeed, artificial introduction of temporal synchrony itself can produce the altered receptive field patterns (Allard et al., 1991). Moreover, synchronization of cortical physiology acquired during training is well correlated with the behavioral performance in a discrimination task. Similar changes in the receptive field patterns of other neocortical areas as a result of specific training experience have also been demonstrated, for example, in the auditory cortex of rats trained in a tone discrimination (Diamond & Weinberger, 1986). Thus these cortical rearrangements may be a general consequence of experiences that support learning and memory. Finally, the changes in sensory representation occur gradually along with increments in discriminative capacity, suggesting they may subserve the alterations in performance supported by procedural memory. These changes, by occurring as tunings or modifications of the actual processing elements in motor and auditory cortices, are dedicated to these particular processing systems and could be expressed only by again engaging the affected processors. These changes would *not* support explicit remembering of the training experiences.

Another example, one that we have cited previously (see Cohen 1981, 1984), concerns effects occurring during certain critical periods in development, specifically, the effects of selective early experience on the visual system of cats. While it is not likely that precisely the same effects occur in adulthood, they nonetheless provide a particularly compelling example of the possible brain changes that could underlie procedural memory. Restricting a kitten's early experience to, say, vertical contours results in modification of the properties of the actual processing elements of the visual system, just as we saw above for the somatosensory system. Individual visual cortex neurons change their orientation selectivity in conformance with their experience, gaining increased sensitivity to vertically oriented lines and losing sensitivity to lines of other orientations (e.g., Blakemore, 1974). This is illustrated in figure 3.6. Recordings from cells in primary visual cortex of normal animals show different neurons with preferences for different stimulus orientations. That is, when the orientation preferences of a substantial sample of visual cortex neurons are plotted, with the orientation to which each sampled neuron is optimally sensitive represented as a line drawn with that orientation, all (or at least many) directions are seen to be represented. However, in animals whose early visual experience is restricted to vertically oriented stimuli, only neurons with a preference for vertical orientation can be found.

In addition to showing the orientation preferences discussed above, cells in primary visual cortex also show a preference in the relative balance given to input from the two eyes. Input from the two eyes is segregated at the stages of processing prior to that accomplished by primary visual cortex; inputs from the two eyes then converge in the input layer of primary visual cortex. However, cells in this processing area differ from one another in how strongly they are driven by one or the other set of inputs (figure 3.7, top). Most neurons are activated equally well, or have equal preference, for the two eyes; others are dominated by one or the other eye, to differing extents, thereby producing a distribution of relative preference or *ocular dominance*. Restricting early visual experience in kittens, by arranging for input to be provided by one eye only, dramatically alters this ocular dominance distribution, as illustrated in figure 3.7 (middle). Suturing closed the *right* eye for a period of training lasting several months early in life produces a pattern of results (in animals tested later with both eyes open) in which neurons respond almost exclusively to the experienced eye: Cells in the left hemisphere are dominated by input from the ipsilateral (*left*) eye, and cells in the right hemisphere are dominated by input from the contralateral (*left*) eye (Wiesel & Hubel 1963, 1965).

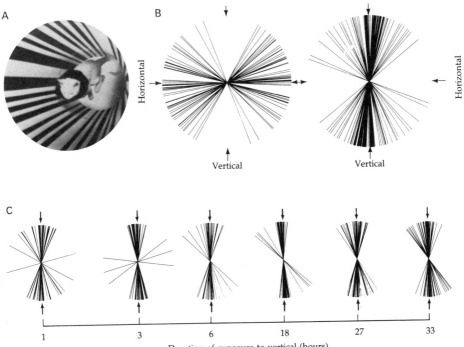

Figure 3.6
Modifications of the receptive field properties of visual cortical neurons by altered early experience. (A) Kittens can be raised in rotating drums in which they see only stripes of one orientation. The kittens wear black collars to hide their bodies and stand on a glass plate; except when in the drum for a few hours each day, they are kept in total darkness. (B) These polar histograms show the distribution of the stimulus orientations eliciting optimal responses in 52 neurons from a kitten that had been exposed only to the horizontally oriented stimulation (*left*) and in 72 neurons from a kitten exposed only to vertical stimuli (*right*). Each line represents the stimulus orientation eliciting an optimal response in a single neuron. (C) Responses of kittens reared in darkness and exposed only to vertical stimuli for the number of hours indicated. As in *B*, each line signifies the optimal orientation for single neuron responses. Evidently, even a few hours of exposure to a particular visual environment can modify cortical connectivity. (From Purves & Lichtman, 1985.)

This tuning and biasing of the processing elements in primary visual cortex can actually be revealed anatomically. Work with normal and monocularly deprived monkeys has permitted anatomical measurements of the relative weight given by primary visual cortex to input from the two eyes (Hubel, Wiesel, & LeVay, 1977). Injection into the eye of slightly radioactive tracers permits visualization of the input converging from different layers of the lateral geniculate nucleus of the thalamus onto the input layer of primary visual cortex. This is visualized as alternating stripes corresponding to the input from the two eyes (figure 3.7, bottom). In normal animals, the stripes of are very nearly equal widths, reflecting the very nearly equal weights given to the two sets of inputs. However, in animals who have had monocularly restricted visual experience, by having had one eye sutured closed, the pattern of striping is dramatically changed: Wide stripes alternate with much narrower ones, showing the marked change in weight given to the input from the experienced eye over the input from the previously closed eye.

These various changes, by occurring as tunings or modifications of the actual processing elements in primary visual cortex, are dedicated to this processor and could be expressed only by again engaging the affected processing elements. These changes would *not* support explicit remembering of the early training experiences. Moreover, although the necessary experiments have yet to be performed, we would make the following pair of predictions about attempts to interfere with this system: Hippocampal system damage would have no effect on the tuning and restructuring of visual cortical cells in the kittens, and blockage of the mechanism by which the visual cortex tuning and restructuring occurs would have no effect whatever on memory for the actual training experiences.

The above described procedural memory systems are only representative of what we presume to be a large number of brain circuits in which performance is tuned or biased through experience. In addition to these cortical systems, a number of subcortical circuits and pathways have been identified that support various forms of conditioning. A few that figure prominently in current research are the following: a system involving the amygdala that supports conditioned emotional responses (e.g., Le Doux, 1991), a system involving the striatum that is critical to learning to approach salient cues contiguous with reward (e.g., Packard et al., 1989), a cerebellar-

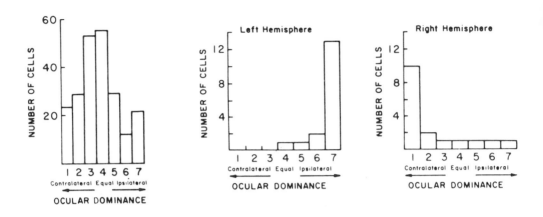

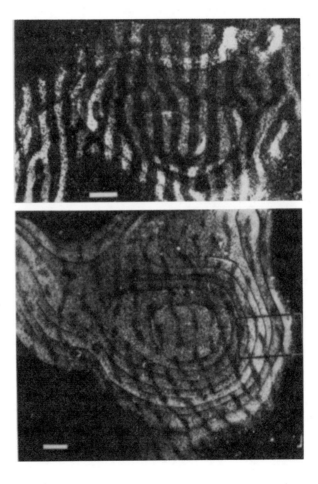

brainstem circuit that supports classical eyelid (and other skeletal muscular) conditioning (Gellman & Miles, 1985), and other forms of simple conditioning such as heart rate, startle reflex habituation, and the vestibulo-ocular reflex (reviewed in Squire, 1987). These systems can extend the kinds of procedural changes discussed above to include the ability to accomplish representations of simple *associations*, in which the characteristics of processing *within* a system or pathway can be changed by training. Thus, for example, specific subcortical circuits are capable of mediating classical conditioning of the nictitating membrane response (NMR) to an air puff, such that when that air puff occurs at a predictable time after an auditory cue, the timing of the NMR is gradually shifted to be emitted prior to the onset of the air puff. This conditioned behavioral change is mediated by modification of the pathways that bring together the auditory information and motor information in the cerebellar and associated brainstem nuclei. Thus, here, tuning of cerebellar networks can bring about representation of simple and highly specific *associations*. But by no means are these the same as the relational representations mediated by the hippocampal-dependent declarative system. The relational representations characteristic of declarative memory can support all manner of conjunctions among all variety of cortical processors, taking advantage of the convergence of cortical processing outcomes onto the hippocampal system, to permit the construction of representations of any conceivable relationship. And these representations are fundamentally flexible and promiscuous in the manner described at length above; they can be accessed under a wide range of testing circumstances,

◄──

Figure 3.7
(*Top*) Distribution of ocular dominance for neurons from striate cortex of normal adult cats (*left*), and for neurons from striate cortex in the left hemisphere (*middle*) and the right hemisphere (*right*) of a cat whose visual experience from 9 weeks to 6 months of age was restricted to the left eye. (From Squire, 1987.) (*Bottom*) Autoradiograph of layer IVc of the striate cortex following injection of radioactively labeled amino acids into one eye of a normal monkey (*upper*) and a monkey whose visual experience from 2 weeks to 18 months of age was restricted to the left eye (*lower*). The white and dark stripes reveal the cortical columns allocated to the left and right eye, respectively. The stripes from the nondeprived left eye are much larger than normal after monocular deprivation. (From Hubel et al., 1977.)

and once accessed can be used completely flexibly. Neither of these is in any way true of the procedural representation of simple associations.

As one looks at the various systems noted above that are capable of supporting procedural-memory brain changes, it seems apparent that the nature of the relevant stimulus and response modalities and operating characteristics might vary considerably among these systems, and in many cases may well be unique. However, they all share fundamental properties that distinguish them from the hippocampal-dependent system—specifically, they each exhibit the dedicated, inflexible form of representation that characterizes procedural memory as distinguished from declarative memory. Accordingly, we treat these various examples of tuning and restructuring of basic processors as all forming a common type or form of memory—procedural memory—by virtue of exhibiting the same kind of representational characteristics, as will be discussed in chapter 12.

Modeling Procedural Memory

The tuning and biasing of various brain processors in accordance with the real-world regularities of the inputs to which they are exposed finds a very comfortable home in current connectionist (or neural network) models. In connectionist models, the knowledge embodied within any given processing system or module is stored in weights on connections among a collection of simple processing elements. The processing elements are typically viewed as being considerably more simple than the nodes of the semantic or propositional networks considered earlier in the chapter, and it is in the connections among them that information is stored. Thus, rather than semantic nodes, each of which individually represents specific objects or features, connectionist models typically (although not necessarily)[4] have a more distributed representation, in which objects and even features of objects are represented across many connection weights, with each of the connection weights contributing to the representation of many different things (McClelland & Rumelhart, 1986; Rumelhart & McClelland, 1986; figure 3.8).

Most important for the present purposes, the connection weights are modifiable by experience, responding to learning rules that ad-

Output Patterns

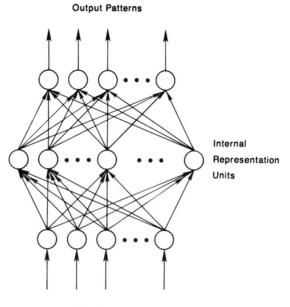

Internal
Representation
Units

Input Patterns

Figure 3.8
A generic multilayer connectionist network, in which there is an input layer of processing units, fully interconnected with an intermediate layer of "internal representation units," in turn fully interconnected with a layer of output units. The connections among the elements across the layers have graded strengths or weights that can be modified by experience. (From Rumelhart et al., 1986.)

just the weights incrementally to reflect the information in the input. As a consequence, such models are superb at capturing the regularities in the information presented; the connection weights will be greatest for those items most often present in the input and smaller for items presented less frequently and less recently. This way of viewing, or modeling, memory seems to nicely capture the examples of procedural memory offered above, including both (1) the superiority in reading or word recognition for the particular words to which subjects were exposed most frequently and recently (e.g., see the word recognition model offered by McClelland & Rumelhart, 1986), and (2) the increased weight accorded to input from the particular eye, and to input of the particular orientations, to which animals' early experience had been restricted (e.g., see the model by Munro, 1984).

Note that there is no mechanism in these simple connectionist networks for reporting on the training experiences, or for otherwise using the knowledge acquired from the experiences in another context. The memory is manifested as changes within the processor (i.e., network) that is engaged by some learning event, and will be expressed when *and only when* the processor is again engaged. Such networks seem to provide a particularly good way of modeling particular processing modules and the plasticities that they exhibit; those within-processor plasticities capture nicely the characteristics we have posited for procedural memory. A few investigators have endeavored to use such networks to model recognition memory performance (hence declarative memory), but to do so have had to appeal to additional mechanisms (Humphreys, Bain, & Pike, 1989; Krushke, 1992; Sloman & Rumelhart, 1991), and even then they fail to capture the full flexibility and compositionality we take to be so central to declarative memory.

Another model for procedural memory in the cognitive literature is that of production systems (Anderson, 1983; Newell, 1973). Production system models assume that knowledge is represented as a set of production rules (or productions) each of which independently inspects the configuration of elements appearing in the input and looks for certain triggering conditions to be met. When a production's triggering conditions are met, it "fires" and thereby initiates some action. The action might be some aspect of a behavioral performance, or it might be a change in the state of the input to the system, which in turn might satisfy the triggering conditions of other productions, and so on (figure 3.9). In such a system, productions are seen as independent and very single-minded processors, each independently searching the common input in an attempt to recognize when its triggering conditions have been satisfied, and each capable of acting independently when its conditions have been met. Learning in such a system includes acquiring new productions, shaping and tuning productions to reflect the actual conditions with which they are likely to be confronted, and modifying the strength or weight afforded to different productions (see figure 3.9). In such

---

RULE 050

PREMISE: (AND (SAME CNTXT INFECT PRIMARY-BACTEREMIA)
                 (MEMBF CNTXT SITE STERILESITES)
                 (SAME CNTXT PORTAL GI))
ACTION: (CONCLUDE CNTXT IDENT BACTEROIDES TALLY .7)

MYCIN's English translation:

IF   1) the infection is primary-bacteremia, and
           2) the site of the culture is one of the sterile sites, and
           3) the suspected portal of entry of the organism is
              the gastrointestinal tract,
THEN   there is suggestive evidence (.7) that the identity of the
           organism is bacteroides.

Figure 3.9
An example of a production rule from the artificial intelligence (AI) expert
system MYCIN, which has a knowledge base made up of production rules
that permits it to diagnose and suggest treatments for infectious diseases.
Such rules are *not* connected to other items in the knowledge base. Note
that this production rule embodies a certainty or confidence factor (in this
case with a value of .7). To the extent that such confidence factors or
weightings can be modified by experience, and thereby change the output
of the production system, it provides a mechanism for memory that does
not rely in any way on recollection or explicit remembering of the learning
event. (From Barr & Feigenbaum, 1982.)

a form of representation, knowledge is clearly embedded in the
procedures for operating on the world; it can be revealed only when
these productions, shaped by experience, are elicited by the appropriate conditions. Furthermore, consistent with the view of procedural memory that we have articulated, there is no mechanism here
for explicitly recalling and reporting the contents of particular learning experiences, nor for using the represented knowledge flexibly.

    The inflexibility of procedural memory representations can be
quite striking. Thus, in some of the examples in chapters 6 to 8 it
will be seen that there are circumstances where "amnesic" subjects—with only procedural memory to draw on—can acquire new
tasks at a normal rate and perform perfectly normally on repetitions
of the learning experience, but fail quite strikingly when asked to

employ their knowledge in even slightly altered circumstances. These circumstances apply to the examples of olfactory and place learning in rats described above and in chapters 6 and 7, and to object discrimination learning in monkeys (see chapter 7). Abundant parallel data exist in examples of preserved skill learning and priming in human amnesics—who also only have procedural memory with which to perform. For example, Glisky and Schacter's (1987, 1989) studies on teaching amnesic patients certain job-relevant terms to use on a computer revealed that patients could, after a great deal of painstaking repetitive practice, learn to enter relevant computer commands, but their knowledge was "hyperspecific"—it would be expressed only when the training conditions were reproduced (see chapter 8). Moreover, skill learning and repetition priming are so sensitive to changes between training and test conditions that the modality of stimulus presentation and even the specific type font of verbal stimuli become critical variables (see chapter 8). All of these exemplify the inflexibility we take to be characteristic of procedural memory. Another way in which we have described this inflexibility is that procedural representations are akin to isolated "snapshots" of experience in the absence of the picture "album" that relates various compositions and elements of the same experience to one another; it is only when representations of experience are stored relationally—that is, declaratively—that they can be used flexibly and generatively (Eichenbaum et al., 1991).

To summarize, procedural memory accomplishes the tuning and modification of various processors in the brain. It is a dedicated representation system; the memory is so closely tied to the processors that it cannot be accessed by other systems, and can be expressed only *inflexibly*, under testing conditions that mirror the circumstances of original learning so closely as to constitute repetitions of the original learning event (i.e., reengagements of the processors used during the original learning event). Procedural memory is invoked whenever there is in place the requisite processing machinery to derive a solution to the problem at hand; with practice, the processing machinery that is used will be tuned and biased by experience, gradually optimizing its performance, producing facilitation when the same processors are again called upon to again derive a solution.

DOES THE PROCEDURAL-DECLARATIVE DISTINCTION MAKE
ADAPTIVE SENSE?: SATISFYING COMPETING DESIGN CONSTRAINTS

Having described the different characteristics we propose for procedural and declarative memory, discussed something of their separate styles of operation, and considered some general models to capture their distinct natures, we might still want to ask whether modularizing memory into at least these two functionally distinct systems makes any adaptive sense. Might there not instead be some way to design a unitary memory system that incorporates both sets of characteristics? This question has led us to consider just what purposes might be served by separate procedural and declarative memory systems, and how well such purposes serve the organism as a whole.

We would like now to introduce the notion of competing design constraints. If we were designing a system of long-term memory to accommodate the range of human performances that we have observed, what are the fundamental capabilities that we would include? And would these separate capabilities be mutually consistent, or would they instead constitute competing demands? The answer, it seems to us, is that the performances considered in this book place at least two competing demands on design of a memory system.

On the one hand, it would be exceptionally useful if memory could be intimately tied to specific processing systems or modules so that experiences can effectively shape and tune these processors to reflect the regularities in the world with which they will be confronted. Capturing the regularities in the input would go a long way toward optimizing their performance in the majority of circumstances. Just as over the course of the evolutionary history of our species, our auditory systems have come to be optimally sensitive to the frequency of sounds occurring in human speech, it would be useful if sensory systems could become optimally sensitive to the objects we encounter most in life, such as human faces, over the course of the lifetime of the individual. If the processors themselves could maintain a form of plasticity that permits them to be shaped and tuned by experience to perform most effectively and most quickly in response to the inputs that are encountered most often, their performance would be optimized for the majority of processing events. By being tied to the processors, memory would permit very rapid and effective responses of the processors to the regularities in the world.

On the other hand, it would be tremendously valuable if memory were fully independent of particular processing systems or modules, so that it could be used in any given situation regardless of how and through what system the information was originally acquired. If memory were accessible to all the brain's processors and could be manipulated and used completely flexibly, then it could support performance in completely novel situations. When new, unforeseen conditions arise, it would be useful if all memory could be accessible to all manner of cognitive operations that might be brought to bear on our attempts to comprehend the situation at hand and construct a plan of action.

It should be clear that these two purposes to which memory could be put constitute competing, and indeed incompatible, design demands. It should likewise be clear that these two purposes correspond to procedural and declarative memory systems, respectively, within our framework. We submit that these competing demands on memory have caused the modularization of memory through evolution along just these lines.

A NOTE ABOUT TERMINOLOGY: HISTORY AND BAGGAGE

The terms *procedural* and *declarative* were adopted by the first author in this thesis work showing normal learning of skills by amnesic patients with profound deficits in recollecting their learning experiences or in introspecting about and reporting the nature of the knowledge underlying their performance (described most fully in Cohen, 1981). The terms were borrowed from the artificial intelligence (AI) literature, because of a strong resonance between issues that were under discussion at about the time these thesis experiments were being conducted and the implications of the amnesia phenomena being revealed in those experiments. Most influential in the choice of terms was Terry Winograd's thesis work with SHRDLU, an early attempt to develop a natural language comprehension system, operating in a simulated "blocks-world" environment. In this system, a user could give verbal commands to a simulated robot arm to manipulate a set of different blocks and could query the system about the blocks-world environment (1972). Winograd's system showed a fundamental dissociation between the ability to perform skillfully in moving blocks around and the inability to articulate or to otherwise gain access to the knowledge mediating its skilled performance.[5]

Consider the following excerpt from Winograd's work with SHRDLU. Items in lower-case text are queries made of the system by a user; items in upper-case text are the responses of the system; items in italics are Winograd's observations:

10. can a pyramid be supported by a block?
    YES
    The deductive system finds an actual example, so it knows this is possible
11. can a pyramid support a pyramid?
    I DON'T KNOW
    The question makes sense, but there is no example in the scene, so there is no easy way to tell without being able to examine the robot's programs
12. stack up two pyramids
    I CAN'T
    The robot tries and fails

What is happening here that when asked about the possibility of stacking a pyramid on top of another pyramid, the system claims not to "know" the answer. Yet, when asked to actually carry out such a stacking operation, the knowledge implicit in its movement production subsystem results in notification that it is not a possible operation. That is, the system does indeed have the requisite knowledge, but it can only express this knowledge when actually engaged in performing, not when engaged in "introspecting" about its knowledge base. The dissociation occurred because of the difference between the procedural representation in which the performance-output abilities of the system had been implemented (in one programming language) and the declarative representation in which the verbal-output abilities of the system had been implemented (in a different programming language). The striking parallel between this dissociation and the one being noted in amnesic patients made adoption of the same terms quite reasonable.

However, it would seem that the choice of terms turns out to be unfortunate, because it carries some unwelcome baggage from the meanings these terms have acquired from AI and from common usage in the language. First, although Winograd's *behavioral* dissociation in the performance of the SHRDLU model provides a good match to the behavioral dissociation seen in the performance of amnesic patients, the procedural-declarative distinction as framed in AI differs significantly from the procedural-declarative distinction offered in Cohen's (1981) thesis, in the presentations of the framework by Cohen and Squire, and in the articulation of the current theory offered in this chapter. The procedural-declarative distinction as framed within AI concerns the difference between that knowledge represented in the form of routines or programs and that knowledge represented as data structures. In Winograd's model, these were instantiated in different computer languages. Subsequent work in AI suggested that the distinction between (knowledge as) programs and (knowledge as) data structures was artificial because more modern computer languages could represent the two "kinds of knowledge" interchangeably; both programs and data structures could be represented in the same code. Consequently, the AI-based distinction, *as framed in that way*, has been abandoned by many within the field.

Second, it carries baggage from common language usage of the terms: Applying Webster's definition of the words "procedural" and "declarative" to the procedural-declarative memory distinction seems to suggest that procedural memory stores knowledge of procedures or rules whereas declarative memory stores knowledge that can be verbally declared. This is *not* the nature of the distinction as articulated here. Declarative memory does provide the only form of representation that is capable of being declared verbally; but, as noted above, declarative memory includes nonverbalizable nondeclarable memory as well, such as visual memories of the appearances of objects and the relations among multiple objects within scenes, or spatial maps of the environment. What defines declarative memory is its relational properties, which in turn give rise to its representational flexibility and promiscuity. As to the other half of the distinction, procedural memory should *not* be equated with memory for procedures. As usually understood, a procedure refers to a method or manner of performing some act, or perhaps a set of rules for performing that act. Some of what would be called procedures under this definition would indeed show the inflexible and dedicated nature that we claim to be characteristic of procedural memory; other examples, however, are likely to be only well-rehearsed ways of acting that are perfectly verbalized and under consciously mediated control, and as such would *not* be procedural in our sense. Certainly we can think of all sorts of rules that we would not consider to be mediated by procedural memory and that would not be learnable by amnesic patients such as H.M. (e.g., "whenever you see the faces of the authors of this book, say 'Hello, Neal and Howard'"—something that, despite our best efforts, H.M. could not be trained to do). Evaluation of the data in terms of the distinction that might be suggested by the dictionary definitions of these terms, rather than the way in which we have defined them, would lead to misunderstanding.

Accordingly, having taken the opportunity in this chapter to finally explicate the theory fully, articulating more precisely the nature and signature of procedural and declarative memory, and having taken the opportunity in the rest of this book to explain the theory in terms of how it accounts for the data, how it can be tested, and how it compares and contrasts with other theories, we hope that the theory will henceforth stand or fall on the merits of the definitions offered here rather than on the unwelcome baggage that the terminology has brought along with it.

4 Anatomical Data Regarding the Procedural-Declarative Distinction

The view of the hippocampal system we have offered as storing the outcomes of the brain's various processing systems and as mediating relational representations requires confirmation from anatomical and physiological data regarding the hippocampal system. We must be able to show that the hippocampal system actually receives the input required by our theory, and that its internal wiring and physiological characteristics provide the requisite machinery for carrying out the functional role we attribute to it. We shall show in this and the next chapter that anatomical and physiological data do indeed meet these challenges, thereby providing converging evidence for our theory.

Even before that, however, we need to specify what we mean by the term *hippocampal system* and describe its anatomical characteristics. It is to this task that we turn now. Hopefully, this will not scare away those readers uninitiated or uninterested in the anatomical details; our presentation here emphasizes the functional implications of the anatomical facts and the way in which these facts provide support for our theory of the role of the hippocampal system in declarative memory. Recent comprehensive and detailed reviews of the anatomy of the hippocampal system (and some functional speculations) can be found elsewhere (e.g., see Amaral, 1987; Squire, Shimamura, & Amaral, 1989; Witter, 1989; our own treatment can be found in Eichenbaum & Buckingham, 1991). Although such detail is critical for formal computer modeling of hippocampal system functions and for understanding the role played by the various components of the hippocampal system (see discussion in chapter 2), it is beyond the scope of what will be considered here. Prefatory to elucidating its functional role in memory, we offer a definition of the hippocampal system and a set of general principles about the flow of information into and out of the components of this system. More details about the structure and connectivity of this system are presented in figures 4.1 to 4.5. Figures 4.1 to 4.3 provide an overview of the morphological structure of the hippocampal system. Figure 4.4 outlines the general stages of hippocampal processing defined in the next section of this chapter. Figures 4.5 to 4.7 offer schematic diagrams of the circuitry connecting these stages and their internal circuitries. Each of these figures is taken from reviews from the literature that focus on different aspects of hippocampal anatomy.

THE HIPPOCAMPAL SYSTEM

What we refer to as the hippocampal system consists of a set of anatomically interconnected and functionally interrelated structures that were all surgically resected in whole or in part in the patient H.M. and are undoubtedly responsible for a set of serial and parallel stages of information processing critical to the accomplishing of declarative memory. The system includes the parahippocampal cortical areas immediately surrounding the hippocampus, several cytoarchitecturally distinct components within what most investigators refer to as the hippocampal formation, and the input and output pathways through which this system communicates

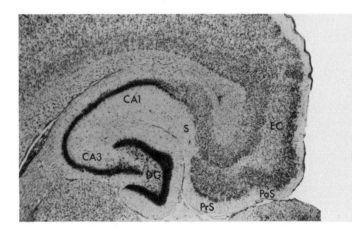

Figure 4.1
Nissl-stained section through the hippocampal region of the rat brain. CA1 and CA3, subdivisions of Ammon's horn (the hippocampus proper); DG, dentate gyrus; EC, entorhinal cortex; PaS, parasubiculum; PrS, presubiculum; S, subiculum. (Courtesy of David Amaral.)

with the rest of the brain (see figures 4.1 to 4.7). In our discussion, we will limit our treatment to presentation of the following three major aspects of hippocampal system anatomy and their functional implications.

First, inputs to the hippocampal system include each of the major association areas of the cerebral cortex plus the amygdala (see figure 4.5). Second, these inputs arrive at a major convergence area that we refer to collectively as the parahippocampal cortical areas, which overlie the hippocampal formation and have several major components that are differentiated by their input and output organizations (see figure 4.6). These components include: the perirhinal cortex and parahippocampal cortex proper that border between temporal neocortex and the entorhinal cortex; the entorhinal cortex, itself composed of multiple subdivisions (primarily the lateral and medial entorhinal areas; Amaral et al., 1987); and the parasubiculum and presubiculum, bordering between the entorhinal cortex and, possibly, the subiculum (see below). Third, the hippocampal formation,

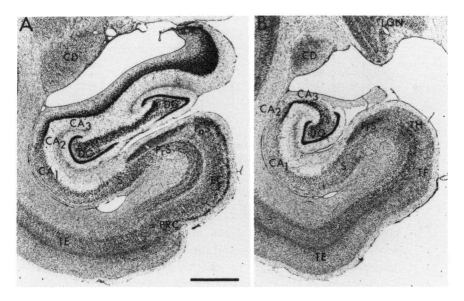

Figure 4.2
Nissl-stained sections through the hippocampal region of the macaque monkey brain. Section *A* is anterior to section *B*. PRC, perirhinal cortex; TE, subdivision of visual association (inferotemporal) cortex; TF and TH, subdivisions of the parahippocampal cortex. See figure 4.1 for other abbreviations. (Courtesy of David Amaral.)

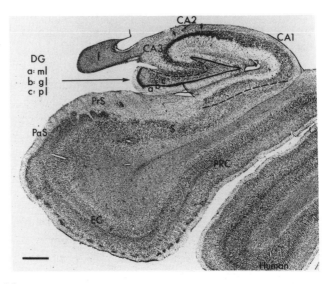

Figure 4.3
Nissl-stained section through the hippocampal region of the human brain. f, fornix; ml, gl, and pl refer to laminae of the dentate gyrus. See figures 4.1 and 4.2 for other abbreviations. (Courtesy of David Amaral.)

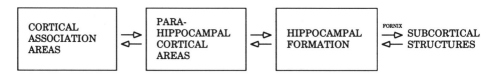

Figure 4.4
Schematic diagram of the bidirectional flow of information between cortical association areas and components of the hippocampal system plus hippocampal connections with subcortical areas.

as we use the term, is itself composed of several closely interacting subdivisions: the dentate gyrus, areas CA3 and CA1 of Ammon's horn, and, possibly, the subiculum. The subiculum is in an ambiguous position with regard to whether it should be considered to be a component of the parahippocampal cortical areas or else part of the hippocampal formation. It has traditionally been treated as a component of the parahippocampal cortical areas because it is *not* part of the trisynaptic circuit of the hippocampal formation (the

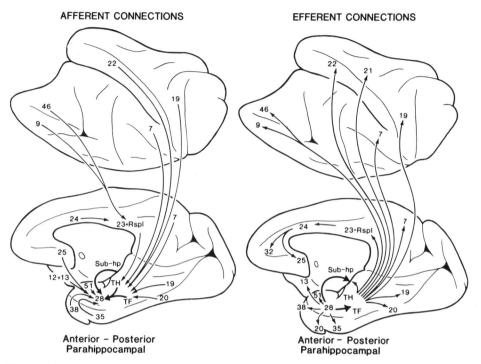

Figure 4.5
Summary of cortical afferent and efferent connections of the rhesus monkey parahippocampal gyrus shown on lateral (inverted) and medial views of the cerebral hemisphere. With regard to afferent connections, the projections from areas 12, 13, 23, 24,
25, 35, 38, 51, retrosplenial cortex (Rspl), subiculum-hippocampus (Sub-hp) and TF-TH
(posterior parahippocampal areas) represent intrinsic pathways within the limbic lobe
that converge on area 28, the entorhinal cortex. The area 51 projections would be
expected to carry olfactory input. Projections from areas 19 and 20 to areas TF-TH are
visual association projections; those from area 22 are auditory association projections;
those from area 7 are visuosomatic projections; and those from areas 9 and 46 are
frontal association projections. Multimodal projections from the cortex in the superior
temporal sulcus are not shown. The heavy-lined arrows from Sub-hp and TF-TH to
area 28 denote that there are two of the heaviest sources of input to this cortex. With
regard to efferent or output projections, note that there is a nearly exact reciprocation
of the input pathways. The heavy line from areas 28 and Sub-hp represents the perforant
pathway. (From Van Hoesen, 1982.)

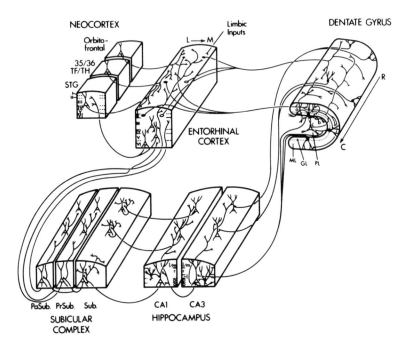

Figure 4.6
Diagrammatic representation of the major intrinsic connections of the hippocampal formation. Much of the sensory input to the hippocampal formation arises in polysensory associational regions of the neocortex such as the orbitofrontal cortex, the perirhinal and parahippocampal cortices (35/36, TF/TH), and the dorsal bank of the superior temporal gyrus (STG). Layer III pyramidal cells in these areas project principally, though not exclusively, to the lateral aspect of the entorhinal cortex. Projection fields from different associational cortices do not have sharp boundaries in the entorhinal cortex and there is substantial overlap. The entorhinal cortex gives rise to the major input to the dentate gyrus, the so-called perforant path, which terminates on the unipolar dendritic trees (located in the molecular layer, ML) of the granule cells. This projection is organized such that cells located laterally in the entorhinal cortex (close to the rhinal sulcus) project preferentially to caudal levels of the dentate gyrus, and progressively more medial bands of entorhinal cells project to more rostral levels of the dentate gyrus. Within the dentate gyrus there are a variety of neurons other than granule cells. Some of these (a, b) are interneurons that give rise to local, inhibitory projections. Other cells (c) located in the polymorphic layer (PL), subjacent to the dentate gyrus, give rise to an extensive associational system of fibers that terminate on dendrites in the inner third of the molecular layer. Associational fibers that arise at any particular level in the dentate gyrus terminate throughout much of the

synapses at the dentate gyrus, CA3, and CA1). However, recent
anatomical data indicate that the subiculum receives cortical connections very similar to those of CA1, and a prominent connection
from CA1, and therefore might be considered as the "fourth stage"
of the trisynaptic circuit.

   The outcomes of neocortical processing make their way through
the parahippocampal cortical areas by multiple routes to be imposed
on these components of the hippocampus and subiculum, as will
be discussed below. Our view is that these can be anatomically and
functionally divided into two main channels of information flow
into the hippocampal formation (Eichenbaum and Buckingham,
1991). Finally, an additional major pathway that connects the hippocampal system with subcortical structures is the fornix (see figure
4.4). This fiber bundle carries inputs and outputs to the hippocampal
system from the thalamus, septum, hypothalamus, and other brainstem nuclei. As we will discuss below, the fornix is a vital connectional pathway for the full operation of the hippocampal system.
However, because little is understood about specific qualities of the
information conveyed by the fornix, we will discuss it further only
in the context of the effects of damage to this pathway (see Amaral,
1987, for a review of these connections).

---

remainder of the structure. The dentate granule cells give rise to a nonre-
ciprocated projection (the mossy fibers) to the CA3 field of the hippocampus. Pyramidal dells in the CA3 field, in turn, originate several intrinsic
and extrinsic connections. Within the hippocampal formation CA3 neurons
give rise to a widespread associational projection to other levels of CA3.
Other collaterals (the Schaffer collaterals) provide the major input to the
CA1 field of the hippocampus. Within field CA1 and CA3 there are also a
variety of interneurons that originate local inhibitory projections. Unlike
the CA3 field, CA1 pyramidal cells do not project to other levels of CA1.
Rather they give rise to a relatively dense and spatially restricted projection
to the subiculum. The subiculum, in turn, projects both to the pre- and
parasubiculum and to the entorhinal cortex. The pre- and parasubiculum
provide a major input to the entorhinal cortex, which terminates principally
in layers III and II. While not yet well studied, there is evidence that cells
located deep in the entorhinal cortex project back to many of the cortical
fields from which it receives input. L, lateral; M, medial; R, rostral; C,
caudal; GL, granule-cell layer; 1/m, stratum lacunosum moleculare; r, stratum radiatum; 1, stratum lucidum; p, pyramidal cell layer; o, stratum
oriens. (From Square et al., 1989).

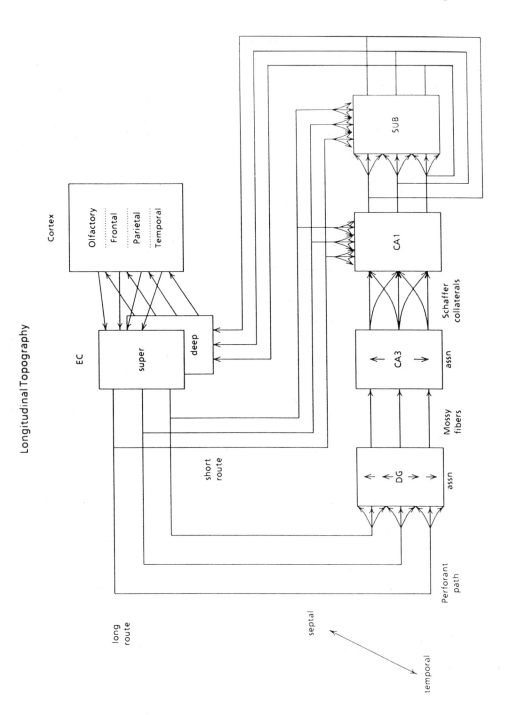

It would be of considerable importance to know how information is transformed as it passes through these stages of hippocampal system processing, that is, to gain a more complete understanding of processing *within* the hippocampal system. Indeed, such information is critical to those investigators interested in modeling hippocampal functioning at the level of mechanism; however, as noted earlier, this is not the goal of the present book. Also, there are few data on the nature of these transformations in the early stages of hippocampal system processing (e.g., in the parahippocampal gyrus and dentate gyrus), and little consensus even on the actual sequence of processing stages in the hippocampal circuit (Witter, 1989). This is in stark contrast to the considerable detail known about the inputs to hippocampus and about the anatomy (and physiology) of the final stage of processing of the hippocampus—the hippocampal field CA1 (the pyramidal cells)—which provide the output of the hippocampus to the remainder of the hippocampal system as well as some of the output from the hippocampus to other brain areas. These data provide important evidence for the role of this brain system in accomplishing relational representation.

CHARACTERISTICS OF THE INPUT/OUTPUT CONNECTIONS OF THE HIPPOCAMPUS

Four general characteristics of the input/output connections of the hippocampal system deserve emphasis:

◄──

Figure 4.7
Schematic diagram of cortical-hippocampal circuits. This diagram focuses on the longitudinal or septotemporal organization and details of the connections of structural areas introduced in figure 4.1. Note the topographic gradients in the organization of cortical inputs to the parahippocampal/ entorhinal cortex (EC), topographic divergence and association systems in the long-route projection to CA1 and subiculum (SUB), and relative topographic preservation in the short-route projection onto CA1 and subiculum. The longitudinal dimension is represented on brain structures on both the vertical axis (top = septal) and the horizontal axis (right = septal). Super, superficial cortical layers; deep, deep cortical layers; DG, dentate gyrus granule cells; CA3 and CA1 are subdivisions of Ammon's horn.

1. Inputs to hippocampus can be characterized as being highly pre-processed outputs of multiple neocortical systems representing meaningful "objects"—that is, what we have called the *outcomes* of processing from each of the higher-order association areas of the brain. This makes the hippocampal system ideally placed anatomically to conjoin, bind, or relate the multiple perceptually distinct objects constituting "scenes" or "events."

2. The input projections from the multiple neocortical association areas are organized by *topographic gradients,* providing for considerable intermixing but not complete overlap of their inputs. This intermixing places the hippocampal network in a position to process the conjunctions or associations of co-active processing outcomes, producing relational representations.

3. Inputs from the parahippocampal area project to hippocampal CA1 neurons by two pathways. The convergence of these two routes onto hippocampal neurons provides for an additional and separate stage of relational processing.

4. The hippocampal system areas that are targets of neocortical projections maintain *reciprocal* connections with the neocortical sources; that is, the processing result is returned to input sites.

Inputs to Hippocampus Are the Outcomes of Processing from Multiple Higher-Order Association Areas of the Brain

Inputs to the hippocampal system, with the exception of olfactory input, come from the highest-order neocortical sensory areas and association areas, providing multimodal sensory information as well as combined sensory, motor, and limbic information. Primary and secondary neocortical processing areas do not project onto the hippocampal gyrus. Rather, they project to higher-order processors that are the substrates for identifying and computing the functional significance of "objects." It is these outputs that are projected onto the entorhinal and parahippocampal areas of the hippocampal system (see figures 4.5 to 4.7).

To illustrate, we need to start by explaining that each of the neocortical sensory processing modules mediate a set of sequential processing stages within a single modality. For example, the primary visual area in the striate cortex projects to secondary visual cortex in the circumstriate belt. Neither of these areas project to the hippocampal system directly, but instead project to higher visual areas in the middle temporal and inferior temporal gyri (see figure 4.5). Similarly, the primary auditory and somesthetic areas are connected with unimodal secondary processing areas in the parietal and temporal lobes. The outputs of each of the sensory modules then converge onto multimodal sensory convergence areas in posterior neocortex, in the posterior parietal lobe and the superior temporal gyrus, and also in prefrontal neocortex, in the dorsolateral and orbital prefrontal areas (Van Hoesen and Pandya, 1975; Van Hoesen et al., 1975). Outputs of these associational systems, in turn, project heavily onto multimodal convergence zones in prefrontal and cingulate cortex, which are highly interconnected with other limbic structures. These various convergence zones provide the major source of inputs to the parahippocampal areas (Goldman-Rakic et al., 1984; Insausti et al., 1987a, b; Van Hoesen et al., 1972). The other inputs to the hippocampal system, the exception to the above scheme, come from the olfactory system—without any further neocortical elaboration—from the olfactory bulb and pyriform cortex (Boeijinga & Van Groen, 1984; Deacon et al., 1983; Habets et al., 1980; Kosel et al, 1981; Room et al., 1984; Turner et al., 1979; Van Groen et al., 1986).

Thus, other than olfactory information, the input to hippocampus can be characterized as being highly preprocessed outputs of multiple neocortical systems. But what is the nature of this information? It is what we have called the outcomes of processing from each of the higher-order association areas of the brain—the objects that collectively comprise the scenes and events encountered during processing episodes. To illustrate, let us again return to the example of the visual system. The visual area that projects to the hippocampal system is the inferotemporal (IT) cortex (area TE), the highest-order visual-object processing area in primates. Behavioral and physiological data indicate that this area accomplishes the identification (and likely long-term memory storage) of visual objects (e.g., Mishkin, 1982). Ablation of this area results in a visual-specific discrimination deficit (agnosia) without impairment in visual fields, acuity, or thresholds. Neurons in the intact inferotemporal cortex are driven by two- and three-dimensional visual stimuli presented nearly anywhere in the visual environment. The visual response properties of these cells are dependent on attentional mechanisms and reward association (e.g., Baylis and Rolls, 1987; Fuster and Jervey, 1981; Gross et al., 1979; Sato, 1988). Most IT neurons respond to many different patterns or objects, but some respond preferentially to particular items, often ones with obvious significance to the animal (Gross et al., 1972). A subset of these cells, for example, respond selectively to faces (Desimone et al., 1984; Perrett, Rolls, & Caan, 1982). See figure 4.8 for an example.

Importantly, the complex response properties of IT neurons are very similar across changes in stimulus size, orientation, and contrast (Baylis et al., 1987; Gross et al., 1972; Miyashita & Chang, 1988; Schwartz et al., 1983), a demonstration of "object constancy" that most feel is essential to support representation of objects. IT neurons, as recorded during the performance of monkeys in visual discrimination and visual delayed-matching tasks, respond preferentially to particular task-relevant stimuli, and respond differentially to the same stimuli when presented as the to-be-remembered cues versus the choice items, or when they were novel versus when they were familiar (Baylis et al., 1987; Mikami and Kubota, 1980). Finally, some of these cells maintain their firing during the memory delay period in short-term memory tasks (Fuster and Jervey, 1981; Miyashita and Chang, 1988).

Clearly, then, input to the hippocampal system from area TE is highly processed, reflecting, it would seem, the outcome of the visual system's processing of object identity. More generally, the information coming from the various higher-order neocortical sensory areas to the hippocampal system is less concerned with particular sensory qualities (such as size, color, texture, etc.) and more with the functional or behavioral significance of the stimuli. Moreover, input from the neocortical convergence zones in the temporal, parietal, and frontal lobes each have mixed multisensory and motor-related components. They are sensitive to changing contingencies and learned behavioral significance, and related to actions taken or about to be taken with regard to environmental stimuli. These conclusions follow from the following observations on each of these areas (see Eichenbaum & Buckingham, 1990 for elaboration): (1) None of these hippocampal sources is topographically organized with respect to simple sensory dimensions, in contrast to the neocortical primary sensory areas. (2) The neurons within each of these source areas are broadly tuned, responding to many different stimuli

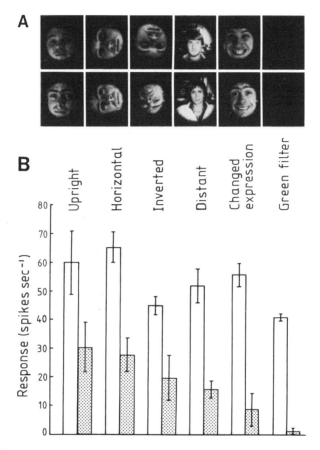

Figure 4.8
Responses of neurons in the inferotemporal cortex of monkeys to faces and face-like stimuli; effects of face identity. (A) Examples of the different views of the faces of the two experimenters P.S. (*upper row*) and D.P. (*lower row*). (B) The mean response to these views (± 1 SE, n = 3–10) is illustrated for cell MO55. The cell responds to the face of P.S. (white bars) under a variety of viewing conditions: when his face was presented upright, horizontal, inverted, at an increased distance, with changed expression, or through a green filter. Comparable views of the face of D.P. (gray bars) produced less response. (From Perrett et al., 1982.)

and having large receptive fields. (3) The neuronal activity in each
of these areas is dependent on attentional variables and/or the behavioral significance of the stimuli. (4) Cells in these areas fire
during the period when responses must be withheld pending instructions, and their activity predicts subsequent behavioral
performance.

Accordingly, the hippocampal network is in a position to receive
the *outcomes of processing* from multiple higher-order neocortical
processing systems, each communicating quite abstract representations of the objects comprising the scenes or events appearing or
occurring in the environment. The important thing here is *not* that
the hippocampal system is unique in receiving such convergence
(it is not; see Damasio's [1989a, b] discussion of convergence zones),
but that it provides the necessary foundation for mediating the
relational representations that we hypothesize.

Topographic Gradients of Overlapping Inputs Support
Relational Representation

Not only is the hippocampal system in a position to receive multiple inputs that can be chunked in relational representations, these
multiple inputs are available simultaneously to the same hippocampal networks (see figure 4.6, 4.7). The input projections from the
multiple neocortical association areas are organized according to
coarse gradients of anatomical topography: More rostral neocortical
areas project more heavily to more rostral portions of the parahippocampal cortex, and more caudal neocortical areas project more
heavily to more caudal portions of the parahippocampal cortex
(Amaral & Witter, 1989; Deacon et al., 1983; Room & Groenewegen, 1986). In turn, the more rostral parts of the parahippocampal
cortex project more heavily to the portion of the hippocampus closer
to the septum, and more caudal parts of the hippocampal cortex
project more heavily to the portion of the hippocampus closer to
entorhinal cortex. Note that this topography is *not* a strict one-to-
one mapping, but rather a fully distributed mapping with a gradient
of connection weightings.

Accordingly, the hippocampal network is in a position to receive
an intermixing of the processing outcomes of the neocortical associational areas, encouraging processing of various conjunctions or
associations of the inputs—namely, relational processing. The

graded distributed input provides the hippocampal network with the means to perform particularly robust or sensitive processing of the various possible relationships among the inputs through the sort of coarse coding scheme discussed in network modeling work (e.g., Hinton, McClelland, & Rumelhart, 1986).[1] That is, any given portion of the hippocampal network would not only receive input from multiple areas, but would actually receive differently weighted inputs from each of the areas to which the hippocampus is connected.

Two Pathways to the Hippocampus: A Further Source of Relational Processing

The parahippocampal and entorhinal areas of the hippocampal system, onto which the multiple neocortical projections converge, in turn send input to hippocampal CA1 neurons via two routes. One is a direct route through projections from the parahippocampal area to the outer parts of the CA1 dendritic zone, and the other an indirect route via sequential hippocampal processing stages through the dentate gyrus and CA3, then to CA1 (the trisynaptic circuit).

Two aspects of the indirect (trisynaptic) pathway should be noted here: A large number of association fibers cross this pathway at different levels, and some of the synapses in this pathway are particularly susceptible to potentiation by patterns of stimulation common during learning events (e.g., Lynch, 1986; see chapter 5). Accordingly, CA1 neurons are in a position to process one further type of relationship, that between the representation of an object or event transmitted directly from the parahippocampal cortex input and the representation of possible learned associations triggered by the same event, being more fully associated with other representations and transmitted through learning-modified synapses reflecting this further level of association in the indirect pathway (see Eichenbaum & Buckingham, 1991). This adds to the variety of high-level relationships of which the hippocampal system seems capable.

Neocortical and Hippocampal System Areas Are Reciprocally Connected

The multiple neocortical processing areas that project to the hippocampal system are themselves recipients of hippocampal output. Thus there is reciprocal exchange of information between neocortical and hippocampal system areas in support of declarative memory. This is important because the neuropsychological data make clear that the hippocampal system cannot be the essential site of long-term memory storage; the fact that H. M. and other amnesic patients with hippocampal system damage have intact remote memories indicates that the hippocampal role in declarative memory is temporally limited.

Accordingly, it is proposed that the hippocampal system does not permanently store the relational representations it helps to mediate, but rather serves to establish, maintain, and, for a time after learning, participate in the retrieval of such representations in the neocortical processors (e.g., Squire, Cohen, and Nadel, 1984). This notion is discussed more fully in chapter 13. The point here, though, is that the presence of reciprocal connections between neocortical and hippocampal system sites is critical to this idea; not only must the hippocampal system be so positioned in the brain as to receive converging inputs from neocortical processors, but it must be capable of affecting memory storage in those same neocortical areas (see chapter 13).

In summary, then, these findings indicate that the input to the hippocampus involves category- and function-specific representations of independent percepts and actions; that these inputs are distributed differentially onto the parahippocampal cortex and thence onto the hippocampal output neurons via two physiologically and anatomically distinct pathways; and that the consequent interactions are transmitted back to the same cortical areas that were the source of hippocampal input. We conclude that the anatomy of the hippocampal system is capable of supporting the functional role in declarative memory that we ascribe to it. We turn in the next chapter from anatomical considerations to physiological ones to show that the neural components of the hippocampal system possess the machinery that the system's proposed role in declarative memory would require.

Physiological Data Regarding the Procedural-Declarative Distinction

In the preceding chapter, we argued that the hippocampal system is ideally positioned anatomically to accomplish the relational processing proposed in our theory: It receives converging inputs from multiple higher-order associational areas that convey information about the functional characteristics of the objects that comprise scenes and events and of the actions taken with respect to the scenes and events. But does the hippocampal system contain the requisite physiological machinery for performing relational processing? This chapter provides evidence that indeed it does. The evidence for this assertion comes from electrophysiological recording of hippocampal CA1 neurons during behavioral performance (we concern ourselves here exclusively with CA1 neurons because in this way we can understand the physiological properties of the output stage of hippocampal processing) and of the synaptic plasticity (long-term potentiation [LTP]) exhibited by hippocampal neurons.

RELATIONAL PROCESSING AND THE REPRESENTATION OF "PLACE"

The first piece of evidence is provided by one of the most striking and widely cited behavioral correlates of cellular activity, the phenomenon of so-called *place cells*. This refers to findings that CA1 pyramidal cells can be found to fire selectively when the animal is in a specific location or "place" in the environment during spatial exploration (e.g., O'Keefe, 1976, 1979; Muller, Kubie, & Ranck, 1987; Olton, Branch, & Best, 1978). Such neurons have been called place cells, and the location of the animal when such a neuron is maximally active is called its place field (figure 5.1). The spatial location being coded by place cell activity is determined by the spatial relationships among salient distal cues. When the salient

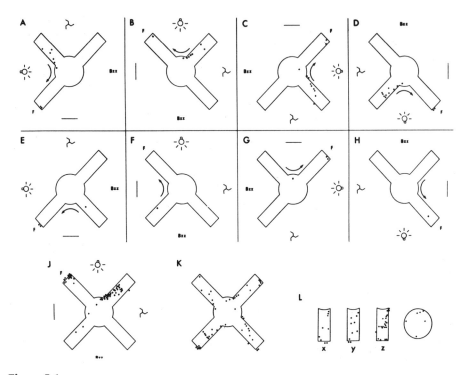

Figure 5.1
Analysis of a hippocampal place cell. The rat was required to move from different start positions in the three-arm maze to find food located at a constant position relative to specific stimuli that were rotated together between trials. Data accumulated from eight trials are shown. (A–H) Individual trials with the start and goal arms in different positions. (J) A–H superimposed by aligning them with respect to distal cues. (K) A–H superimposed without rotation. (L) Each of the maze components superimposed as in K. This cell has two distinct place fields in different arms. (From O'Keefe, 1976.)

visual cues are rotated, place fields are found to rotate (Miller & Best, 1980; Muller et al., 1987; O'Keefe and Speakman, 1987); and when the testing environment itself is changed by enlarging or shrinking, at least some place fields scale up or down accordingly (figure 5.2; Muller and Kubie, 1989).

Furthermore, activation of these cells is not dependent on any particular one of the environmental stimuli, but rather on the relationships among them. Place fields, once established through the animal's exploration of its environment, persist despite removing a

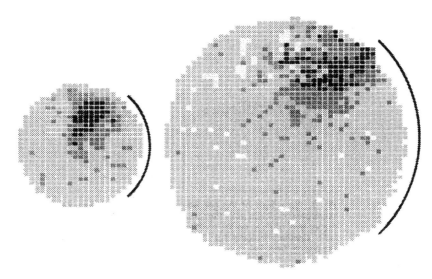

Figure 5.2
The place field of this cell, indicated by darkest areas, enlarges when the rat is taken from a small cylindrical area (*left*) in which to navigate to a large cylindrical area (*right*), although the scaling is not linearly related to the change in size of the environment. The arc at the circumference indicates the position of an orienting cue card. (From Muller et al., 1987.)

subset of the cues (Hill & Best, 1981; O'Keefe and Conway, 1978) or even all of the cues after the animal is oriented within the environment (O'Keefe & Speakman, 1987; Quirk et al., 1990), as shown in figure 5.3. Thus, the cells are not coding for specific sensory properties, but rather more abstract spatial relationships representing where in the environment the animal "thinks" it is (see Eichenbaum & Cohen, 1988, for discussion).

So compelling are these place field phenomena that, taken together with findings that animals with hippocampal system damage are markedly impaired in spatial learning tasks (see chapter 7), they have formed the basis for the claim (O'Keefe & Nadel, 1978) that hippocampal function specifically supports the construction and storage of spatial (or cognitive) "maps" of the environment and enables "place learning" (see chapter 11). However, as shall be seen below, spatial relations are just one example of the relational processing encoded by hippocampal neuron activity; and, as shall be

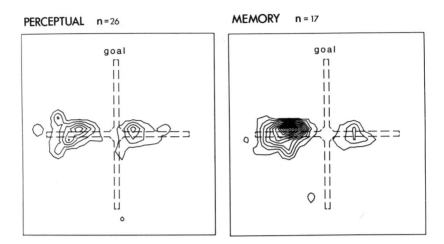

Figure 5.3
Place fields of this cell, indicated by the areas within the densest contour
lines, were very similar when various cues were present in the environment
surrounding the maze (perceptual trial) and after they were removed (memory trial). The apparent higher level of firing on the memory trial was not
a consistent finding across cells. Contours indicate 1.5 spikes s^{-1} steps in
firing rate. (From O'Keefe & Speakman, 1987.)

seen in chapters 7 and 8, impaired spatial learning is just one example of the behavioral deficit that follows hippocampal system
damage.

RELATIONAL PROCESSING IS NOT EXCLUSIVELY SPATIAL

As we have discussed elsewhere (Eichenbaum & Cohen, 1988; Eichenbaum, Otto, & Cohen, 1992), "place" is not the only deter-
minant of CA1 cell firing rate; other relationships in addition to
spatial relations are encoded by hippocampal CA1 neurons. Thus,
whereas such cells have place fields in spatial exploration tasks,
there is more encoded by the cells' firing than the "place" of the
animal. Describing these cells as "place cells" gives too narrow a
view of their functional role. Rather, they should be viewed as
"relational cells," as they seem to encode various relationships
among critical cues and their relations to specific behavioral events.
Four different lines of evidence substantiate this claim:

1. Cells with place fields are often sensitive not only to the animal's spatial location but also to second-order spatial variables, such as direction and speed of movement through the preferred location.

2. Many CA1 neurons are activated by various conjunctions of spatial and nonspatial variables, such as the presentation of a particular stimulus in a specific location.

3. Hippocampal neurons are active in any number of nonspatial tasks, firing to various nonspatial task-relevant stimuli and conjunctions of such stimuli.

4. The same hippocampal neurons have different preferred stimuli in different task environments, for example, having place fields in a spatial task and some other task-relevant correlate in a nonspatial task.

Hippocampal Neurons Are Sensitive to Second-Order Spatial Variables

The initial reports of hippocampal cells with place fields suggested that it was the location of the animal in space and not the particular behaviors the animal was producing that determined neuronal activity. It is now clear that the activity of hippocampal neurons can be highly dependent on movement (or second-order spatial) variables, including direction, speed, and turning angle of the animal's trajectory through the preferred location (McNaughton, Barnes, & O'Keefe, 1983; Wiener et al., 1989), as well as the destination of the movement (Muller & Kubie, 1989). Figure 5.4 provides an example. This cell was recorded in a rat placed in a square arena performing a spatial memory task similar in demands to Olton's radial-arm maze. The rat was required to move to and remember its visits to each of the four corners of the arena. The cell had a clearly defined place field near the center of the arena. But the cell's firing rate when the rat was in the place field was also highly dependent on the following movement variables: It fired selectively when the rat was moving at higher speeds, in the northerly direction, and turning to the right. Furthermore, the activation of the cell was clearly time-locked to the approach to the northeast corner of the arena. The point is that place-related hippocampal activity, at least in some behavioral situations (see also Muller & Kubie, 1983; Foster, Castro, & McNaughton, 1990), can be characterized by actions in space rather than by passive registration of location—a higher-order relationship between the relationships defining spa-

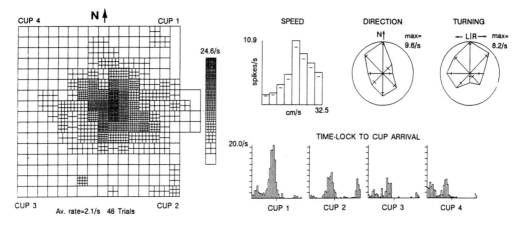

Figure 5.4
Example of analyses of unit activity in relation to spatial variables and goal-directed movements. The activity of this cell was recorded as an animal performed a task requiring it to remember the locations of rewards retrieved at each corner of an arena. (From Wiener et al., 1989.) The analysis is composed of: (1) at the *left*, a firing rate map, indicating the firing rate at each pixel and outlining the boundaries of the place field; the firing rate scale is to the right of the map; (2) *bottom right*, four histograms showing unit activity time-locked for ± 2 sec around the arrival at each reward cup during the same session; a tic mark on the abscissa indicates arrival time; tic marks on ordinate indicate multiples of the average firing rate; and at the *top right* (from left to right): (3) a histogram showing the average firing rate at different speeds of movement within each subfield; bars indicate standard error, (4) a polar plot showing the average firing rate for different directions of movement within each subfield; cross bars indicate standard error; no line is plotted for directions with fewer than 5 data samples, and (5) a polar plot showing the average firing rate at different turning directions during movement within the place field.

tial location and those defining behavioral activity in space. More speculatively, these data suggest that in such situations hippocampal neuronal activity may be reflecting the registration of behavioral events that are defined both by the spatial location in which they occur and by the actions taken, one of the various *conjunctions* that CA1 neurons seem capable of encoding.

Hippocampal Neurons are Activated by Various Conjunctions of Spatial and Nonspatial Variables

Moreover, the relational processing determining place fields often also includes a further, or higher-order, relationship involving the conjunction of place with particular task-relevant objects or events. Figure 5.5 illustrates this for rats performing in our odor discrimination learning tasks. In the simultaneous odor discrimination paradigm, a number of hippocampal cells fired maximally only during sampling of a specific left-right configuration of a particular pair of odors, that is, when one odor was delivered from the left-hand port and the other odor was simultaneously delivered from the right-hand port, and not for the alternative configuration of these odors nor for either configuration of a different pair of odors (see figure 5.5A).

Similar results have now been reported in other modalities. Some hippocampal cells were specifically active in relation to conjunctions of goal-box color and position in a spatial delayed response task in rats (Wible et al., 1986), and to conjunctions of two-dimensional patterns and their spatial positions within a stimulus array in visual recognition tasks in monkeys (Cahusac, Miyashita, & Rolls, 1989; Ono et al., 1991; Rolls et al., 1989). In some experiments, unit activity in relation to task events has been recorded as monkeys have been moved to different locations within a test room. For some cells the allocentric position of the animal influenced cellular activity, but neuronal reponses were also always closely linked to the onset of particular stimuli and/or behavioral responses (Ono et al., 1991; Rolls and O'Mara, 1991).

Hippocampal Neurons Fire in Association with Various Nonspatial Task-Relevant Stimuli and Conjunctions of Such Stimuli

The above findings clearly indicate that relational processing by hippocampal neurons is not exclusively spatial. Other findings reveal relational processing that is thoroughly nonspatial. Simply stated, when placed in task environments or confronted with paradigms in which nonspatial processing is required, nonspatial relational processing is very clearly observed in the activity of CA1 neurons. This can be seen in classical conditioning tasks and in discrimination and delayed matching tasks, where the relevant cues are presented successively in a single spatial location and thus spatial cues are not predictive. Perhaps the most striking example is in classical conditioning of an eyeblink response in restrained rabbits (Berger et al., 1983). During the course of conditioning, CA1

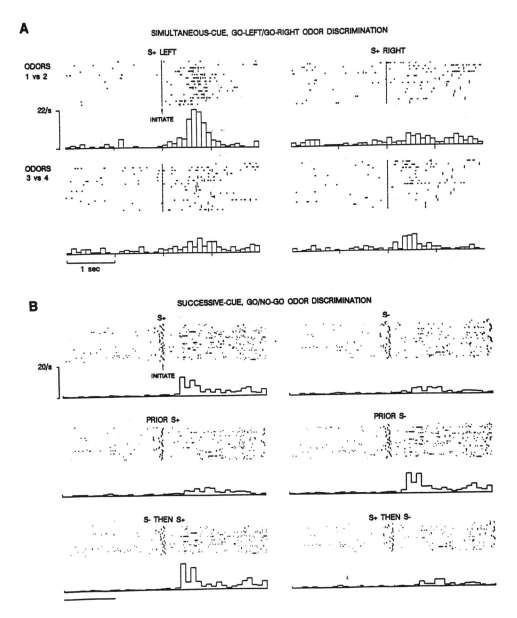

Figure 5.5
Examples of analyses of hippocampal unit activity in rats performing odor discrimination tasks. Each analysis consists of a raster display of sample trials and below it a
summary histogram of unit activity from all trials 2 sec before and after odor onset.

cells fire just prior to and then throughout the conditioned response movement. These behavioral correlates of hippocampal neuron activity are every bit as striking as the place field correlates, yet are often ignored in theorizing about the functional role of the hippocampal system in memory. This is in large measure because of behavioral work indicating that damage to hippocampus does not impair basic eyelid conditioning in rabbits; in other words, the integrity of the hippocampal system is not required for performance of this task, while the hippocampal system certainly is necessary for spatial learning. We will have more to say about this issue in chapter 10. But, for now, let it suffice to say that this nonspatial correlate of hippocampal firing is just as robust and significant as spatial correlates of firing observed in tasks which do not require hippocampal function (Muller et al., 1987) and cannot be ignored; it is one of many well-documented examples of physiological evidence for relational processing in the hippocampal system.

In instrumental paradigms, some CA1 neurons have been observed to fire in association with discriminative stimuli in any sensory modality—auditory (Foster, Christian, Hampson, Campbell, & Deadwyler, 1987; Segal, Disterhoff, & Olds, 1972), visual (Brown & Horn, 1978; Cahusac et al., 1989; Heit et al., 1988; Ono et al., 1991; Rolls, 1987; Wible et al., 1986; Wilson et al., 1987), or olfactory (Eichenbaum et al., 1987; Wiener et al., 1989). Others have found CA1 cells to fire in relation to conditioned appetitive movements (Cahusac et al., 1989; Cahusac & Miyashita, 1988; Eichenbaum et al., 1987; Sakurai, 1990; Watanabe & Niki, 1985; Wilson et al., 1987). For example, in our successive odor discrimination paradigm, the firing of a number of hippocampal cells was dependent on the specific temporal sequence of odor presentations, e.g., the nonrewarded odor (S−) followed by the rewarded odor (S+) (see figure 5.5B). This observation of cells whose activity depended on both current and previous stimulus valence in odor discrimination is similar to observations by Deadwyler and colleagues of "sequential dependencies" of hippocampal unit activity across trials in a tone-cued discrimination (e.g., Foster et al., 1987), and may share a common basis with the P300 phenomenon recorded from the scalp in humans, in that the cell activity is responsive to unusual or unexpected changes in the pattern of stimuli delivered. In humans, hippocampal and hippocampal gyrus cells fire selectively during presentation of words or pictures for which a memory choice had to be made (Halgren et al., 1978; see also Heit et al., 1988).

In all of these experiments, CA1 cells are *not* firing in relation to simple sensory or motor events. In the classical conditioning paradigm, the cells did not fire during spontaneous or reflexive blinks; they fired only to conditioned responses. In the instrumental paradigms, CA1 firing was dependent on various relationships, such as those between current and previous stimuli (Brown, 1982; Eichenbaum et al., 1987; Foster et al., 1987; Watanabe & Niki, 1985; Wible et al., 1986; Wilson et al., 1987), or particular combinations among or conjunctions of multiple stimuli and/or responses (Halgren, 1984; Port, Beggs, & Patterson, 1987; Rolls, et al., 1985; Watanabe & Niki, 1985; Wiener et al., 1989; Wible et al., 1986). The optimal "trigger features" of hippocampal cells therefore seem to reflect higher-order relationships, beyond the multimodal processing of the neocortical areas that project to the hippocampal system. They seem to be *supramodal*, in the sense that they encode the significance of the stimuli and/or actions taken in respect to them rather than the specific sensory characteristics of the stimuli or the specific movements involved. To our way of thinking, this reflects the processing of relationships among the task-constrained objects or events with which the animal is confronted, the task-defined relevance or significance of those objects or events, and the behavioral responses made under these constraints. This is truly relational processing, providing support for the theoretical framework offered here.

The Same Hippocampal Neurons Have Different Preferred Stimuli in Different Task Environments

One further piece of evidence for relational processing by CA1 neurons comes from the fact that virtually all of the cells that have place correlates in spatial paradigms also have nonspatial relational processing correlates of the sort seen in the conditioning or discrimination learning tasks just described. Thus, on different occasions or in different task environments, the same neurons may code different types of relationships among task relevant stimuli. Figure 5.6 shows an example of one of the hippocampal neurons from Wiener et al. (1989) that fired while sampling odor cues in the course of performing in the odor discrimination task, but also had a place

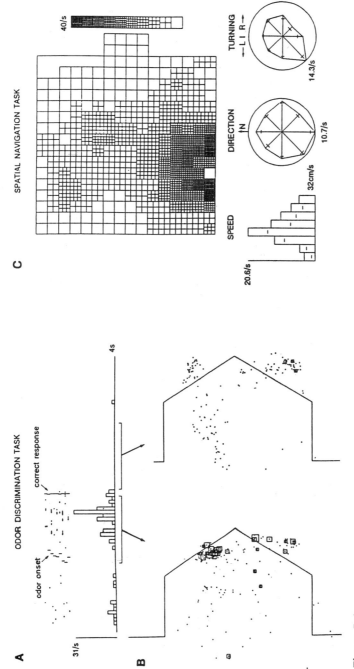

Figure 5.6
Example of analyses of the same cell recorded while the rat performed an odor discrimination task and then a spatial memory task in the same environment. (*A*) Raster display and summary histogram of firing time-locked to the discriminative response. (*B*) Spatial analysis of the position of the rat's snout in 50-msec samples (dots) and firing indicated by squares plotted around the dots. (*C*) Activity of the same cell as the rat performed the spatial memory task (see figure 5.4 for explanation of analysis).

field (as well as other spatial movement correlates) at a different location within the same physical environment when performing a spatial memory task. Kubie and Ranck (1984) had shown earlier that hippocampal neurons could have quite different place fields when alternately placed in different task environments within the same room location, and have more recently shown such "remapping," as they have termed it, to occur in a variety of situations where environmental cues are substantially altered (Bostock et al., 1986; Muller & Kubie, 1987).

These physiological properties, as unusual as they appear from the perspective of the orderliness apparent in sensory systems, conform nicely with the predictions drawn above from the anatomical facts about the hippocampal system, and, as we shall see, with the role we attribute to it in supporting declarative memory. Placed in a position of receiving inputs from multiple cortical processing modules, hippocampal CA1 neurons do indeed process a variety of different relationships among environmental stimuli. Confronted with different task environments on different occasions, the same hippocampal networks process different relationships among the events and objects they receive as inputs. Moreover, presented with a gradient of weighted and highly preprocessed information, the relationships coded by CA1 neurons may be quite abstract and multidetermined.

RELATIONAL PROCESSING AND THE FUNCTIONAL ORGANIZATION OF THE HIPPOCAMPUS

Additional information about whether the physiological machinery of the hippocampus supports relational processing, and how it might do so, comes from the simultaneous recordings we have obtained from multiple distinct CA1 neurons in rats performing our odor and place learning tasks (Eichenbaum et al., 1989). These findings provide a preliminary insight into the functional organization of this system. We investigated first the relational processing that permits the representation of "place" in the hippocampus during spatial tasks. Electrodes each consisting of a bundle of fine wires whose recording surfaces were distributed over a 1-mm diameter area were used, one per recording session, to record the activity simultaneously of an ensemble of hippocampal cells in the CA1 pyramidal cell layer while a rat performed a behavioral task. In our initial analyses of hippocampal ensemble activity, we determined the relationships among place fields of 3 to 11 cells while rats performed a spatial memory task. The spatial distribution of place fields within such cell ensembles was quantified by two measures: (1) the average distance between nearest neighboring place fields, and (2) the ratio of overlap of all the place fields recorded compared to the amount of the environment that could conceivably be covered by place fields of those sizes. This ratio permits an estimate of place field overlapping independent of place field size—that is, across ensembles with place fields of different sizes. Statistical analyses of these measures of nearest-neighbor distance and overlap ratio were based on Monte Carlo simulations designed for each ensemble of cells. Each Monte Carlo simulation sample used a set of place fields identical in size and form to that of the place fields in the recorded ensemble, but each of the simulated place fields was positioned and oriented randomly within the environment (the orientation and distances among subfields within a given place field were maintained). For each recorded ensemble, 1000 Monte Carlo samples were run, and nearest-neighbor distance and overlap ratio were calculated. The percentile rank of each of these two measures for each recorded ensemble was determined from the distribution of the corresponding Monte Carlo simulations. Findings from this study are illustrated in figure 5.7.

The findings indicated that the representation of space in the hippocampus involves a local order; but, unlike the representation of visual space in the primary sensory neocortex, hippocampal spatial representation does not reflect a systematic topography of environmental locations mapping onto neuroanatomical structure. Instead, place fields of neighboring neurons tend to overlap and are found in multiple clusters of redundant representation of some places and underrepresentation of other places.

Further analyses were employed to assess the extent to which place field distance and overlap were associated with differences or similarity of the movement correlates of cellular activity as the rat passed through the fields and subfields. Cells with overlapping or nearby place fields tended to have similar speed, direction, and

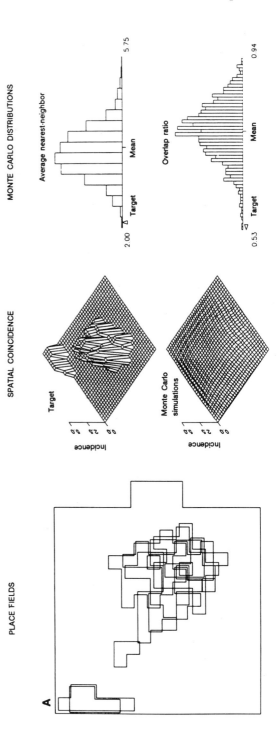

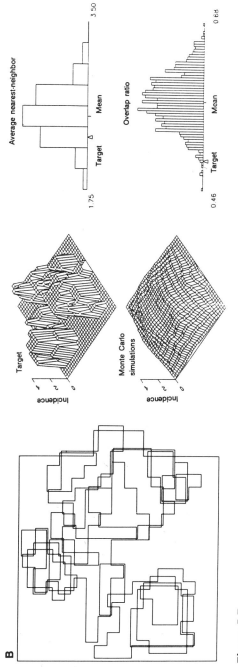

Figure 5.7

Analyses of ensemble activity (reproduced from Eichenbaum et al., 1989). Distinct place fields and multiple subfields that could be recorded from single cells were clustered in recorded ensembles. (A) An ensemble of 7 cells had 9 subfields that clustered in two distinct areas of the maze. (B) An ensemble of 9 cells had 16 subfields that clustered in three separable areas of the maze. For each ensemble analysis: *Left*, an outline of the experimental chamber is shown from a top view of the environment; the location of the cul-de-sac is indicated on the right side. The boundaries of the place field of each cell are outlined with overlapping edges of place fields shifted slightly to aid their visualization. *Center*, the three-dimensional graphs indicate the spatial coincidence of pixels, i.e. the number of times a given pixel was included in a place field, both for the target recorded ensemble (above) and the average spatial coincidence for the 1000 Monte Carlo runs (below). *Right*, the distributions of average nearest-neighbor and a measure of overlap for the Monte Carlo runs are shown, with the arrowhead indicating the value of each measure for the target recorded ensemble. The range of the Monte Carlo distributions was determined by the size and number of the place fields used in the simulation: larger and more numerous ensembles were more constrained by the size of the apparatus than were smaller ensembles. The range of each Monte Carlo distribution is noted numerically and illustrated by the width of the bars in the figure.

turning angle correlates. Combined, these data indicate a "patch-wise" representation of multiple aspects of particular loci in the environment.

What about the functional organization of hippocampus in representing *non*spatial relations? Compilation of data from individual electrode penetrations in each rat performing a simultaneous odor discrimination task allowed a preliminary survey of the behavioral correlates of large groups of neighboring hippocampal neurons. For this compilation, each cell was categorized by one of five functional identifications that Wiener et al. (1989) found useful in previous electrophysiological recording studies of rats performing our odor discrimination tasks: *port-approach* cells, that fired primarily as the rat approached the odor sampling area; *cue-sampling* cells, that fired preferentially during odor sampling; *reward-approach* cells, that fired as the rat approached the water cup; cells that *decreased firing* during the performance of discrimination trials; and cells with no identified behavioral correlate in this task environment.

To determine if the behavioral correlates were "clustered" in the same way as were the place fields discussed above, the distribution of these five categories of neurons in each penetration was compared to that expected from a random distribution of those neuron categories based on their frequencies of occurrence recorded across all subjects. Most penetrations demonstrated a striking clustering of behavioral correlates. For example, as shown in figure 5.8, in one penetration there was a predominance of cue sampling (middle panel), whereas in another penetration there was a predominance of port- and reward-approach cells (bottom panel). These findings indicate that, as is the case with spatial task environments, hippocampal neurons activated in nonspatial tasks seem to have a patch-wise representation of task-relevant objects or events, with neighboring groups of cells tending to overrepresent some of the relevant stimuli and underrepresent others.

Interestingly, recent computational modeling work with neural networks suggests that the sort of functional organization exhibited by the hippocampus might be common to networks with massively parallel processing and distributed representation. Like the place fields exhibited by hippocampal neurons in spatial task environments, the hidden units of a simple three-layer network memory trained in a place learning task demonstrated activation that was

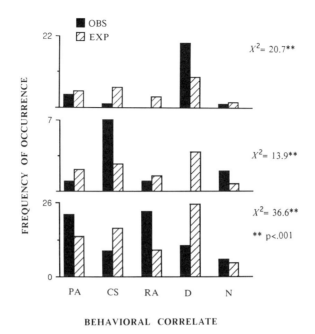

Figure 5.8
Distributions of firing correlates of cells recorded in single penetrations through hippocampal area CA1 as rats performed an odor discrimination task. PA, port-approach; CS, cue-sampling; RA, reward-approach; D, decreased firing; N, no identified correlate.

reliably associated with particular locations in the environment (Shapiro et al., 1990; Sharp, 1991). But, it is the functional organization of the artificial hidden units that is of particular note here: In the Shapiro et al. work, these hidden units developed place fields that were complexly shaped and clustered in ways that closely approximate what we observed in the actual hippocampal neural ensembles described above.

These findings suggest that nontopographic organization in the hippocampus is the product of competitive interactions among the elements of a large distributed representation substrate (Mc-Naughton & Morris, 1987; Rolls, 1989; see Eichenbaum & Cohen, 1988 and Eichenbaum & Buckingham, 1991). The absence of a systematic relationship between places in the environment and the anatomical organization of the hippocampus, on this view, occurs because the entire hippocampal network is seen as participating in representing each significant aspect of space. Such a representation of space does not seem the most obviously intuitive or straightforward, contrasting sharply with the topographic representation of space that have been so clearly documented in primary sensory cortices. But such a nontopographic distributed representation seems an ideal organization for this system, given that it receives inputs from multiple cortical processing modules—not only spatial ones—and it must be able to participate in the processing and storage of a variety of different relationships among the events and objects to which it is exposed. The same network of hippocampal neurons must handle all manner of relationships within and across different learning events, including relationships that have no spatial component and for which no preexisting spatial structure could have been anticipated. Clearly, there is no simple spatial topography onto which all of these various relationships might be mapped. Accordingly, the nontopographic distributed organization suggested by the above findings, while counterintuitive if one starts with a spatial mapping view of hippocampal system function, makes good sense given the role we attribute to the hippocampal system in supporting the relational representation characteristic of declarative memory. Accordingly, we take these findings as providing further converging evidence in support of the procedural-declarative framework we have offered here.

LONG-TERM POTENTIATION

So far we have shown that the hippocampal system is anatomically positioned in such a way as to receive converging inputs from the brain's various processing modules, and that hippocampal neurons are engaged in encoding and otherwise processing these converging inputs, thereby providing the substrate for the relational form of representation that we have attributed to hippocampal-mediated declarative memory. One final piece of this argument is provided by the finding that the hippocampal system possesses (not exclusively) a particularly robust form of synaptic plasticity called long-term potentiation (LTP), that can support the storage of such conjunctions and relations and that exhibits properties paralleling (at least some of) those of declarative memory.

LTP in the hippocampus is probably the best known and most widely studied example of activity-dependent synaptic plasticity in the brain. Following a brief stimulating burst to any one of several pathways in the hippocampus (e.g., the perforant path into the dentate gyrus of the hippocampal system) the responsiveness of target cells (the dentate granule cells, in this example) to a subsequent single shock of the same pathway is enhanced for an extended period of time, of up to hours, days, or even weeks. Although the details of the mechanisms, properties, and sufficient conditions for producing LTP are certainly beyond the scope of this book, a few words are in order here to understand how well the presence of this type of plasticity in hippocampus conforms to our theory about the relational nature of declarative memory mediated by this system.

LTP is widely thought to depend critically on the presence of two classes of glutamate receptors, NMDA and non-NMDA receptors, on the same dendritic spines of the target neurons. This complex of receptors truly seems to serve as conjunction detectors. The NMDA receptor is voltage and chemical sensitive; its channel is opened (activated) only by the simultaneous occurrence of transmitter binding to the receptor (as is the case for the typical chemical-sensitive receptor, such as the non-NMDA glutamate receptor) *and* a sufficient level of depolarization of the membrane (in response to another, preceding or simultaneously present, input) (Wigstrom & Gustafsson, 1985). This physiology provides an ideal mechanism for detecting converging inputs arriving in close temporal contiguity.

Hippocampal LTP exhibits properties that are much like those of (behavioral) declarative memory. Due to the above-described physiological mechanism, hippocampal LTP exhibits the "associativity" and "specificity" of memory. McNaughton et al. (1978) demonstrated the associative nature of LTP by independently stimulating different components of the perforant path that project to different regions of the dendritic tree of cells in dentate gyrus. Near-simultaneous activation of both pathways produced LTP far more robustly than did stimulation of each path separately—a clear example of conjunction detection or relational processing. LTP shows specificity in that only those fibers that participated in the induction of LTP (i.e., that were actually stimulated in producing potentiation in the target neurons) display lasting potentiation. Similarly encouraging is that hippocampal LTP can be induced rapidly with brief episodes of stimulation (Diamond et al., 1988; Larson & Lynch, 1986), is strengthened by repeated episodes of stimulation (Barnes, 1979; Bliss & Lomo, 1973), and decays over several days or weeks in the absence of repeated stimulation (Barnes, 1979; Racine et al., 1983).

A current question of importance, before leaving this topic, is whether the natural physiological activity of the hippocampus is likely to produce the necessary conditions for LTP. The question of the role of hippocampal firing in memory processes requires consideration of the temporal patterning of neuronal activity in the hippocampus during behavior. Several recent studies have indicated that LTP is induced preferentially by patterns of electrical stimulation that have the following three qualities: high-frequency bursts of stimulation, repetition of bursts at frequencies corresponding to the theta rhythm or preceding activation at corresponding latencies, and activation at the peak of the dentate theta rhythm (Larson et al., 1986; Larson & Lynch, 1986; Pavlides et al., 1988; Rose & Dunwiddie, 1986). Our recent examination of the firing patterns of putative hippocampal CA1 pyramidal cells in rats engaged in hippocampal-dependent spatial and olfactory learning tasks has revealed that all three of these necessary characteristics of patterned stimulation occur simultaneously and selectively during the critical behavioral events associated with memory processing. It was found that during the course of hippocampal-dependent memory processing, hippocampal neurons did discharge in high-frequency bursts, were preceded by neural activity preferentially at intervals corresponding to the theta rhythm, and were phase-locked to the positive peak of the dentate theta rhythm (Otto et al., 1991).

Figure 5.9 illustrates these patterns during significant behavioral events associated with likely periods of stimulus analysis, selection, or storage in a hippocampal-dependent odor discrimination task. It thus shows that the optimal conditions for inducing hippocampal LTP are indeed present in animals engaging in the relational memory processing functions we attribute to the hippocampal system. Accordingly, it appears that the hippocampal system possesses exactly the kind of physiological mechanism, sensitive to converging inputs arriving in close temporal contiguity, required by our procedural-declarative theory. This is not to say that LTP is found *only* in the hippocampal system, or that the data in any way *prove* the procedural-declarative theory. However, these and the above data suggest that the system does indeed have the machinery to accomplish the processing role we attribute to it, and hence are taken as providing further converging support for our theory.

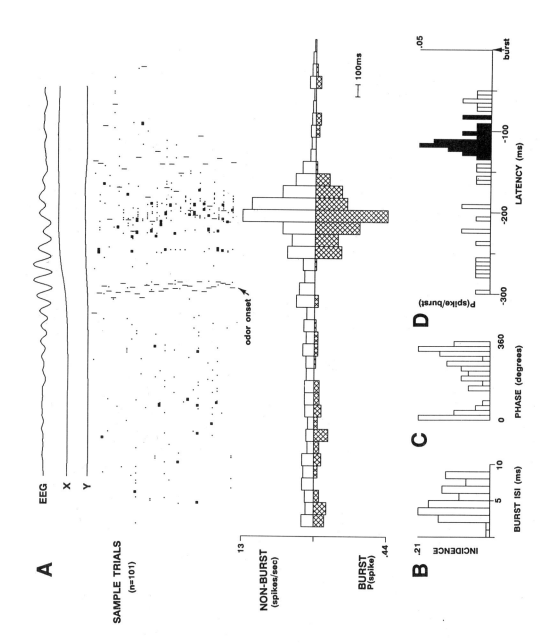

Figure 5.9
Firing patterns of a CA1 pyramidal cell in a rat performing an odor discrimination task. (*A, top to bottom*) EEG, movement (separately as X and Y dimensions), and unit activity across trials time-locked to the first dentate theta peak after odor onset. EEG was first normalized then averaged across trials; movement was averaged across trials as well. EEG (upward deflections reflect positivity) was first normalized within the 4-sec sampling period, then averaged across trials. Separate X and Y movement traces respectively indicate averaged head movements toward the sampling ports and to the left (up) or right (down). Rasters show single spike (small dots) and burst (large dots) for a subset of analyzed trials. Note that spike and burst activity are aligned to the cycles of averaged EEG across trials. Histograms indicate the incidence of single spikes (open bars) and bursts (shaded bars). P(spike) refers to the probability of burst-related spike activity within each 100-ms bin. (*B*) Distribution of within-burst interspike intervals. (*C*) Distribution of the incidence of burst onsets across phases of the theta cycle. Zero and 360° indicate successive positive peaks of dentate theta rhythm. (*D*) Distribution of latencies of unit activity prior to identified bursts. Darkened bars indicate latencies corresponding to 7 to 12.5 Hz. P(spike/burst) refers to the probability of a spike occurring during each 10-ms bin prior to an identified burst.

Accounting for the Behavioral Data

Having described a theory of hippocampal-dependent declarative memory, articulating the features that distinguish it from memory mediated independently of the hippocampal system, we can now show how our account permits us to understand and to predict the pattern of sparing and loss in amnesia. This discussion will be presented in two parts. The first part, presented in this chapter, applies the procedural-declarative account to three sets of data: our own olfactory discrimination work, the O'Keefe and Conway (1980) maze learning experiment, and the Graf et al. (1984) word-stem completion study. These are the data mentioned earlier as examples where either impairment or sparing can be observed in amnesia for the same behavioral paradigm depending upon the precise details of testing, and as such provide a challenge for any theory of memory and amnesia.

The second part of our discussion, presented in chapters 7 and 8, extends our account to seven behavioral paradigms that enjoy especially widespread use in the human or animal amnesia literatures and that figure particularly prominently in various theoretical accounts of amnesia. These paradigms are as follows: delayed nonmatch to sample (DNMS), spatial learning, conditional discrimination, sensory discrimination, skill learning, repetition priming, and recall and recognition. We document the ability of the account to handle the full range of performances across all of these paradigms and across the various animal species to whom these paradigms have been administered, thereby fulfilling our promise of a comprehensive, rather than a limited-domain, account.

Regrettably, our presentation here cannot be completely inclusive with respect to explaining the findings from every paradigm in the literature and every study ever conducted in amnesia. For example, the literature on conditioning in animal models of amnesia receives relatively less attention here than the more cognitively based literature, although conditioning phenomena are represented in the book and their implications are considered. The seven paradigms that are discussed in detail here account for the overwhelming majority of studies on amnesia across species; we deem it critical for the theory to get these phenomena right.

For each of the paradigms to be considered, the performance of subjects with hippocampal system damage relative to that of control subjects turns out to depend on the specific testing conditions imposed by different variants of each task. (Note here that we have distinguished between *paradigms*, such as olfactory discrimination learning, and *tasks* or *task variants*, such as the simultaneous odor discrimination learning task used in Eichenbaum et al. [1989] and discussed below.) Performance of amnesics relative to control subjects depends on the extent to which variants of each task encourage or actually require the use of hippocampal-dependent declarative memory for successful performance.

Understanding the full pattern of spared and impaired memory performances following hippocampal system damage—accommodating performance across not only different paradigms but also across different variants of each paradigm—thus becomes a major challenge. The successful theory of amnesia must go beyond general predictions of impaired performance on some memory paradigms and intact performance on other memory paradigms. It must also be able to account for the sensitivity of each paradigm to task manipulations that alter the pattern of sparing and loss in amnesia. Holding theories of amnesia to this criterion ups the ante considerably. We shall endeavor to show that the procedural-declarative account fulfills this higher criterion.

The theory proposed here will be shown to have one further virtue, or to handle one further significant challenge, namely the ability to accommodate certain "odd" results that were heretofore difficult to understand because of lack of correspondence with other results from the same paradigms. That is, in several paradigms for which there exist multiple reports of impairment in subjects with hippocampal system damage, the presence of one or a few reports of sparing has been treated as "noise" in the data or has been attributed to some peculiarity of test administration. Deeming such experiments as somehow involving "nonstandard" variants of the task has seemed to justify ignoring the conflicting data. Unfortunately, this is tantamount to employing a rule of *psychoarithmetic* to judge the adequacy of theories: Apparently, for a given paradigm, you just take a head count of the number of studies showing impairment and the number of studies showing sparing, and then let majority rule; if the majority of studies with paradigm x show impairment, then you assert that performance on paradigm x is impaired in amnesia. But this goes against the best tradition of scientific inquiry. Unlike politics, science does not and should not proceed in purely democratic fashion. Even a single counterexample could be cause for rejection of a theory or abandonment of an empirical generalization if it cannot be adequately explained. That is, if performance on paradigm x is only impaired in amnesia some of the time (or most, or even almost all of the time), then it is *not* appropriate to ignore the counterexamples and make sweeping generalizations. Rather, a new empirical generalization is needed—one that explains why, and the precise circumstances under which, performance on paradigm x varies.

There is another, alternative approach that is equally worthy of blame. That approach correctly eschews psychoarithmetic, but goes too far: If there are any counterexamples to a finding of preserved learning on a given paradigm, then just reject (and ignore) the initial claim. This is a mistaken view for the same reason that the "majority rules" criterion is mistaken. What is needed is a way to understand all of the findings with a given paradigm—providing an account of the variance as well as of the main effects.

Our account rejects these two approaches. Instead, it offers an explanation of how the different task variants give rise to different behavioral outcomes. Thus, the account is comprehensive in this sense as well.

It turns out that manipulation of task conditions—producing different variants of a given paradigm—serves to change the nature of the representational demands placed on subjects. This in turn leads to sometimes revealing and sometimes obscuring the differences in representational systems between amnesic patients versus normal subjects. Differences across the task variants emerge in two general ways: in the extent to which the task variants depend on hippocampal-mediated declarative representations for successful performance; and in the extent to which they encourage or discourage the use of performance strategies dependent on declarative representations.

DEPENDENCE ON DECLARATIVE REPRESENTATION

Some task variants absolutely require declarative memory; successful performance of these tasks depends on flexible, promiscuous representations of the outcomes of particular previous processing events. For these, the inflexible and dedicated procedural representations available to amnesic subjects will not suffice, and so amnesic performance will be grossly impaired. Other task variants might confer a relative advantage on performance that is guided by hippocampal-dependent declarative memory; on these, the memory systems to which amnesic subjects have access are adequate for successful performance but cannot support *optimal* performance. Accordingly, the performance of amnesic subjects will be impaired relative to that of normal subjects, or at least relative to the performance of those normal subjects who choose strategies making use of declarative memory (see below). Still other task variants neither require nor confer any advantage on performance strategies supported by declarative memory; these can be supported by either hippocampal-dependent or hippocampal-independent memory systems. On these variants, the performance of amnesic subjects can be fully comparable to that of control subjects *quantitatively*, but the nature of the representations guiding performance would be quite different for the amnesics versus the controls. We shall show examples of each of these different outcomes.

ENCOURAGING OF PERFORMANCE STRATEGIES SUPPORTED BY DECLARATIVE MEMORY

Some tasks suggest or otherwise encourage the use of declarative memory, even if strategies based on procedural memory are available. In encouraging subjects to make use of declarative memory, such tasks permit normal individuals to take advantage of the representational system that distinguishes them from amnesic patients, thereby serving to increase the likelihood that differences between the groups will emerge in their overt performances. We cannot overemphasize the point that such differences will be observed either in terms of (quantitatively) impaired performance by the amnesic subjects or in terms of (qualitative) differences in the characteristics of the representations they store.

Accordingly, in the discussion that follows, evidence for our theory about declarative memory, amnesia, and the hippocampal system will be adduced in two ways: (1) on task variants for which performance requires or at least is facilitated by the availability of declarative representations, amnesic subjects will show impaired performance; and (2) on task variants for which performance can be mediated by either hippocampal-dependent or hippocampal-independent memory systems, but use of hippocampal-mediated declarative memory is encouraged, amnesic subjects will differ from normal subjects *not* in their performance level but in the flexibility and promiscuity of the representations of experience they store. Both of these outcomes are documented below.

OLFACTORY LEARNING STUDIES

We turn now to consideration of how this description of hippocampal-dependent and hippocampal-independent memory representation accounts for results from the Eichenbaum et al. (1988) study discussed above and from our other supporting work in rodents. The study was designed to offer a set of conditions that, while holding the learning materials constant, varied the representational demands to encourage or hinder dependence on declarative memory representation. Additional *probe studies* were performed to assess the kinds of representation actually used by the animals, with particular attention paid to the flexibility with which the representations could be used (see Eichenbaum et al., 1989). The necessity of conducting probe studies in order to evaluate the nature of representation used by animals in various memory studies is another way in which the theoretical position we have offered here "ups the ante" for conducting work in this area.

In the successive-cue condition of the Eichenbaum et al. (1988) study (see right panels of figure 3.1), the two odors in each problem were presented successively on separate trials, and the animal simply had to learn which odor was the one for which they should stay in the odor port to receive reward. Successful performance on each problem could be achieved by coming to appreciate that one of the odors was "good" and choosing to stay in the odor port for it, or that one of the odors was somehow undesirable and choosing not to stay around in the odor port upon its presentation. The animal would *not* have to be capable of making comparative judgments about the *pair* of odors, or have any sense of the relationship of that problem to any other problem presented previously. In such a case, the representation guiding performance need *not* be flexible or promiscuous, in that it need only be expressed in testing situations that are repetitions of the original learning situation. Accordingly, successful performance on this variant of the task would be capable of being mediated by the inflexible, dedicated representations we attribute to procedural memory systems functioning independently of the hippocampal system. And, indeed, the performance of rats with hippocampal system damage following fornix lesions was at least as good as that of control animals.

Some of our other olfactory learning data provide insights about the representations actually used by normal rats versus rats with hippocampal system damage, making clear that representation of the same learning materials differed between the two groups. Consider a study that probed representation of odors learned in the successive odor discrimination task by challenging rats with reversal learning following the end of discrimination training (Eichenbaum et al., 1986). In this study, a new odor discrimination problem was presented on each of three days, and animals exhibited acquisition of a learning set, learning each problem more quickly than the previous one. On the fourth day, animals were presented with the reversal task, in which the odors from the previous day were re-presented but with reversed reward assignments (the previously rewarded odor becoming non-rewarded and vice versa). As shown in figure 6.1, normal rats required many more trials to learn the reversal problem than they had needed to learn the previous discrimination problem, suggesting that they recognized the relationship between odors presented on the two days (i.e., recognized the odors from the previous day) and were "confused" by the difference between days in reward assignments. This requires the sort of flexible, declarative representation we attribute to the hippocampal-dependent memory system in order to judge relationships and make comparisons among multiple stimuli. By contrast, rats with hip-

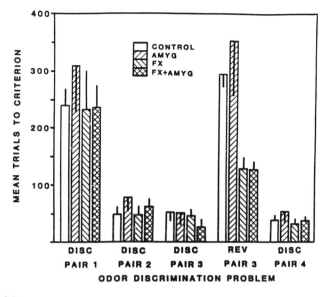

Figure 6.1
Performance of control and brain-damaged rats on discrimination (DISC)
and reversal (REV) problems with successive pairs of odors. Groups are
identified by locus of bilateral lesion: CONTROL, normal and sham-
operated; AMYG, amygdala; FX, fornix; FX+AMYG, combination fornix
and amygdala. Vertical bars indicate standard error. Amnesic animals with
damage to the hippocampal system (FX or FX+AMYG) performed as well
as did controls on the discrimination problems, and showed facilitation
with respect to controls on the reversal problem.

pocampal system damage (fornix lesions), although influenced to
some degree initially by the previous day's reward assignments,
acquired the reversal nearly as quickly as they had learned the
previous discrimination problem. We infer that they failed to perceive the relationship between the odors and reward assignments
from day 3 and the odors and reward assignments from day 4, and
consequently treated the reversal problem as just another discrimination. A quite similar pattern of results also has been observed
for monkeys with object discrimination reversal (Zola & Mahut,
1973). This is just what would be expected in the absence of flexible,
declarative representations. (For a more comprehensive review of
the role of the hippocampal system in reversal learning see Eichenbaum et al., 1986.)

In the simultaneous-cue condition of the Eichenbaum et al. (1988) study, the two odors in each problem were presented simultaneously and a discriminative choice had to be made between two possible active responses, a situation designed to encourage making (and remembering the outcome of) comparisons among multiple stimuli and response choices (see left panels of figure 3.1). Representing such relationships requires the hippocampal-dependent declarative memory system, and thus would confer a performance advantage on normal animals relative to animals with hippocampal system damage. The results conformed with this prediction: Animals with hippocampal system damage following fornix lesions exhibited performance that was markedly impaired compared to the performance of normal animals. Moreover, several additional results lend credence to this account of their performances. First, in a subsequent study of simultaneous odor discrimination performance (Eichenbaum et al., 1989), we found a qualitative distinction between normal and amnesic animals in their response latencies. Normal animals had bimodal distributions of latencies, with one peak corresponding to left-port responding and the other peak to right-port responding, suggesting that the animals sample both ports and make some comparative judgment at the time of their response decision. By contrast, the responses of animals with hippocampal system damage had shorter latencies and a single-peaked distribution, suggesting that these animals made their choices without comparative judgments at the time of their response decision (figure 6.2).

Further insight into the determinants of the performance of the two groups, and the nature of their underlying memory representations, comes from a subsequent condition of the Eichenbaum et al. (1989) study. Following training on two different problems, animals were given probe trials in which the odor pairings were changed so that each odor from the first problem was re-paired with an odor from the second problem, but all odors maintained their original reward assignments (figure 6.3). Normal rats had no difficulty in choosing the S+ odors in the novel pairings of the probe trials, in line with our proposal that they acquire flexible representations of their experiences with the various odors; their declarative memory permits them to make comparisons among the different odors between and within trials, and to express their learning flex-

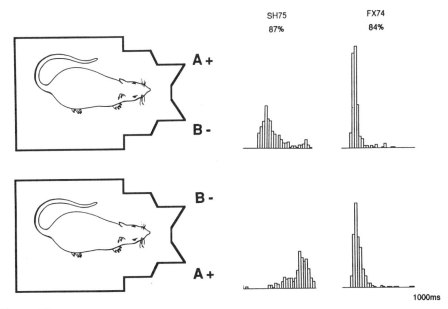

Figure 6.2
The distributions of response latencies for a sham operated rat (SH75) and a rat with a fimbria/fornix transection (FX74) on odor discrimination trials given during over-training, where performance was similar for both subjects (87% for SH75 and 84% for FX74). Separate distributions are shown for correct responses when the S+ odor and response was on the left versus on the right. The distribution of response latencies differed for the sham operated rat, as a function of where the S+ was presented and which response was made. In contrast, the response latencies of the FX rat had a single mode more rapid than even the early mode of the sham operated rat. (From Eichenbaum et al., 1989.)

ibly in novel situations. In the absence of such a declarative representation system, however, animals with hippocampal system
damage were markedly impaired on the novel pairings, initially
treating the probe trials as though they had never experienced the
familiar odor stimuli at all.

THE O'KEEFE AND CONWAY (1980) STUDY

This study involved spatial learning of the location of the goal arm
in a plus-shaped elevated maze surrounded by a plain curtain, with
a small set of stimulus cues visible to help guide performance (see
figure 3.2). Rats were trained in one of two ways: Either the stim-

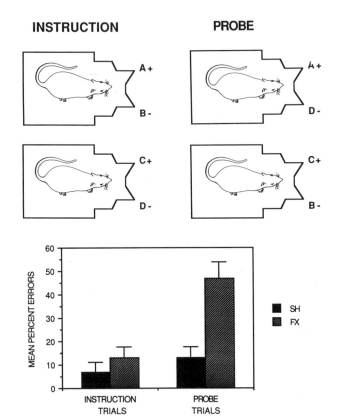

Figure 6.3
Assessment of flexible use of odor memory representations in sham operated rats (SH) and rats with a fimbria/fornix transection (FX). (*Top*) Schematic diagrams of the odors presented on instruction and probe trials.
(*Bottom*) SH and FX rats perform equivalently well in overtraining on
instruction trials. SH rats continue to perform well on probe trials made
up of mispairings of odor cues from the instruction trials, but FX rats made
as many errors as would be predicted by chance. (Data taken from Eichenbaum et al., 1989).

ulus cues were spatially dispersed around the testing environment, or the same stimulus cues were concentrated at the goal arm. For rats trained with the first method, hippocampal system damage markedly impaired performance; however, for rats trained with the second method, hippocampal system damage had no effect.

Our analysis suggests that the critical difference between the two conditions producing impaired versus spared learning in amnesic animals concerns the extent to which flexible encodings of the relationships among multiple stimuli are required for performance. Thus, when trained with a set of cues dispersed around the testing environment and with various starting locations across trials, it is the spatial relations among the cues and the maze arms that specify the goal arm. Such relational information about the goal arms' location with respect to all of the other cues, and with respect to each of the possible starting locations, must be represented across trials and must be capable of being flexibly expressed. These are precisely the properties we have proposed as fundamental to declarative memory. Given disruption to this system following hippocampal system damage, performance on this task would be expected to be severely compromised. By contrast, when trained with the same set of cues concentrated at the goal arm, all that is required for successful performance is learning to go toward the compounded set of cues or any individual cue element, independent of their location in the same environment or of their positions with respect to one another. Such a strategy does *not* require the declarative memory system; rather the ability of procedural memory to support the acquisition of a bias or preference, in this case toward a particular portion of the spatial environment or compound cue, would be sufficient to guide performance. Accordingly, animals with hippocampal system damage would be expected to show intact performance on this variant of the task.

THE GRAF ET AL. (1984) WORD-STEM COMPLETION STUDY

In the Graf et al. (1984) study, involving two different measures of retention of words presented during an earlier study phase, the critical difference between conditions producing impaired performance and those producing intact performance in amnesic patients is the presence of flexible and relational representations. In the test phase of this study, subjects were presented with initial-letter word stems and their memory probed in one of two ways: In a *word-completion* condition, they were instructed to report "the first word that comes to mind" that completes each three-letter stem; in a *cued-recall* condition, they were instructed to use the three-letter stems as cues to help them recall specific items from the list of studied words (see figure 3.3). Let us consider the representational demands of these two conditions. When given cued-recall instructions, subjects are basically encouraged to compare each of the three-letter stems to the stored representations of the particular (whole) words that were together on the study list. This requires the representation of the relations among these arbitrarily associated words, conveying their conjunction on the same list during a particular learning event in a psychology experiment; and it requires the flexible manipulation of these representations to permit their comparison with each of the word-stem cues. These are cardinal features of the declarative memory representation we claim to be mediated by hippocampal system functioning. Accordingly, amnesic patients with damage to the hippocampal system would be expected to exhibit impaired performance.

The representational demands of successful performance when given word-completion instructions are quite different. Performance here could be accomplished through a facilitation of the word-identification process for the previously presented words, expressed when (and only when) producing those words again. This facilitation would not require that the subject be capable of judging that the words had been previously presented, or be capable of reporting anything about previous experiences with the words, or indeed be able to express a memory representation of the learning experience in any other way. What is required is that the word-recognition device or system have been slightly tuned or biased by the recent experience with the words on the study list, giving rise to a priming of the studied items in response to the word-stem cues.

This could easily be understood as recent-experience-induced changes in the weights or connection strengths between letter-level and word-level representations in a connectionist model such as that offered by McClelland and Rumelhart (1986), noted in chapter 3. In such a model, the ability of a given word input to be correctly identified depends on the learned associations among letter features (line segments), letters, and words, represented in the network as differential connection strengths or weights. Exposure to particular words will serve to modify the weights between those words and their constituent letters and letter features, biasing or tuning the network in the direction of better performance (due to stronger weights) for those items, at least until subsequent exposure to different words biases the system in a different direction. Thus, for a time after exposure to the items presented in the study phase, those items could be expected to show some amount of priming when the same network is again engaged. Connectionist models of word priming along just these lines have recently been offered (e.g., Rueckl, 1990). The point is that successful word-completion performance could be supported by the kind of inflexible, dedicated representations that we attribute to procedural memory. Accordingly, amnesic patients with damage to the hippocampal system would be expected to show no deficit.

To the extent that this explanation of priming in word completion in correct, it should be possible to show that the representations driving performance are actually inflexible and inextricably tied to word recognition processes. That this is indeed the case will be documented extensively in chapter 8. For the moment, perhaps an example here will suffice. The inflexibility of the representations driving word-completion performance can be seen by running the experiment slightly differently. If, in the study phase, the words are presented auditorily rather than visually, and then the word-stems are presented visually as usual, it is possible to determine just how closely tied the representations of the earlier exposure are to visual word-identification processes. The results, shown in figure 6.4 from a study by Graf et al. (1985), are quite clear: Word-completion to the visually presented stem cues is dramatically reduced when the initial exposure to the words is in a different modality, and hence activates a different processor, than the modality/processor that was engaged at test time. This inflexibility of the representations underlying word completion performance is exactly as predicted by the procedural-declarative account. By contrast, cued-recall performance is not affected at all by changing modalities between study and test, a flexibility that provides support for our claim that performance in the cued-recall condition depends critically on declarative memory.

DIVISIONS OF LONG-TERM MEMORY

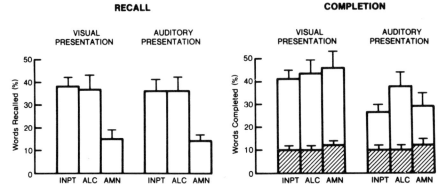

Figure 6.4
Word stems were presented visually to amnesic patients (AMN) and control subjects
(ALC, alcoholic controls; INPT, inpatient controls) as cues to recall words from an
earlier study list (RECALL) or as cues to generate the first word that comes to mind
that completes each stem (COMPLETION). The previous study list was presented
either visually or auditorily. Word-stem completion priming (priming effect = the
difference between completion of baseline stems, striped bars, and completion of stems
corresponding to previously studied words, open bars) was as good for amnesic patients
as for control subjects, and for all groups was poorer when the modality in which the
stems was presented differed from the modality in which the words were initially
presented. (From Graf et al., 1985).

THE ROLE OF PROCEDURAL AND DECLARATIVE MEMORY SYSTEMS
IN BEHAVIORAL PERFORMANCE

These examples help us to illustrate the claim that procedural and
declarative memory systems ordinarily act in parallel, each contributing to behavioral performance to the extent that they are able.
Thus, *in the normal course of affairs, a given learning event leads*
both to storage of the outcomes of processing, through the media-
tion of the declarative system, and tuning of the actual processors
themselves, through the participation of the procedural system.
Declarative memory of the processing outcomes, because of the
relational form of its representation and its representational flexibility, is capable of being used by any number of the brain's processing systems, permitting manipulation of and comparisons
among aspects of stored information, and the expression of this

information in novel situations—the essential requirements in those task variants just discussed that are impaired in amnesia. Procedural memory, by contrast, because it is fundamentally inflexible and tied to the particular processors engaged during the original learning event, will contribute to performance or be revealed only to the extent that the testing situation reengages the original processors. The task variants discussed above for which amnesic performance is intact have just this character. If the tuning or priming of the processors engaged during initial learning are *not* sufficient to guide performance, however, as when relations among multiple stimuli must be computed and stored, or when novel testing situations are imposed, then procedural memory will have little to contribute and its operation will go largely unnoticed.

QUANTITATIVE DIFFERENCES IN THE STRENGTH AND PERSISTENCE OF MEMORIES IN HIPPOCAMPAL-DEPENDENT AND HIPPOCAMPAL-INDEPENDENT SYSTEMS

The fundamental differences between procedural and declarative memory as outlined above concern the nature of the representations supported by these two systems. However, in addition to these qualitative differences in representation, there are other differences of importance between the two memory systems in terms of their operating characteristics. They differ, too, in terms of the incremental strength of the memory "trace" produced by exposure to each to-be-remembered item (learning rate) and in the persistence (decay rate) of such traces. But these differences are not always reliable in distinguishing between the memory systems. In general, the declarative system is apparently capable of adding full-fledged memories or at least of making relatively large-scale changes to declarative memory organizations after but a single exposure, with such memories persisting for variable durations (minutes, hours, days, or more, depending on many factors—see below). Furthermore, the functional persistence of declarative memories can apparently be significantly increased with repeated exposures to the same item. By contrast, procedural representations are most typically acquired as relatively small, incremental tunings, biasings, or primings of various processors, and the persistence of each individual change potentially can be quite substantial, depending upon the degree to which the tunings, biasings, or primings produced in the same processor by subsequent processing events pushes the system in a similar direction. If, however, subsequent processing events tend to bias the system in competing directions, tuning it toward optimization for different stimulus items, then the persistence of the original trace will be quite temporary.

Also, in a few specialized adaptive learning situations, such as the acquisition of flavor aversions or conditioned emotional responses and in some cases of verbal or perceptual priming, robust procedural learning can occur in a single trial. Thus strength and persistence characteristics by themselves do not always distinguish the two memory systems. Nonetheless, they can be, and indeed often have been, exploited in experimentally dissociating hippocampal-dependent and hippocampal-independent memory. Moreover, it turns out that work on humans, monkeys, and rats have differed with regard to which aspect of the distinction between procedural and declarative memory has been tapped by the experimental manipulations. Most of the recent work on amnesia in monkeys has focused on the issues of strength and persistence differences; most of the work on amnesia in rats has focused on relational versus individual representations; and most of the recent work on human amnesia has focused primarily on the flexibility of memory in normal subjects versus amnesic patients. This state of affairs has understandably contributed to some of the confusions and lack of comparability of the findings across species. Nevertheless, in all three literatures, there are both examples of dissociations based on strength and persistence differences between the systems, as well as more illuminating dissociations between normal and amnesic memory abilities that are explained in terms of the nature of representation and representational flexibility between declarative and procedural memory.

In the next two chapters we will illustrate further how the differences we have proposed between procedural and declarative memory systems can explain the pattern of spared versus impaired memory performances in amnesia, by applying the theory more generally to the seven most widely used behavioral paradigms in the human and animal amnesia literatures.

Generalizing to Other Paradigms: Animal Studies

For each of the three paradigms considered in the previous chapter, manipulations of the task conditions or instructions changed the nature of the representational demands placed on the subjects, and therefore changed the performance of amnesic subjects with respect to that of control subjects. Amnesic subjects were impaired whenever task conditions required declarative representation, or whenever conditions conferred an advantage on performances based on such representation. With an intact declarative system, subjects could take advantage of relational representation to permit promiscuous access and manipulation of stored memory, and to permit flexible expression of memory in a variety of novel situations. By contrast, amnesic subjects were intact whenever the task conditions permitted successful performance to be accomplished based on an *in*flexible, dedicated form of representation, such as when subjects had only to adapt their behavior to a repetition of the original learning situation.

Accordingly, we have documented the ability of our multiple memory system account to span across three very different tasks, across sensory modalities, and even across species. To further document the generality of our account, we next consider its applicability to each of several paradigms used by investigators studying the effects of hippocampal-system damage. Seven different paradigms are addressed in detail in the course of this and the following chapter, including the four major paradigms (plus brief accounts of several other related paradigms) in the animal model work (in this chapter) and the three paradigms receiving the most attention in the human amnesia literature (chapter 8). This discussion has been divided across the two chapters because the human work and animal model work remains largely segregated in the published literature and, on the surface at least, the methods, data, and issues of concern to most researchers differ in accordance with the species studied. Accordingly, we confront those issues separately and show how the present articulation of the procedural-declarative framework handles them. However, because the theory offered here aspires to be comprehensive and, we claim, succeeds in accounting for both the human and animal model findings, we encourage the reader to tackle both chapters and see the commonalities that illustrate our point.

DELAYED NON-MATCH-TO-SAMPLE (DNMS)

In the version of this task that has become so widely used in studies of monkeys (Gaffan, 1974; Mishkin & Delacour, 1975), each trial consists of a sample phase and a match phase. In the sample phase of each trial the animal is exposed to one of a large set of objects; it is placed in the center position of a three-position display, and the animal is to displace it to receive a reward (figure 7.1, top). Following a variable delay interval, the match phase occurs. As depicted in figure 7.1, the object from the sample phase is presented together with another from the set of available objects; they are placed in the two outside positions, and the animal is to displace the object that was *not* previously presented in order to receive reward.

Similar tasks have been created for rats, some using conventional objects as cues (Mumby, Pinel, & Wood, 1990; Rothblatt & Kromer, 1991), others using a two-alley Y-maze apparatus in which removable visually and tactually distinct maze arms serve as the "objects" (Aggleton, 1985; Gaffan, 1972; Rafaelle & Olton, 1988), and others that employ identical Y-maze arms and use spatial position of the sample as the memory cue (Olton, Becker, & Handleman, 1979; Thomas & Gash, 1988). The animal is forced to run down one or another of the arms in the sample phase and then to choose an arm during the match phase. That choice is either to the arm in the other direction from the one in the sample phase (in the "spatial" variant of the task), or to the arm whose visual characteristics or textural covering differs from the one in the sample phase, independent of its spatial position (in the "cued" variant of the task). In the spatial version of the task, as well as in one object-cued version (Rafaelle & Olton, 1982), the same cues are used repetitively

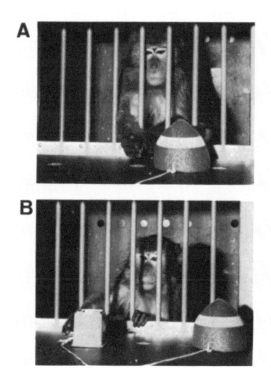

Figure 7.1
A version of the delayed non-matching-to-sample task. (*A*) The monkey displaces an object presented alone over the center foodwell to receive a food reward. (*B*) After a delay period, typically of seconds to minutes, during which the monkey's view of the foodwells is obscured, the old object is re-presented along with a new one over the two outside foodwells. The monkey must displace the novel object in order to receive a food reward. (From Zola-Morgan et al., 1982.)

on each trial. Most recently Otto and Eichenbaum (1992) have developed a continuous-matching variant of this paradigm using odor cues. In this task a series of up to 16 odors are presented individually in sequential trials; animals are selectively rewarded for responding appropriately when the current odor is different from the immediately preceding odor (a non-match).

This test has been particularly successful in revealing impaired memory following extensive hippocampal-system damage both in monkeys (Gaffan, 1974, 1977; Gaffan & Saunders, 1985; Mishkin, 1978, 1982; Zola-Morgan & Squire, 1985) and, in more recent work, in rats (Aggleton et al., 1989; Otto & Eichenbaum, 1992). Performance is normal in short-delay conditions, becoming manifested only with longer delays; thus, as with humans, the impairment is one of long-term memory. The magnitude of the impairment of long-term memory is directly related to the length of the variable delay interval between the sample and match phase, with performance approaching chance levels as the delay interval increases to 60 seconds. Also, in monkeys, when several sample trials are presented in rapid succession, as a list of to-be-remembered objects, and subjects are then presented with a series of choice tests, the impairment is exacerbated.

However, even animals performing at chance levels following extensive hippocampal system damage demonstrate intact learning and retention of the procedures for performing the task. Monkeys learn to displace the centrally placed object and rats run down the offered maze arm or sample an odor to receive reward in the sample phase; and they learn to respond differentially and then search for their reward in the match phase. Their only problem is in knowing which of the choice objects, maze arms, or odors is to be rewarded, and that is only the case if there is a sufficiently long interval since presentation of the sample that is to guide their choice. The preserved learning and remembering of the task procedures, together with the delay-size and list-length–dependent impairment that characterizes performance on this task, model very closely the performance of amnesic patients on tests of recognition memory.

This paradigm is not without findings in need of explanation, however. Some findings of little or no impairment following damage to the hippocampal system must be considered. One controversy involves the critical locus of the lesion within the hippocampal system. This issue, as we discussed in chapter 1, will not be considered here. More related to the nature of memory representation in DNMS, there are now reports that varying the task so that the correct response in the match phase is to choose the object that had been previously presented in the sample phase (delayed match-to-sample [DMS]), rather than the DNMS rule of choosing the novel object, dramatically reduces the effects of hippocampal system damage in both rats (Rawlins et al., 1988) and monkeys (Gaffan et al., 1984).[1] Such a difference in results between these two task variants cannot be understood in terms of differences in whether or not they result in a deficit in recognition of the objects but rather in the demands they place on expression of memory.

Consideration of the task demands of DNMS versus DMS permits an understanding of how the procedural-declarative framework accounts for the observed pattern of performance following hippocampal system damage. What kind of memory for the sample-phase cues is required for successful DNMS performance? As is the case for recognition memory (and other tests of explicit remembering) in humans (see chapter 8), performance here needs to be supported by declarative representations of the cues encountered during the previous phases (and trials) of the task. The representational flexibility and promiscuity that characterize declarative memory are necessary to permit comparisons to be performed between stored representations of the sample phase cues and the items actually present in the match-phase displays, and are required to support the expression of the stored memory in a test situation that is *not* a repetition of the original acquisition event. Whereas the to-be-remembered cues are initially presented as single, centrally positioned items to which the animal is to respond, when they are represented in the match phases they appear (typically) in two-choice displays positioned laterally to the original displays, and now animals are *not* to respond to them. Removing this non-match response requirement in the DMS variant reduces the demand for representational flexibility and thus its dependence on the hippocampal declarative system. The fact that the deficit caused by hippocampal system damage is less in the DMS variant is in complete conformance with this view.

It must be kept in mind, though, that a significant impairment is observed even on the DMS variant of the paradigm. This, we believe, is due to operating characteristics of the hippocampal system that confer an advantage to normal subjects over the capabilities of subjects with hippocampal-system damage. It will be suggested below that differences between hippocampal-dependent and hippocampal-independent systems in the strength and persistence of memory traces for single presentations of objects are the basis of the observed dissociations in performance (see section on Sensory Discrimination), applicable here to DMS and contributing significantly to the dissociations in DNMS as well.

SPATIAL LEARNING

Largely because of the findings indicating that many hippocampal neurons exhibit place fields when placed in spatial tasks, the effects of hippocampal system damage on spatial learning and memory has been explored extensively, at least in rats. Two major paradigms have been employed, each of which will be discussed in detail.

Water Maze

This task, developed by Morris (1981) and now employed by several investigators, uses a 2-meter diameter circular tank (or pool) filled with opaque fluid (milk or colored water) and an escape platform slightly submerged under the water surface at a constant location relative to various extramaze visual cues. In the standard version of the task (figure 7.2, top left panel), the rat is placed into the tank at various locations around the circumference of the pool on successive trials. The animal swims around until it finds the platform and can escape from the water. Across trials, normal animals come to locate the platform increasingly rapidly, and eventually learn the spatial location of the platform sufficiently well to permit them to navigate directly to it from any start location. On later trials, they may be presented with the platform in a different location and again placed into the tank at various locations around the circumference of the pool, thus having to learn a new escape location from any start location.

Hippocampal system damage has been found to impair the ability to learn the location of the escape platform (figure 7.2, bottom left panel). Placed into the pool at various starting positions, rats with hippocampal system damage are *not* able to swim directly to the platform, instead being forced to search exhaustively for its location each time, with the result that their escape latencies are abnormally long (DiMattia & Kesner, 1988; Schenk & Morris, 1985; Sutherland, Wishaw, & Kolb, 1983).

Despite their profound impairment on the task, however, animals with hippocampal system damage do become efficient swimmers and do learn to climb up onto the platform (and thereby escape from the water) when they finally locate one. Across trials they may also acquire a strategy of swimming a circular path around the pool at a certain distance from the pool wall that corresponds to

PLACE LEARNING

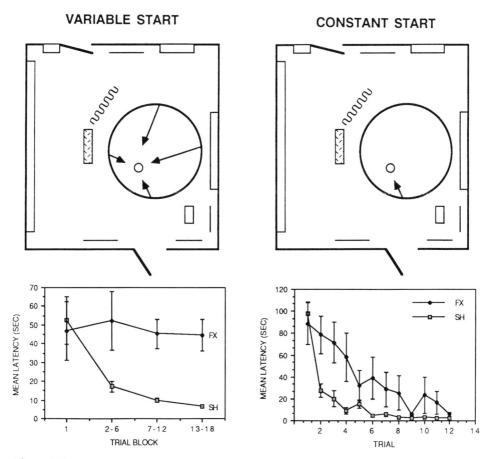

Figure 7.2
Performance of sham operated rats (SH) and rats with transection of the fimbria/fornix
(FX) on two variants of the Morris water maze task, one using variable start locations
and the other using a constant start location. Arrows indicate starting positions in
each task variant. Symbols represent various objects visible from the surface of the
maze. (From Eichenbaum et al., 1990.)

where platforms tend to be located (on different sets of trials, the platform may be located in different quadrants of the pool but at a constant distance from the pool wall). Thus, rather than swimming directly toward the appropriate (or any other) platform from the various starting positions, as do normal animals who remember the specific platform location, animals with hippocampal damage may just circumnavigate the pool at the appropriate radius until encountering a platform (Morris, 1984). By so doing, they never achieve the same escape latencies as normals, whose straight-line paths produce very short latencies, but they demonstrate the ability to learn and retain the procedures of the task, and to generate and use adaptive strategies. This pattern of impairment and sparing seems to have the very same form as that seen in human amnesia.

One variant of the water maze task fails to produce the pattern of performance considered thus far, however. In a recent study by Eichenbaum, Stewart, and Morris (1990), hippocampal system damage did *not* prevent rats from learning the location of the escape platform. For the animals in this study, a constant starting location was used throughout training; that is, animals were to learn to navigate to the escape location from a *fixed* starting location (figure 7.2, right panels). The fact that hippocampal system damage did not produce the same impairment on this variant of the water maze as it produces on the standard variant of the task is particularly revealing about the nature of hippocampal-dependent memory. Accordingly, we turn now to consideration of the difference in the demands that these two task variants place on memory and how this fits into the procedural-declarative framework.

The processing and memory demands of the standard variable-start-location variant of the water maze task appear very similar to those of the distributed cues condition of O'Keefe and Conway's (1980) maze experiment, both of which are sensitive to hippocampal-system damage. Animals in the water maze must learn the spatial location of the escape platform across trials, just as animals in O'Keefe and Conway's maze must learn the location of reward. For both tasks, learning the goal location depends on the use of cues that are distal from the site of reinforcement rather than on cues proximal to that locus. This is particularly true of the water maze, in which the proximal surroundings of the site of reinforcement are particularly variable. More importantly, perhaps, both tasks employ multiple starting locations that involve overlapping perspectives of the same perceptual stimuli. These overlapping perspectives would generate conflicting behavioral responses (go to the right of a particular cue under certain circumstances and to the left under others) unless performance is based on a flexible response guided by spatial relations among the cues and the position of the subject, rather than by a rigid approach trajectory guided toward a particular cue or compound set of cues. The need of animals to build a representation of the position of the platform in relation to the various visual cues arrayed in the room, independent of particular swimming routes, and to flexibly express this stored information regardless of where in the pool the animal is placed at the time of test, is precisely met by the characteristics of the hippocampal-dependent declarative memory system. Indeed, the task seems an excellent probe of representational flexibility and relationality, and therefore of the integrity of the hippocampal-dependent declarative system. Animals with damage to the hippocampal system would certainly be expected to fail on this task.

But what about the constant-start-location variant of the water maze task? The demand for flexibility and relationality in the standard variant is removed in this variant of the task. By training animals with a constant start location, the emphasis on representation of spatial relations among the distal cues is eliminated and animals can demonstrate successful performance by instead learning a rigid approach trajectory guided toward a particular cue or cue complex. Accordingly, successful performance in no way depends on the integrity of the hippocampal system, and the failure of hippocampal-system damage to interfere with performance on this variant of the task is thus precisely what would be expected on our procedural-declarative account.

This interpretation was tested in the Eichenbaum et al. (1990) study by assessing the flexibility of the representations used by animals with hippocampal-system damage in probe tests conducted after training. The probe testing assessed the ability of animals to navigate to the escape location when presented with novel start positions. Intact animals readily navigated to the platform from novel starting positions. In contrast, under these testing conditions, animals with hippocampal system damage who had been trained with just the single start location required much longer to find the platform, sometimes never finding it during the probe trial (figure 7.3). That is, although the animals succeeded in learning a direct approach to a specific "place" in the initial testing, they lacked the representational flexibility required when the test was other than a repetition of the original acquisition situation. This failure to exhibit the necessary representational flexibility mirrors their problem on the standard version of the task. Thus their success on the (initial phase of the) constant-start-location variant is to be attributable to learning to navigate based on an *inflexible*, dedicated representation such as what would be used to learn a rigid approach trajectory guided toward a particular cue or cue complex. This kind of learning strategy and underlying representation is precisely the type we have attributed to procedural memory systems operating *independently* of the hippocampal system.

Note that while declarative memory was *not necessary* for successful performance in the constant-start-location task variant, *normal* animals acquired a declarative representation nonetheless. It was their ability to acquire a declarative representation that permitted them to successfully navigate to the escape location from novel start positions in the probe testing. This tendency of normal animals to acquire and rely on the use of declarative representations even in the absence of any explicit demand for such memory for successful performance was raised in the context of our odor discrimination learning work, in chapter 6, and will be a recurring theme in our discussion of the different paradigms in the literature.

Another recurring theme illustrated in this example is the importance of probe testing as the means to understand the nature of the representations being used to drive performance, and, by gaining such an understanding, to permit the testing of our theory.

One final point deserves discussion. Results of the above study highlight the fact that there are various types of "spatial" representations or various representational bases for supporting "spatial" performance, only a subset of which depend on declarative memory. The cognitive maps to which O'Keefe and Nadel (1978) referred as mediating the representation of "places" in the environment certainly entail the relational representations that are central to our notion of declarative memory. However, as indicated by the Eichenbaum et al. (1990) study, "places" can also be defined by the set of cues local to, or forming the background of, a location (see

INSTRUCTION   PROBE

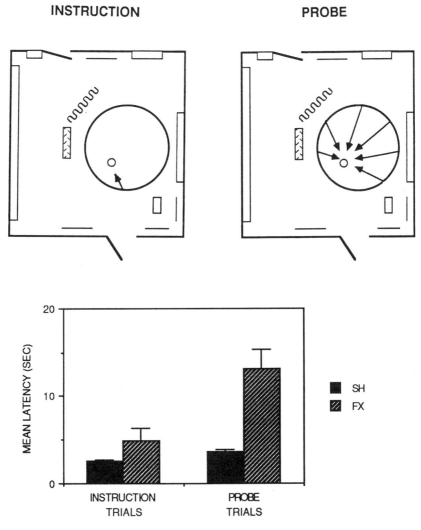

Figure 7.3
An assessment of flexible use of place memory in sham-operated rats (SH)
and rats with a fimbria/fornix transection (FX). SH and FX rats performed
equivalently well in overtraining on instruction trials (the task variate
shown in figure 7.2, right panels). Intermixed among repeats of the instruction trials, one of six "probe" trials was presented; in each of these trials
the subject was required to swim starting from a position at the circumference of the maze at which it had never started before. SH rats performed
well on these probe trials, but FX rats had difficulty finding the platform
from novel start positions. (From Eichenbaum et al., 1990.)

also Eichenbaum et al., 1991, 1992; O'Keefe and Conway, 1980). The animals with hippocampal-system damage in the constant-start-location variant of the task learned the "place" where the escape platform was hidden in the water maze, but did not know the place in the same way as did normal animals; they did not know it in terms of its relations to various other objects within the same environment (or at least had no way of expressing that aspect of their knowledge of place). This suggests at least two ways of representing allocentric space.

In addition to allocentric space, there are types of egocentric spatial representations that are referenced to the body axis and that can specify the body with respect to objects in space (e.g., being to the left of A). Tasks involving spatial processing can typically be solved in multiple ways, invoking different ones of these various types of spatial representations. Animals can learn to "go left" in a Y-maze, or learn to orient or be guided toward a particular cue, without requiring the relational representations of declarative memory. Alternatively, they can learn the relations among a whole set of cues in order to guide their behavior, thereby becoming dependent upon declarative memory. In simultaneous discrimination tasks, animals could learn about the different cues in their respective positions, or about the specific "places" in which they appear, or about exclusively nonspatial characteristics of the cues individually; and they could base their performance on one or more of these sources of information. Clearly, each of these different encoding (and performance) strategies would lead to different patterns of expectations about hippocampal-system involvement. It behooves those who wish to speak about spatial memory and spatial processing, therefore, to be clear about whether or not any given example entails relational representations, and hence whether or not it requires declarative memory.

Radial-Arm Maze

In this widely used test of memory in rats (first discussed by Olton & Samuelson, 1976), training occurs in an elevated maze composed of a starting platform and a number (e.g., 4, 8, or 17!) of goal arms extending out radially from the starting platform (an 8-armed maze is depicted schematically in figure 7.4). The ends of the arms are baited with food at the beginning of each trial (and not replaced

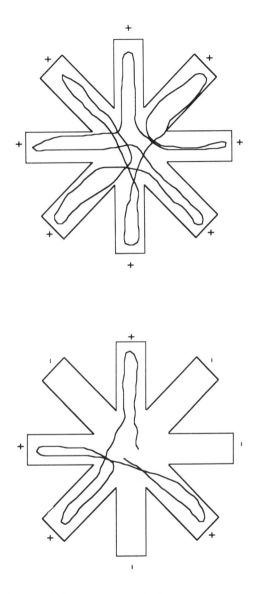

Figure 7.4
Two variants of the radial-arm maze task. (*Top*) All arms are baited (+) at
the outset of a trial. The rat's movements (tracing) indicates that it samples
each of the arms once to maximize the efficiency of its food retrieval.
(*Bottom*) Four of the arms are never baited (−) and four baited (+) only at
the outset of each trial. The rat ignores the unbaited arms and samples
each of the baited arms only once.

during a trial) and animals are allowed to explore the maze until all of the food has been obtained from the arms. Alternatively, the number of arm visits is restricted to a maximum corresponding to the total number of maze arms (e.g., in an 8-arm maze only 8 arm visits would be permitted per trial), and the number of food rewards actually obtained is recorded. With practice, normal animals learn to obtain the food in the minimum possible number of arm visits, entering each arm only once, even if they are prevented from using the strategy of systematically turning into consecutive adjacent arms (figure 7.4, top panel).

Rats with hippocampal system damage are found to be impaired on this task. They make multiple visits to maze arms within a trial. Thus, they require extra entries to obtain all of the food, and they fail to obtain all of the food rewards if the maximum number of arm visits is limited by the experimenter. Yet, as in the other tasks we have considered, animals successfully learn and retain the procedures of the task. They learn to run the radial-arm maze in a procedurally appropriate manner, running down arms in search of food rewards and eating whatever food they find. This is just the pattern of impairment and sparing seen in the other tasks we have considered. It is interesting to note that the arm sampling behavior of rats with hippocampal system damage rapidly becomes abnormally stereotyped and more limited than that of normal rats (Devenport et al., 1988). This "rigidity" in their performance on the radial-arm maze, like that on other tasks, reflects the inflexibility of what is learned by amnesic animals in the absence of hippocampal-dependent declarative memory.

There are variants of the radial-arm maze task for which performance is often *not* impaired, however. Olton and Pappas (1979) created a variant of this paradigm in which only a subset of the arms are baited at the beginning of each trial (figure 7.4, bottom panel). Across trials, intact animals learn to avoid entering the never-baited arms, and to enter the once-(per-trial) baited arms only one time per trial. Animals with hippocampal system damage were able to learn to avoid the never-baited arms, although they could *not* learn to avoid multiple entries into the once-baited arms. Packard, Hirsch, and White (1989) reported that rats with hippocampal-system damage also showed intact learning in a *cued* variant of the task, in which the arms to be approached were signaled by a light cue.

Consideration of the memory demands of the radial-arm maze task clearly suggests the requirement for the declarative form of representation we claim is mediated by the hippocampal system. This requirement comes from two critical aspects of the task that are functional analogs of those already discussed in our treatment of the water maze and DNMS. First, the task requires the ability to navigate around the maze, disambiguating among and remembering the various reward locations (maze arms). Because there is no fixed path through the maze for the animals to run, animals could base their identifications of the maze arms on their representation of the spatial relations among extramaze cues as seen from different perspectives in the choice area. This imposes a demand for relational representation that is functionally comparable to what we have suggested is required in the water maze; in both tasks, it is a requirement that can only be met by hippocampal-dependent declarative memory.

Second, the task requires the ability to keep track of the arms already visited on each trial in order to guide subsequent choices *away* from those arms. This too is a demand for representational flexibility of the sort that is only provided by hippocampal-dependent declarative representations. Such representations would provide the animal with the means to compare each alternative arm choice with a continually updated representation of the arms already visited on that trial. Furthermore, in a functionally comparable manner as that required in the DNMS task, declarative representations would permit the flexible expression of the stored information in the form of a non-match response, that is, a response to arms other than those experienced earlier in the trial.

On our account, then, the sensitivity of radial-arm maze performance to hippocampal system damage comes from the above two demands on representation flexibility. Reduction of these demands on representational flexibility would be expected to reduce the dependence of task performance on hippocampal system functioning and hence reduce the likelihood of observing impairment following damage to the hippocampal system. Indeed, the failure to see impairment on the variant of the task with never-baited arms (Olton

& Pappas, 1979) would seem to provide evidence for just such a claim. This variant removes the second demand for representational flexibility considered above. This is because learning to avoid entries into the never-baited arms only requires that subjects repeat the same avoidance behavior across trials; there is no need for a continually updated representation of the arms already visited on that trial nor for the ability to express memory flexibly in the form of a non-match response. At the same time, the variant of the task involving cuing removes the first demand for representational flexibility, by providing an individual signal that need not be compared and related to any other stimuli in order to successfully guide navigation.

Other investigators have reported results at variance with Olton's findings of spared performance for never-baited arms, instead reporting impairment for *both* once-baited *and* never-baited arms (see Jarrard, 1986, Jarrard et al., 1984, and Barnes, 1988 for reviews). An explanation for these conflicting findings may lie in differences in the qualities of the distal cues available to subjects that serve to emphasize or de-emphasize the spatial relationships among the cues. The nature and distribution of these cues is highly variable across laboratories and is seldom adequately described. As we have already seen in the O'Keefe and Conway (1980) experiment, the distribution of cues can be critical to the behavioral outcome, determining whether hippocampal system damage produces impaired or spared performance. Jarrard and colleagues showed that eliminating distinctive guidance cues on the arms increases the impairment due to hippocampal-system damage on choices for once-baited versus never-baited arms. Within the perspective of our procedural-declarative account, we see this manipulation as having the effect of increasing the demand for declarative representation needed to capture the spatial relationships among distal cues by eliminating cues within the arms whose presence would allow animals to navigate based on an approach toward individual cues or cue compounds. Increasing the demand for declarative representation would on our view increase the dependence on the hippocampal system, here producing impairment even on the never-baited arms. Thus, when performance can only be guided by the organization of distal cues, as in the appropriate condition of the O'Keefe and Conway (1980) maze experiment and in the standard version of the water maze, marked impairment of performance is observed—for all aspects of the task. In the absence of normal hippocampal system function, rats become rigid in their solution strategies and fail to acquire the task (Okaichi, 1987).

CONDITIONAL, CONFIGURAL, AND CONTEXTUAL DISCRIMINATION

In this class of tasks, which has received a good deal of attention recently (e.g., Gaffan & Harrison, 1989b; Hirsch, 1980; Ross, Orr, Holland, & Berger, 1984; Sutherland & Rudy, 1989), animals must learn to choose their responses to discriminative stimuli in conjunction with some other (conditional) stimulus. Although there are several variants of these tasks, the common fundamental representational demand is that accurate responses be guided by such conditional logic rather than by the accumulated associative strength of a set of stimuli. One example of conditional discrimination is serial feature–positive conditioning (Loechner & Weisz, 1987; Ross et al., 1984). In this classical conditioning task, animals have to learn that presentation of a tone stimulus (A) is followed by a food reward as the unconditioned stimulus (US) only when it is preceded by presentation of a visual stimulus (X); that is, the tone-food association is conditional on the tone being preceded by the visual stimulus (figure 7.5, top). A second example is the negative patterning problem (e.g., Sutherland & Rudy, 1989), an operant version of conditional discrimination in which a tone or light signifies the availability of reward but the combination of tone plus light signifies the absence of reward (figure 7.5, middle). This version of conditional discrimination is a more compelling demonstration of conditional logic, because unlike feature positive conditioning, the problem cannot be solved by summing separate associative strengths accumulated for the stimulus elements. A third example, well represented in the literature, is what we shall call contextual discrimination (figure 7.5, bottom). This type of conditional discrimination task involves training animals on a discrimination in which the correct choice between two discrete cues (e.g., three-dimensional objects, visual patterns) is conditional on more diffuse environmental cues such as different spatial locations of the discrete cues relative to the animals (Gaffan & Harrison,

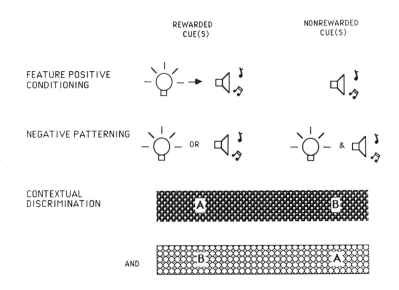

Figure 7.5
Schematic illustrations of three conditional discrimination paradigms. In the example of feature positive conditioning, presentation of a light followed by a tone predicts reward but tone alone does not. In the negative patterning example, presentation of a light *or* a tone predicts reward, but the combined presentation of both cues is not associated with reward. In the example of contextual discrimination, which of two background patterns is presented determines which of the two discriminative cues (A or B) is the one associated with reward. Across trials the left-right positions of A and B vary randomly in both background contexts.

1989a; Murray, Davidson, Gaffan, Olton, & Suomi, 1989); different "scenes" behind the discrete cues (Gaffan & Harrison, 1989b); distinct experimental chambers where the discrimination is performed (Good & Honey, 1991; Isaccson & Kimble, 1972; Winocur & Olds, 1978); different stimuli sampled prior to the choice (Gaffan et al., 1984; Sutherland, Macdonald, Hill, & Rudy, 1989); and different experimenter-induced internal cues (e.g., hunger, thirst—Hirsh et al., 1979; Hsiao and Isaacson, 1971).

There are now reports of impairment following hippocampal system damage on each of the above examples of conditional discrimination tasks. Ross et al. (1984) found that rats with lesions of the hippocampal system failed to acquire the conditional discrimination in the serial feature–positive conditioning task, although they did learn to respond appropriately to the individual (i.e., *noncon-ditional*) cues that were presented intermixed with conditional discrimination trials. On the negative patterning problem, rats trained to treat the presence of a tone or a light as a positive stimulus could not learn to withhold responses to the joint presentation of light and tone following hippocampal system damage, although they could withhold responding to other, nonconditional cues (Sutherland & Rudy, 1989). Hippocampal system damage also results in impairment in each of the contextual discrimination tasks discussed above. Finally, animals with hippocampal lesions are also impaired in learning stimulus chains that lead to reinforcement (Port, Beggs, & Patterson, 1987; Leaton & Borszcz, 1990); this kind of learning would seem to require the acquisition of sequential predictive relations among a set of arbitrary stimuli, just as do formal conditional logic tasks.

As was the case for the other tasks discussed in this section, animals who failed these conditional discrimination tasks following hippocampal system damage were nonetheless capable of learning and remembering the task procedures. They had no difficulty when the tasks were run in an identical manner but with only nonconditional discriminations required, and even when conditional discriminations were required the animals still proceeded to make a choice between objects or response alternatives and then look for food reward. Accordingly, the pattern of impairment and sparing seems to take the same form as in human amnesia.

As was also the case for the other tasks discussed thus far, there are findings that disagree with the basic pattern and that must be understood. There are a number of reports of intact performance on conditional discrimination learning tasks. Jarrard and Davidson (1990; Davidson & Jarrard, 1989) failed to find the impairment observed by Ross et al. (1984) in a version of the serial feature–positive conditioning paradigm that had fewer concurrent contingencies and slightly different stimuli. Also, Markowska et al. (1989) found intact performance in rats with hippocampal system damage in learning to respond discriminatively to two objects dependent on the place in a test room where the task was performed or on the animal's orientation when observing the discriminative cues. Finally, Gaffan et al's (1984) and Gaffan and Harrison's (1989a,b) work with monkeys showed intact performance after hippocampal-system damage in a variety of contextual discrimination tasks.

In several cases, investigators found either impaired or spared performance depending on the task conditions. Gaffan and Harrison (1989b) and Murray et al. (1989) found either impaired or spared learning in monkeys with fornix lesions in different forms of conditional place-object discrimination. For example, the monkeys were impaired in learning to choose between a pair of objects conditional on the place they appeared to occupy within a "scene" (i.e., a particular arrangement of background stimuli), but they performed normally when their choice was conditional on which of two different background "scenes" resulted when the monkey was located in different places in the test area. Loechner and Weisz (1987) showed that rabbits with hippocampal system lesions either failed or succeeded in learning a serial feature–positive discrimination depending on whether the tone or the light was more salient to subjects prior to training and then whether it served as the conditional cue as opposed to the discriminative cue. The fact that hippocampal system damage may or may not produce impairment on conditional discrimination tasks depending on the specifics of the experimental procedures is reminiscent of the three paradigms discussed at length in the previous chapter, and it provides important constraints on an account of hippocampal mediated memory. We shall try to show next how the procedural-declarative account offers an explanation of impairment in some conditional discrimination tasks and sparing in others.

Conditional discrimination tasks seem to place strong demands on representational flexibility and relationality, just those characteristics of representation we have attributed here to the hippocampal-dependent declarative system. Solving these tasks through the application of conditional logic requires making judgments based on the (spatial or temporal) relationship among independent stimuli and requires responding flexibly to the stimuli depending on the conditional associations that were learned. Accordingly, damage to the hippocampal system would certainly be expected to produce impairment on conditional discrimination tasks.

However, this expectation comes with the proviso that subjects actually employ conditional logic in order to solve the tasks. That is, performance on conditional discrimination tasks, just like performance on the other tasks we have considered, can frequently be solved in numerous ways that place different demands on memory systems. Not all conditional discrimination tasks actually require conditional logic for solution; hence not all such tasks require the declarative memory system. Although all of these task variants can be *described* in terms of conditional logic, animals may actually treat them differently as a function of the way in which the stimuli are presented to and are perceived by the subjects, significantly influencing the form of representation relied on by animals, and hence the demands placed on hippocampal system functioning.

To be more specific with respect to the procedural-declarative framework, a declarative representation would be essential if the cues are treated as a set of perceptually independent stimuli whose significance depends on a learned conditional relationship—for example, object A when standing in location 1 is to be distinguished from *the same* object A standing in a different spatial location 2; this is the key to what we meant by *compositionality* in chapter 3. When approaching the problem in this way, hippocampal system damage should cause impairment in learning. Alternatively, at least for some conditional discrimination tasks, animals may treat the cues as a perceptually linked *compound* stimulus that can be used as a unique cue associated with reinforcement (thus, scene X [consisting of object A in location 1] versus scene Y [consisting of object A in location 2]). If approached in this way, the requirement for conditional logic, and hence relational representation, is removed. Learning should then be spared despite hippocampal system damage. Note that the need for hippocampal system involvement is dependent on the nature of prior perceptual analyses; perceptual analyses that combine the stimuli into compounds—and performance strategies that encourage and make use of such analyses—obviate the need for hippocampal-dependent representation of the conditional relationships among the stimuli. That stimulus compounds can form unique "configurals" with properties separate from those of the relevant stimulus elements has been demonstrated in normal animals (Rescorla, 1973).

Note that this account contrasts directly with the hypothesis offered by Sutherland and Rudy (1989) that the function of the hippocampal system is to form such compounds or "configurals," as they refer to them, to resolve the ambiguous significance of conditional cues. On their view (described in more detail in chapter 11), animals with hippocampal system damage would be *unable* to form configurals. Yet, a number of studies have now shown that, in several different conditional or contextual discrimination situations, animals with hippocampal system damage are more likely than normal animals to form configurals—even when unnecessary—as a solution for their learning (see chapter 11).

The interpretation of the conditional discrimination data that we have offered in the context of our procedural-declarative framework receives support from findings that animals with hippocampal system damage unnecessarily "fuse" multiple cues into compound stimuli. Winocur et al. (1987) and Schmajuk and Isaacson (1984) found increased conditioning to background (i.e., contextual) cues in addition to the explicitly conditioned stimuli in a classical conditioning situation. Contextual cues can become "fused" with the differentially rewarded cues in discrimination learning: Winocur and colleagues (Winocur & Gilbert, 1984; Winocur & Mills, 1970; Winocur & Olds, 1978) found that rats with hippocampal system lesions who were trained on a visual discrimination in one apparatus performed abnormally poorly when transferred to a discrimination of the same visual cues in another apparatus, and showed better than normal performance on a reversal of the discrimination in the new apparatus. The discriminative cues themselves can become fused in conditional discriminations, just as in our own work on sensory discriminations (Eichenbaum et al., 1989). Thus, Saunders and Weiskrantz (1989) found that monkeys with hippocampal system damage could learn as rapidly as intact monkeys to discriminate object pairs containing common elements, but unlike intact animals they could *not* match the elements when the pairs were separated in a subsequent probe test.

As an addendum to our suggestion that the formation of compounds or configurals provides a solution to conditional learning for amnesic animals, let us suggest that when conditional stimuli *precede* the cues that are ambiguously associated with reward, the conditional cues may not be part of a representation of relations between specific cues, but instead act as general "facilitators" of any partially reinforced stimuli—the mechanisms of such generalized facilitation also seem to be supported outside of the hippocampal system (Jarrard & Davidson, 1991), and thus offer another alternative nonhippocampal representational strategy for some types of conditional learning. Finally, at least some of the discrepancies in this literature are likely related to locus of lesion (Jarrard & Davidson, 1991), with various investigators differing significantly in the size and approach of their lesions.

On our view, in the absence of a hippocampal-mediated representation system for storing relationships among multiple stimuli, animals must adopt the strategy of fusing the stimuli into compound cues. To the extent that they are successful in constructing perceptually unique compound cues, the conditional discrimination task reduces to a sensory discrimination task. As was shown earlier in the discussion of our olfactory discrimination learning work, and will be elaborated in the next section, sensory discrimination performance can proceed normally despite hippocampal-system damage.

SENSORY DISCRIMINATION

For each of the previous paradigms discussed in this chapter, animals with hippocampal-system damage were typically impaired compared to intact animals, although their ability to learn and retain the task procedures remained intact. On this paradigm, however, sparing of performance despite hippocampal system damage is the typical result. Yet, just as there are exceptions to the "typical" result with the previous paradigms, with some variants producing intact rather than the usual impaired performance after hippocampal system damage, there are variants of this paradigm that behave "atypically" and thus produce impaired rather than the usual intact performance. Both outcomes will have to be accommodated in a successful account of the role of the hippocampal system in memory.

Our own sensory discrimination work with odors has clearly documented that either sparing or impairment can result from hippocampal system damage, depending on certain procedural variables of test administration. Review of the burgeoning literature on the effects of hippocampal system damage on acquisition of a large variety of sensory discriminations indicates that the results are similarly "mixed." Many experiments have found intact simple-discrimination learning in rats (e.g., Eichenbaum et al., 1986, 1988) and monkeys (e.g., Malamut, Saunders, & Mishkin, 1984; Zola-Morgan & Squire, 1985). Yet there are numerous variants of sensory discrimination learning in which impairment has been found in rats (e.g., Eichenbaum et al., 1988; Staubli et al. 1984; Wible & Olton, 1988) and in monkeys (Zola-Morgan & Squire, 1985; Mahut & Moss, 1984; for a listing of earlier studies on rats and monkeys see table A17 of O'Keefe and Nadel, 1978). Some reports even observed facilitation of discrimination learning (Eichenbaum et al., 1988; Otto et al., 1991).

Sensory discriminations would be expected to be acquired without the declarative system. As observed in our earlier discussion of olfactory discrimination learning, successful performance can be achieved by coming to appreciate that one of the objects was somehow "good" or by developing a "bias" toward it and therefore choosing it. The acquired knowledge is assessed only in trials that continue to repeat exactly the same stimuli with exactly the same reward assignments, and there is no requirement either for making comparative judgments about the pair of objects or for appreciating the relationships of the current objects to any other presented previously. Thus, there is no need for the flexibility and relationality provided by declarative representations, and performance can be supported by nonhippocampal systems. Strategies based on nonhippocampal systems can be encouraged in subjects by explicitly separating presentations of the individual stimuli, as we did in the successive-cue variant of our olfactory discrimination learning task (see right panel of figure 3.1).

In simultaneous-cue variants of discrimination learning (see left panel of figure 3.1), the same strategy of acquiring positive or negative approach tendencies to each cue separately might be used. Alternatively, animals could learn the appropriate response to the compound stimulus composed of the spatial arrangement of the discriminative cues, as was observed in our own work with simultaneous odor discrimination learning (Eichenbaum et al., 1989; see above) and was also considered in discussing conditional discrimination tasks. As long as performance could be guided without mediation by declarative representations, no deficit will be observed following hippocampal-system damage.

What about those variants of discrimination learning for which deficits are observed? One view taken by some was that impairment is observed on successive but not simultaneous discrimination. This suggestion was based on Kimble's observations that hippocampectomy resulted in impairment on a successive brightness discrimination (Kimble, 1963) but not simultaneous brightness discrimination (Kimble & Kimble, 1970) in rats. Attributing the observed pattern of spared and impaired performance solely to the simultaneous-successive variable is in direct contrast to our own observations on odor discrimination (Eichenbaum et al., 1988), suggesting some other explanation must be sought.

Two further points are relevant in the Kimble data. First, the similarities in Kimble's and our successive discrimination paradigms are deceptively superficial. Kimble's successive discrimination required rats to chose one arm in a Y-maze when the maze was white and the other arm when the maze was black. While this paradigm indeed involved a successive presentation of the two mazes, the task seems more reasonably characterized as a conditional color-spatial discrimination (see above for a discussion of conditional discrimination) and not the learning of individual associations for sequentially presented cues in the way that our successive odor discrimination could be characterized. Second, in the simultaneous brightness discrimination, even though the rate of learning by hippocampal rats did not differ from that of intact rats, their sampling strategies were abnormal, reminiscent of our findings of occasionally successful simultaneous odor discrimination in rats with fornix lesions. Both of these observations underline the need to avoid using formal characterizations of tasks, such as "simultaneous" and "successive," as opposed to representational or processing characterizations, and to carefully examine both the representational demands made by tasks and the learning strategies actually used by animals attempting to solve the task.

Although no single parameter ties together all variants of discrimination learning that are impaired by hippocampal system damage, two factors are prominent. One consistent factor, noted by Gray (1982), is that impairment frequently results when the training procedures include a form of pre-training capable of influencing animals to adopt a representation counter to that most optimal for successful performance on the subsequent discrimination. The most explicit variant of this is reversal learning, in which the animal is "pre-trained" on a discrimination with one set of reinforcement assignments and then "trained" with the same cues now having opposite reward assignments. Impairment nearly always results under these circumstances, with the exception of our results in rats (Eichenbaum et al., 1986) and Zola and Mahut's (1973) results in monkeys, in which facilitation occurs. (The way in which these exceptions actually provide strong evidence in favor of the procedural-declarative theory was discussed earlier). These findings serve to highlight the inflexibility of animals with hippocampal system damage in using previously acquired information in ways other than simple repetition of the original learning events—our very definition of a declarative memory impairment.

The other consistent factor is that impairment commonly results on task variants requiring that a number of discriminations be learned concurrently (e.g., Moss et al., 1981; Zola-Morgan & Squire, 1985). The concurrent discrimination requirement may serve to encourage the construction of a representation of the entire set of stimuli, that is, a declarative representation including the relationships among the various items. Our electrophysiological recording work with rats learning olfactory discriminations certainly suggests that hippocampal neurons come to be activated by certain relations among the discriminative stimuli, even when the storage of such relations is unnecessary for successive performance (see chapter 5). Animals with damage to the hippocampal-dependent declarative system would be unable to store such relational information, and they would show impaired performance relative to normal subjects to the extent that such information contributes to successful performance.

It is notable that the specific pattern of sparing and loss on many sensory discrimination learning tasks, just as for some object memory (DNMS and DMS) tasks (see the first part of this chapter), owes much to the selection of testing intervals that take advantage of differences between hippocampal-dependent and hippocampal-independent systems in the strength and persistence of memories for specific sensory cues. To the extent that this is the case, the data say as much about these characteristics of declarative memory as about the qualitative nature of declarative representation. Three properties seem critical here: First, both intact and amnesic animals can make use of hippocampal-independent immediate or short-term memory (working memory) to support performance across short delays. Hippocampal amnesia spares such performance across species. Second, the hippocampal-dependent memory system also develops a strong representation of sensory cues lasting for up to hours after only a single exposure. This is profoundly impaired in amnesic subjects. The hippocampal-independent system, preserved in amnesia, develops only a weak representation after a single exposure to stimuli, although its maintenance can outlast that for the hippocampal-dependent trace in these paradigms. Third, both forms of memory are enhanced in strength by repetitions given within their survival time, although the benefit shown by the hippocampal-independent procedural system is only gradually incremental in most traditional discrimination tasks. These increments are reflected both in terms of performance level and persistence.

These memory strength and persistence characteristics permit us to understand the specific pattern of sparing and impairment observed on discrimination tasks in animals with hippocampal damage: Normal performance would be expected in many sensory discrimination tasks with discrimination intertrial intervals or recognition delays short enough to be supported by immediate or short-term memory, which is intact in amnesic patients; impairment in performance at longer delays (30 to 60 seconds or more) for which the maintenance of hippocampal-dependent memory would confer an advantage to normal subjects over amnesic patients; and no impairment in performance when the stimuli are repeated at delays longer than the period effectively bridged by hippocampally mediated representation. Let us consider the empirical findings. In various tests of delayed (non)matching, amnesic animals and intact animals perform comparably in "remembering" novel objects across delays of several seconds; but, lacking a hippocampally mediated memory that persists for many minutes or hours, amnesics show impaired performance for the longer-delay conditions (Aggleton et al., 1989; Gaffan, 1974; Mishkin, 1978; Otto & Eichenbaum, 1991). Likewise, on concurrent object-discrimination learning with massed practice, amnesic animals, with no hippocampal-mediated capacity for maintenance of object memory between repeated exposures to cues spaced at a few minutes (well within the persistence characteristics of that system), show impaired acquisition compared to normal animals (Moss et al., 1981; Wible & Olton, 1988; Zola-Morgan & Squire, 1985). Furthermore, even a small amount of

massed practice on single object discriminations results in strength-
ening of hippocampal-dependent memory, extending its duration to
the periods required for success in delayed testing; amnesic animals,
with only a gradually incrementing hippocampal-independent
memory, are impaired (Zola-Morgan and Squire, 1985). Finally, in
one experiment that involved very long delays (24 hours) between
repetitions of cues in spaced concurrent object-discrimination learning in monkeys, (i.e., when practice was spaced too far apart for the
advantage usually conferred by the hippocampal system in memory
maintenance to be applicable), amnesic monkeys performed as well
as normal animals (Malamut et al., 1984).

The magnitude of differences in the strength and persistence of
hippocampal-dependent versus hippocampal-independent memory
is likely to vary significantly across learning materials and across
species. Thus, within monkeys, these differences may be much
smaller in discrimination learning involving two-dimensional patterns than in discrimination learning involving three-dimensional
objects; for object discrimination learning, these differences may be
much larger for humans than for monkeys (see Squire et al., 1988).
In rats, the persistence of memories for single exposures to colors,
local environmental cues, odors, and spatial positions differs for the
hippocampal-dependent and hippocampal-independent systems
(Aggleton et al., 1989; Kesner, 1991; Raffaelle & Olton, 1988; Winocur, 1990). In addition, the degree of preoperative training may be
an important factor even in tests of recent memory (e.g., Bachevalier
et al., 1985; Barnes, 1988).

OTHER PARADIGMS

A wide variety of additional learning and memory paradigms, as
well as assessments of nonlearned behaviors, have been examined
in animals with hippocampal system damage (for some listings see
O'Keefe & Nadel, 1978; Gray, 1982). Some of these have been
considered briefly above in the course of discussing the more widely
explored paradigms. For example, the effects of hippocampal-system
damage on reversal learning was considered in the context of sensory discrimination, and exploratory behavior strategies in animals
with hippocampal-system damage was considered in the context of
place learning and of sensory discrimination. Here we will make

brief mention of two other sets of findings that, while representing only a small fraction of the overall literature on the effects of hippocampal system damage, must nonetheless be accounted for by any theory of memory, amnesia, and the hippocampal system. We shall show how our theory does so. Unlike our strategy above, these paradigms are not grouped according to formal task descriptions but according to what we believe are the common factors that make these dependent on or independent of the integrity of hippocampal system function.

Phenomena Related to Differences in Strength and Persistence Characteristics

Animals with hippocampal system damage are impaired on two tasks not described above that might seen to be outside the province of explanation by our (or other prominent) accounts of hippocampal function—classical eyelid conditioning in the "trace" but not "delay" format, and timing tasks. We propose that each of these phenomena is based on the different operating characteristics (strength and persistence) of the declarative and procedural systems.

Hippocampal lesions have differential effects on different versions of classical eyelid conditioning in rabbits. Thus, following hippocampal system damage no impairment is observed in "delay" conditioning where the auditory conditioned stimulus (CS) and the airpuff unconditioned stimulus (UCS) are contiguous (e.g., Schmaltz & Theios, 1972). This finding is entirely consistent with our claim that acquisition of representations of the significance of (or tuning for and biasing toward) individual stimuli is within the province of the hippocampal-independent, procedural memory system. As with some other sensory discrimination paradigms, reversal learning of discriminative conditioning in the eyelid conditioning paradigm is impaired by hippocampal system damage (Berger & Orr, 1983). However, in apparent contradiction to this account, hippocampal system damage produces a striking impairment in "trace" conditioning, which involves the same individual association of CS and UCS as in delay conditioning, but in which the CS and UCS are separated by a fraction of a second (Moyer et al., 1990). The temporal delay in trace conditioning is well within the scope of short-term (or working) memory processes ordinarily supported by hippocampal-independent systems, so it seems inappropriate to attribute these findings to rapid decay of the CS-UCS association. Nevertheless, these results do indicate that the persistence of some hippocampal-dependent representation serves to make trace conditioning possible. It would appear that the hippocampal-independent systems, such as cerebellar-brainstem circuits, that ordinarily support classical conditioning require CS-UCS contiguity; that is, they cannot support conditioning even for brief trace periods interposed between the CS and UCS. This contiguity requirement can, however, be circumvented in the trace paradigm when a *persisting declarative representation of the CS* is contiguous with the UCS; the declarative representation can be employed to make the classical association with the UCS in the extrahippocampal system. After hippocampal system damage, the declarative representation is eliminated, no other form of contiguity with the CS is preserved, and impairment in trace conditioning is observed. The same explanation accounts for deficits observed after hippocampal system damage in instrumental conditioning situations where a delay is interposed between predictive stimuli (Rawlins, Feldon, & Butt, 1985).

Animals with hippocampal system damage perform poorly at tasks that require timing, including duration discrimination tasks (Meck, Church & Olton, 1984; Olton Meck, & Church, 1987) and an operant timing paradigm known as differential reinforcement for low rates of response (DRL) (e.g., Sinden et al., 1986; Rawlins et al., 1983). In duration discrimination tasks, rats are given a long-lasting signal indicating they may begin to press a bar. On some trials a reward is given for the first bar press after a fixed duration has elapsed; on other test trials no reward is given. Normal rats' response rate increases to the time associated with reward, then decreases in the no-reward tests. Rats with hippocampal system damage underestimate the time of reinforcement and cannot sustain timing when a brief gap is imposed in the otherwise continuous signal. In DRL, rats are rewarded with food for operant bar pressing with the contingency that reinforcement is provided only for bar press responses separated by a specific minimum period. Rats with hippocampal system damage can perform a DRL when the minimum period is 5 seconds but their accuracy declines with longer timing requirements; a severe impairment is typically observed for 20-second delays.

Such timing tasks seem not to require relational representation and thus seem to lie outside the range of our account. However, as was the case with some variants of classical conditioning and sensory discrimination, we believe the critical factor relates to differences in the strength and persistence characteristics of the procedural and declarative memory systems. The neural basis of the capacity for timing in the above described tasks is unclear, but might depend directly on the animal's ability to perceive the strength of the memory trace for the events surrounding the last rewarded response. If so, the abnormally rapid decay of such traces in animals with hippocampal system damage would seem to put them at a severe disadvantage in timing when the requirements exceed the capacity of their intact hippocampal-independent short-term memory. In line with this interpretation (and, admittedly, others), it has been shown that the DRL performance of rats with hippocampal system damage is selectively improved when an external cue is added midway through the delay (Rawlins et al., 1983). Also, the observation that rats with hippocampal system damage specifically underestimate the passage of time is consistent with the notion that the strength of their hippocampal-independent memory trace is decaying more rapidly than that of normal subjects.

Phenomena Related to Abnormally Rapid or Strong Procedural Conditioning in the Absence of a Declarative Representation

Above we cited a number of cases where learning in animals with hippocampal system damage is observed to occur more rapidly than in intact subjects (i.e., to cause facilitated learning), for example, in some cases of successive odor discrimination and reversal (Eichenbaum et al., 1986; 1988; Otto et al., 1991) and object reversal in monkeys Zola & Mahut, 1973). There are similar observations for various forms of learning ranging from simple classical conditioning (e.g., Port et al., 1985) to light-cued radial maze learning (Packard et al., 1989), and many investigators have casually observed that animals with hippocampal system damage "shape" more quickly than intact animals when preparing them for various formal learning tasks. There are a variety of related observations on animals with hippocampal system damage: They adopt response strategies abnormally rapidly and rigidly adhere to initially acquired responses and sampling strategies (e.g., Blue, 1983; Devenport et al., 1988; Hirsh, 1970; Osborne and Black, 1978; Suess & Berlyne, 1978), and they fail to reverse and resist extinction abnormally long after partial reinforcement (Feldon et al., 1985).

Other situations in which animals with hippocampal system damage are observed to condition abnormally well, or condition to stimuli in situations where intact animals would not, include examples of overconditioning to context (see above) and demonstrations of deficient latent inhibition, overshadowing, and blocking in classical conditioning paradigms (cf. Solomon et al., 1986). In the latent inhibition paradigm, when animals are repeatedly preexposed to a stimulus without reinforcement before training with the same stimulus as the conditioned stimulus, acquisition is retarded in normal but not hippocampally damaged animals (Solomon & Moore, 1975). Blocking and overshadowing are related paradigms in which some stimuli normally come to predominate over others due to prior exposure. In blocking, animals are trained in two stages, initially with a single stimulus (CS1) and later with a compound stimulus including the original CS1 plus another stimulus (CS2). In later testing with individual stimuli, normal animals, but not those with hippocampal system damage, respond relatively weakly to CS2, which has no added predictive value (Rickert et al., 1978; Solomon, 1977). In the overshadowing procedure, animals are trained on a discrimination of compound cues containing a common element. In later testing with individual stimulus elements in this paradigm normal animals, but not animals with hippocampal damage, respond poorly to the common element (Rickert et al., 1979; Wagner, 1968). Of course, as has been the case with the paradigms discussed above, not all of the data come out in the same way. In some training conditions, normal overshadowing and blocking are observed (Garrud et al., 1984); however, the procedures involved in these paradigms differ along many dimensions, precluding an analysis of those conditions under which the phenomena are or are not observed. Nonetheless, we can note that each of these paradigms has at least some conditions under which animals with hippocampal system damage are unable to perceive as irrelevant poorly predictive contextual or redundant stimuli.

The "irrelevance" of contextual or redundant stimuli, as raised just above, is in each case *relative* to that of the designated or preceding CS. For each phenomenon, our interpretation is that a reduced level of responding to such cues comes about as a consequence of hippocampal-mediated comparisons between the relative predictability or coincidence of different cues and reinforcement, or the relative added predictability of sequentially presented cues. Without these mechanisms for comparison, hippocampal-*independent* processing for each cue would be expected to go on individually, resulting in increased conditioning to these cues, as observed.

8 Generalizing to Other Paradigms: Human Studies

The starting point of our treatment of memory, amnesia, and the hippocampal system was the set of findings demonstrating preserved skill learning and repetition priming effects in amnesic patients who were profoundly impaired on tests of explicit remembering such as recall and recognition memory. Some of the empirical findings that illustrate preserved learning and memory in amnesia were presented in chapter 2. In this chapter, we present additional findings on spared and impaired memory performances and demonstrate how our procedural-declarative theory accounts for these phenomena, extending and elaborating the discussion we offered in chapter 6 concerning Graf et al.'s (1984) report of intact repetition priming despite impaired cued recall. In covering the human literature, we cannot be fully inclusive. What we shall do here is consider examples of all those empirical phenomena that bear most critically on the theoretical account of memory, amnesia, and the hippocampal system that we have proposed and show how the procedural-declarative distinction permits us to understand the resulting pattern of impaired versus spared memory abilities in amnesia.

Normal learning by amnesic patients occurs on those tasks that can be mediated by the inflexible, dedicated memory representations we attribute to procedural memory, which are still available after hippocampal system damage. That is, spared learning is seen when successful performance can be mediated by the tuning or biasing of processors and the incremental adaptation of behavioral performance in accordance with the regularities across learning events. These conditions are met in skill learning and repetition priming tasks, in which there is repetition of the original processing circumstances, and when experience-based modifications of these processors (mediated by procedural memory) can influence subsequent performance. By contrast, those tasks or components of tasks that depend on or benefit greatly from the ability to manipulate and flexibly express memory in novel situations, or from the ability to learn new relationships, cannot be handled successfully by amnesic patients. Impairment occurs because of the loss of the flexible, relational representations of hippocampal-mediated declarative memory.

As with the data we considered earlier, however, particularly the animal model data in chapter 7, there are reports of sparing and reports of impairment following hippocampal system damage on nearly every paradigm, despite broadly consistent patterns of sparing and loss across the various categories of tasks. Consistent with the view we expressed earlier, our theory—any theory—that seeks to explain the pattern of sparing and impairment in amnesia must account for both the broad patterns and also the specific deviations of the data. Accordingly, we shall endeavor to show how the procedural-declarative theory deals with both normal and less-than-normal performances of amnesic patients in these categories of tasks. To do so for skill learning and for repetition priming, we shall first outline the data indicating spared performance, then the data suggesting some impairment, and then attempt to reconcile the differences. At the end of the chapter we go on to consider the tasks on which impairment is found universally in patients with hippocampal system damage, and discuss these findings too in the context of the procedural-declarative theory.

SKILL LEARNING

In skill-learning tasks, subjects are challenged on multiple occasions to solve some type of problem or perform some repetitive task, and the speed and efficacy of their solution performance is evaluated across trials. Amnesic subjects have been challenged to learn perceptual-motor, perceptual, and cognitive skills, and their performance has been evaluated with respect to that of control subjects.

Perceptual-Motor Skills

The performance of amnesic patients has been evaluated in several tests of perceptual-motor skill learning. In *mirror tracing,* subjects trace the outline of a five-pointed star that can be glimpsed only in a mirror. Thus, the only visual information about the position of the hand and pen with respect to the star is through mirror reflection (see figure 2.4). Subjects are asked to accomplish this task several times on each of several successive days. H.M.'s dramatic improvement across trials on this task, despite his profound amnesia, provided the first indication of preserved learning abilities in amnesia (Milner, 1962). In *rotary pursuit*, subjects maintain contact between a hand-held stylus and a small disk mounted on a revolving platter. As with mirror tracing, subjects are challenged with this task multiple times per session in each of several sessions. Following Corkin's (1968) report that H.M. showed improved performance across trials on this task (as well as on a test of *bimanual tracking*) several investigators (Brooks & Baddeley, 1976; Cermak et al., 1973; Cohen, 1981) showed that amnesic patients of various etiologies could acquire and express the perceptual-motor skills necessary for rotary pursuit as well as could control subjects—that is, their learning was fully preserved, as illustrated by the time-on-target scores shown in figure 8.1.

In Nissen and Bullemer's (1987) *serial reaction time* task, subjects see a light appear on each trial at one of four possible locations on a computer monitor, and press as quickly as they can that one of the four response keys that corresponds to the location of the light. The locations at which the light appears form a repeating pattern across trials. That is, trials are organized into a 10-trial sequence that repeats 10 times in each block of 100 trials, with no indication given of the end of one repetition of the sequence and the beginning of the next one. Subjects participate in four such blocks, followed by a fifth block in which the locations are arranged randomly. Amnesic patients with Korsakoff's disease could perform equivalently to (at least some) control subjects on this task, showing the same increased speed of responding across the four experimental blocks, followed by the same sharp falling off of this trend in the control block (figure 8.2).

Data from monkeys with hippocampal system damage also suggest the ability to learn skills despite amnesia. Because such data come from paradigms that are more akin to those used in human studies than in the animal models literature, they are included here rather than in the preceding chapter. Challenged on the *barrier* and

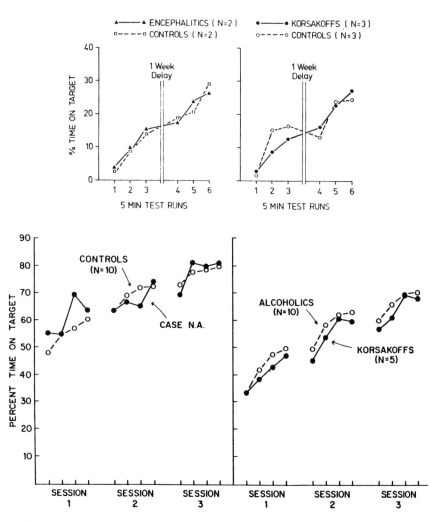

Figure 8.1
Normal perceptual-motor learning by amnesic patients of various etiologies on the
rotary pursuit task, depicted as an increase across trials and sessions in the percentage
of time per trial spent on target. (From Brooks & Baddeley, 1976 [*top*] and Cohen, 1981
[*bottom*]).

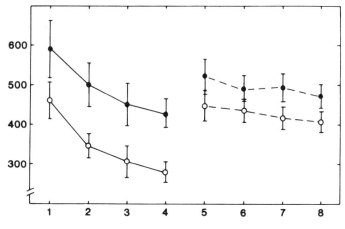

Figure 8.2
Learning in the serial reaction time task by patients with Korsakoff amnesia
(filled circles) compared to normal controls (open circles), depicted as a
decrease in latencies for correct responses to items in the repeating sequence (solid lines, *left*) as compared to latencies for correct responses to
items in the random (untrained) sequence (dashed lines, *right*). (From Nissen & Bullemer, 1987.)

lifesaver motor skill tasks designed by Zola-Morgan and Squire
(Zola-Morgan & Squire, 1984; Squire & Zola-Morgan, 1985), such
monkeys have shown fully preserved learning. In the barrier task,
monkeys have to reach a hand through a barrier of vertically oriented Tinkertoy sticks arranged in three rows, then pick up a breadstick, and then navigate their way back through the Tinkertoy
barrier with the breadstick without it breaking or dropping. Monkeys with hippocampal system damage showed a normal increase
across sessions in the number of trials in which they successfully
navigated the breadstick through the barrier. In the lifesaver task,
monkeys have to maneuver a Lifesaver candy along a bent metal
rod and slide it off the rod. Monkeys with hippocampal system
damage showed a normal decrease across sessions in the time taken
to get the Lifesaver candy off the rod.

Perceptual Skills

Amnesic patients have also been found to show normal learning of
skills beyond the motor domain, as first documented by Cohen and

Squire (1980) for the reading of mirror-reversed text (illustrated in figure 2.5; see also Martone et al., 1984; Moscovitch et al., 1986). In the Cohen and Squire (1980) *mirror reading* task, subjects see words presented as unrelated word triplets in mirror-reversed form, with the task of reading each word aloud as quickly as possible. Subjects see several blocks of triplets in each of several sessions; reduction across blocks in the average time required to read each triplet serves as the measure of learning. Normal learning and 13-week retention were seen in several different etiologies of amnesia: patients with Korsakoff's disease, the diencephalic case N.A., and patients who had just completed a course of bilateral electrocon-vulsive therapy (ECT) treatments.

Cognitive Skills

Amnesic patients have also been challenged with the learning of cognitive skills, including solving the Tower of Hanoi puzzle, and learning simple arithmetic algorithms including the Fibonacci rule and a procedure for mentally squaring two-digit numbers. The *Tower of Hanoi puzzle* is a problem in which subjects are confronted with a set of five blocks arranged in size order on one (the leftmost) of three pegs, and must restack them into a different (the rightmost) peg, while only moving one block at a time and never placing a larger block on top of smaller ones (figure 8.3). This task is difficult, and subjects are asked to attempt it on multiple occasions, with the goal of solving the puzzle in the shortest number of "moves." Optimal solution requires 31 moves.

Work with normal subjects has shown that there are a number of different solution strategies for solving the puzzle that differ in

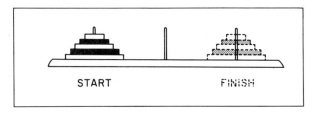

Figure 8.3
Schematic of the Tower of Hanoi puzzle.

their memory and processing demands, and subjects differ in the strategies they choose and in the way the choice of strategies changes with practice (Karat, 1982; Simon, 1975). The number of moves required for solution is too large to permit a strategy based exclusively on rote remembering. In general, over successive trials subjects' performance gradually approaches the optimal solution, requiring fewer moves and involving fewer "detours" in the optimal "solution path" (Cohen et al., 1985). We have found that amnesic patients, including H.M., are capable of learning to produce the optimal solution normally (Cohen, 1981; Cohen et al., 1985; figure 8.4). A subsequent study by Saint-Cyr et al. (1988) also found robust learning despite amnesia in patients with Korsakoff's disease.

Learning in two tasks involving simple arithmetic algorithms, including the Fibonacci rule (Kinsbourne & Wood, 1975) and one for mentally squaring two-digit numbers (Charness et al., 1988; Milberg et al., 1988) has also been reported for amnesic patients. Finally, learning in two computer-based skill tasks, the "sugar production" and "computer person" tasks of Berry and Broadbent (1984), has been reported in amnesic patients (Squire & Frambach, 1990) as well.

There is evidence of what might plausibly be considered cognitive and/or perceptual skill learning in animals, explored in the context of learning set—the phenomenon of progressively faster learning of new discrimination problems. That is, just as amnesic patients get faster at reading new examples of mirror reversed text (see above), rats (Eichenbaum et al., 1986) and monkeys (Murray & Mishkin, 1986) have demonstrated the ability to get faster at solving new olfactory or visual discrimination problems, respectively, after hippocampal system damage. It is not entirely clear what is being learned by the animals as they gain more "skill" across trials in these tasks, but it is likely to include learning to tune in to the perceptual characteristics of the discriminanda and to become increasingly sensitive to, i.e., biased toward, those stimulus dimensions most relevant for making the discriminations (Zola-Morgan and Squire, 1984). As with the motor skill learning phenomena in monkeys considered above, these findings seem better discussed along with comparable human data than with the bulk of the findings with animals using very different paradigms.

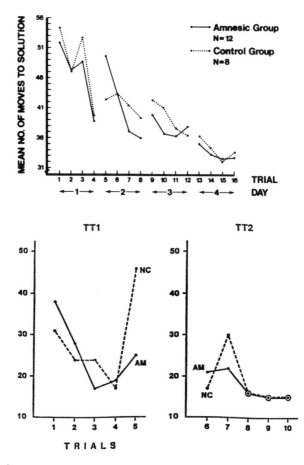

Figure 8.4
Performance of amnesic patients on the Tower of Hanoi puzzle (*top*) and the somewhat simplified Tower of Toronto puzzle (*bottom*). Subjects (12 amnesic patients and 8 control subjects) solved the Tower of Hanoi puzzle four times on each of four consecutive days. Subjects (2 amnesic patients and 24 control subjects) solved the Tower of Toronto puzzle five times in each of two sessions. Learning is expressed as a decrease in the number of moves per trial required for solution. The amnesic patients showed normal learning.

Dissociations

The preserved acquisition of these skills by amnesic patients, as we noted in chapter 2, occurs despite a profound impairment (1) in recalling and recognizing the very materials on which the patients are demonstrating their increasingly skilled performance, (2) in recollecting the training experiences themselves, and (3) in accessing the knowledge underlying their increasing expertise in these very tasks. The fact that normal acquisition and expression of skilled performance on a given task is accompanied by otherwise impaired memory for other measures on the same task is a point that we have emphasized strongly in previous writings (Cohen, 1981, 1984) and shall do so again here. The sparing as well as the impairment must be explained.

For example, as we have noted in our previous descriptions of H.M.'s learning of the optimal solution to the Tower of Hanoi puzzle (Cohen & Corkin, 1981; Cohen et al., 1985), successful performance occurred despite profound memory impairment for the task and for his training on it: He could not recollect any prior experiences with the task, had no sense of familiarity with the puzzle, had no sense of getting better on the task across trials, and had no insight into the nature of his increasingly skilled performance. Indeed, this last point is illustrated by the following excerpt from transcripts of the sessions, in which he claimed that he saw no way for it to be solved despite having himself already solved it four consecutive times on that day.

H.M.: And, naturally, I think of just the opposite of . . . It would be just opposite.

N.C.: Where? What do you mean that they would be opposite?

H.M.: Because your small one would have to be over here [on the middle peg]. If it was here, it would have to be over here—down at the bottom.

N.C.: Do you think you had them all piled up with the smallest one on the bottom?

H.M.: . . . You would have to.

N.C.: But, it [the diagram] says that you can never put a larger block on top of a smaller one. Right? So you couldn't have had the smallest one on the bottom and the others on top.

H.M.: (silence)

N.C.: . . . Do you have a feel for what it is that you did that enables you to get them [all five blocks] there [on the goal peg]?

H.M.:   If you can only move one block at a time . . . No, I couldn't figure it out.

N.C.:   But, you did! See, you just—

H.M.:   (interrupts) I did?

N.C.:   And you did it very well, too.

H.M.:   Funny, I was trying to figure it out, and I couldn't.

Basically, at this point in his training (the end of the first of his four sessions), H.M.'s verbal reports were in stark contrast to his actual performance: He suggested that the only way to solve the puzzle was to make moves that were not allowed by the rules of the game (i.e., placing the four smaller discs upside down on the middle peg in order to get the largest disc over to the rightmost goal peg), despite the fact that he had already solved the puzzle multiple times within the rules.

The dissociation here between skilled performance and poor insight into the knowledge mediating performance is strongly paralleled by the one demonstrated by Terry Winograd's AI blocks-world system (SHRDLU) discussed in chapter 3. This parallel was one of the factors originally motivating our thinking about amnesia in terms of the procedural-declarative distinction (Cohen, 1981; Cohen & Squire, 1980). A further parallel, this time involving the behavior of intact control subjects, will become clear below.

This pattern of sparing and loss is the mirror-image of the pattern shown on the DNMS, the spatial learning, and the conditional, configural, and contextual discrimination tasks by animals with hippocampal system damage, in which impaired performances occurred in the context of preserved learning of the test procedures on the same tasks. This relationship between impaired and spared aspects of memory must also be explained.

Less-than-Normal Performance

Before turning to the ability of the procedural-declarative theory to account for the dissociations, however, there have been reports of less-than-normal learning of skills by amnesic patients on some of the above paradigms. In contrast to the findings of normal learning of the Tower of Hanoi puzzle by amnesic patients (Cohen et al., 1985; Saint-Cyr et al., 1988), there are reports by Butters et al. (1985) and Gabrieli et al. (1988) that the learning on this task is not fully preserved. Likewise, Charness and Milberg's (Charness et al., 1988; Milberg et al., 1988) work on learning of an algorithm for squaring two-digit numbers in amnesia reveals normal performance only for a component of the task, and not for all amnesic patients tested. Moreover, in conflict with the results of Kinsbourne and Wood (1975) and of Squire and Frambach (1990), neither the Fibonacci rule nor the computer-based "sugar production" task of Berry and Broadbent (1984) could be learned normally by H.M. (Gabrieli and Corkin, in preparation). These findings, too, must be accommodated by a complete account of preserved skill learning in amnesia. The account provided by the procedural-declarative framework is the topic to which we turn now.

Explaining the Phenomena: Preserved Skill Learning

Preservation of skill learning in amnesia can occur, on our view, because skill learning can be fully supported by procedural memory, through its mechanisms for tuning and modification of the various processing modules that support information processing in the brain. Successful acquisition of skills does *not* require the representational flexibility and relationality usually provided by the hippocampal-dependent declarative system; thus, failure of the declarative system, as occurs in amnesia, does *not* interfere with the ability to learn skills. To explain, a characteristic of skill-learning tasks in general, and certainly of those we have been considering here, is that performance is assessed in repetitions of the original learning situation; the same problem is presented on multiple occasions, and learning is indexed by increasing success across those occasions. For example, the performances include an increase in speed across trials in the mirror tracing, mirror reading, and sequential reaction time tasks, and a decrease in errors across trials in these tasks and on the Tower of Hanoi puzzle or the numerical rule problems. There is no need for the information acquired during training to be carried over to other domains or to novel situations outside of the original training context, and hence no need of the representational flexibility and promiscuity mediated by declarative memory.

The learning that occurs through the procedural system is, we have argued, dedicated to the particular processes or operations that were engaged by the particular task—such as visual pattern analysis, word recognition, and text comprehension processes engaged during mirror reading; or cognitive problem solving and sequential planning procedures engaged during the Tower of Hanoi task. When these processes or operations are once again engaged, the procedural tuning caused by training can be expressed. From the perspective of the processors engaged in performance, each trial in training is a repetition of the original learning event. This is why there is no need to carry over the training to novel contexts and why the representational flexibility and promiscuity mediated by declarative memory is not required here.

Let us consider the example of mirror reading in somewhat more detail at this juncture. The various processing systems engaged during mirror reading would be tuned by the action of procedural memory, shaping these processors in accordance with the particular regularities of this text. These processors, have been organized by past experience, continue to be shaped and molded by new experiences, making and keeping them maximally tuned to the inputs they actually receive most frequently and recently.

Each time these processors are re-engaged in reading, they reveal the way in which they have been shaped and tuned by experience via procedural memory. The well-known effects of word frequency on reading speed provides evidence for this view: Words with higher frequency of occurrence in the language are read more quickly than are words with lower frequency of occurrence in the language. For mirror reading, there must be learning of the mapping of the mirror reversed letter forms onto the letters of our alphabet. One way to think of this is in terms of McClelland and Rumelhart's (McClelland & Rumelhart, 1981; Rumelhart & McClelland, 1982) interactive activation model of reading and its successors, connectionist models in which the knowledge supporting reading is represented in the connection weights that capture the learned associations among letter features (lines, curves, etc.), letters, and words. The connection weights are modifiable by experience, responding to learning rules that adjust the weights incrementally to reflect the regularities in the input. In models of this sort, learning of mirror reading could be understood as tuning and modifying the network(s) that implement(s) word recognition, in order to capture the regularities between the mirror-reversed letter features and the usual letter forms associated with English words. This learning would be contained wholly within the word recognition network(s), reflecting a procedural-memory supported tuning of the processor itself.

Investigations of skill learning in normal subjects further suggest the inflexibility of the representations mediating this form of learning, supporting the procedural memory interpretation we have offered. For example, Kolers's (1979) work with college students has shown that learning to read mirror-reversed, geometrically inverted, or otherwise transformed text is specific to the particular transformation of the text, showing limited transfer among different ones. A further dimension of this specificity in normal subjects has been demonstrated by Masson (1986): When trained to read mirror-reversed text comprising word triplets presented with mixed upper- and lower-case letters, subjects showed more performance facilitation for subsequent repetitions of the triplets when they were presented with the same alternating pattern of upper- and lower-case letters as in training than if they were presented with a different arrangement of the cases.

The procedural-memory explanation of learning mirror-reading skill that was offered above in terms of an interactive activation model seems to provide a straightforward account of this inflexibility, as well. Exposure to mirror-reversed letter-forms tunes the network, to capture the new regularities between mirror-reversed letter-features and the usual letter-forms associated with English words. On this particular procedural account, the mirror-reading skill that is being acquired can be specific to the particular letters actually trained, and yet still be general to all words containing those letters.

Another example comes from work with college students learning the Tower of Hanoi puzzle, in which the inflexibility, or context specificity, of the representations underlying this example of skill learning is demonstrated. The inflexibility is revealed in the difficulties of transferring the learning to formally identical "problem isomorphs" of the puzzle in which the surface similarity among variants is well disguised (Hayes & Simon, 1977; Simon & Hayes, 1976). It is important to be very clear here about the level of processing at which, or about the processor(s) in which, the cognitive skill learning for the Tower of Hanoi is presumed to occur, and the implications this has for transfer to other variants of the task. We presume that the effects are at the level of problem solving and the organization of behavioral plans or sequences, processes usually attributed to the executive functions of the frontal lobes. Thus, this learning is thought to be associated with a processor(s) that handles information that is considerably more abstract than the sensory features of the discs and pegs used for the puzzle, or than the actual motor commands issued to physically make the moves in solving the puzzle. We think that the tuning or other procedural modifications act to change the efficacy with which subjects search the problem space for this puzzle, that is, change the way in which they explore various move options in attempting to derive the next move. What this means is that changing the size or color of the disks and pegs would not be expected to have any impact on performance, nor would changing from a wooden version of the puzzle to a computer-based version. Such changes would be opaque to the processor in which the learning effects reside. The problem isomorphs to which learning does *not* transfer are those where it is not obvious how to apply the biases or tunings of search strategies or move options acquired during training.

Explaining the Phenomena: Impaired Recall, Recollection, and Introspection

Moving now to the impairment in amnesia, whenever the performance requirements are changed such that the information acquired during training must now be carried over to other domains or to novel situations outside of the original training context, then the *lack* of representational flexibility and promiscuity of procedural memory is manifested by the *deficits* shown by amnesic patients in recalling or recognizing the stimulus materials on which they trained while learning their new skills, in recollecting the training experiences that gave rise to their skill learning, and in introspecting about the knowledge underlying their newly acquired expertise. These three types of memory performance are impaired in amnesic patients because they require declarative representations and cannot be supported by procedural memory. Each of these types of memory performance will be considered in turn.

Recall and recognition of the materials presented during skill learning inevitably depend on processes that can inspect the data structures derived from (i.e., the outcomes of) the processes performed during the initial presentation of those materials, and then require the ability to express the accessed information flexibly. The relevant processes are not those originally engaged and modified during learning, but are instead processes that must compare the relative level of familiarity or strength of various items in memory (i.e., is this item more "familiar," or "stronger," or more "fluent" than its usual base rate would suggest—and hence likely to have been presented recently?), or else processes that are capable of determining which items are associated with which contexts (i.e., did this item occur in the test list?). The testing context differs from the original learning context, and the presentation of the materials for test involves a different format—indeed, recall is assessed in the absence of the test materials altogether. Similarly, verbal recollections of previous training experiences and verbal introspections about the knowledge underlying skilled performance requires that memory of the outcomes of the learning events be promiscuously accessible to the processes that mediate conscious introspection, and they must be expressed in a context completely outside of the original learning situation. Thus, rather than again engaging the processes used and modified by experience in attempting to read mirror-reversed text or attempting to solve the Tower of Hanoi puzzle, subjects are instead to talk about their experiences, evaluate their performance, and consider the nature of their expertise. Such performances clearly require the particular representational properties that characterize declarative memory.

The ability of procedural memory to mediate skill learning but not explicit remembering of the training experiences or their contents is seen in normal subjects as well, but in a different way. Unlike amnesic patients, normal subjects do have explicit remembering of their training experiences, can successfully recall or recognize the materials presented during original training, and can recollect the prior training sessions. But these examples of explicit remembering need not have any causal role to play in the acquisition and expression of skilled performance. For example, Kolers reported that skilled performance in reading geometrically inverted and otherwise transformed texts was not predicted by recognition memory for the contents of the texts (Kolers, 1979). Likewise, we found that solution performance on the Tower of Hanoi puzzle was not reflected by recall, recognition, and verbal recollection performances (Cohen et al., 1985; Cohen, Gabrieli, & Corkin, in preparation). As we had noted in Cohen et al. (1985), "skilled performance on the Tower of Hanoi puzzle depends no more upon the explicit remembering of specific puzzle configurations or moves than skilled performance in tennis depends upon the explicit remembering of specific arm movements or arm trajectories" (pp. 68–69).

Although procedural and declarative memory systems are seen as independent, with functionally distinct contributions to make to memory performance, they may both affect task performance, particularly for complex cognitive tasks. Thus, for example, Ross (1984, 1987) has shown that normal cognitive problem-solving performance is aided considerably when subjects are "reminded" of previous experiences with similar problems. In such cases, rather than deriving a solution to the problem at hand, subjects may instead use their declarative memory for explicit remembering of some previous related learning event, remember the strategy used for the previous event, and adopt it for the present problem. A good deal of attention has been generated recently in the potential for such instance-based approaches to skilled performance (e.g., Logan, 1988).

Another example comes from mirror reading. In the Cohen and Squire (1980) study, subjects were presented with word triplets (see figure 2.5) of which some repeated in each block of the experiment, while others appeared only once. Normal subjects, but not amnesic patients, were able to recognize the repetitions and were eventually able to recall whole (repeated) triplets. Although normal subjects and amnesic patients had equivalent reading speeds for the nonrepeated triplets and equivalent speed-up across trials, normal subjects showed an additional facilitation in reading the repeated word triplets—relative to nonrepeated triplets—that was significantly greater than that seen in amnesic patients. (This additional facilitation for repeated over nonrepeated items is an example of repetition priming, and thus apparently more appropriate for the immediately following section of this chapter. But the explanation of the failure of amnesic patients to show the full effect of the repetitions in the context of their normal skill learning speaks directly to the interaction of procedural and declarative memory, and thus is highly relevant here.) It seems reasonable to suppose explicit remembering of the triplets contributed to the performance of control subjects and explained their superiority over the amnesic patients for the repeated items. That is, subjects who have an intact declarative memory system are capable of learning the relationships among the words of the oft-repeating triplets. Hence, upon reading the word CAPRICIOUS, they are capable of gaining access to representations of the appropriate triplet and could *generate* the next two words—GRANDIOSE and BEDRAGGLE—rather than actually having to read all three words. Accordingly, they would surely be capable of responding faster to that triplet than would a subject who actually read through all three words (this point was discussed in Cohen, 1984; also see Masson, 1986; Moscovitch et al., 1986; Musen et al., 1990).

A third relevant example comes from the work with serial reaction time (Nissen & Bullemer, 1987; Nissen et al., 1989; Willingham et al., 1989), in which it has been made clear that control subjects, but not amnesic patients, can sometimes gain conscious awareness of the repeating sequence through declarative-based remembering. Under these circumstances, such subjects are removed by the investigators from further comparisons with the patients. Otherwise the patients would show impairment in performance *not* because they are incapable of showing incremental motor-sequence learning but because they are unable to take advantage of the opportunity for declarative memory to contribute to performance.

Explaining the Phenomena: The Interaction of Procedural and Declarative Memory Systems, and Apparent Discrepancies in the Data

The point is that in tasks where the two memory systems—if intact—can interact to support performance, amnesic patients with damage to the declarative memory system would be expected to show impairment (provided that control subjects use the two systems to good advantage). This state of affairs creates the possibility of substantial interpretive difficulties for researchers attempting to infer the componential organization of memory from patterns of impaired versus spared memory abilities in amnesia. The way in which the task is structured and, consequently, the extent to which the use of the different memory systems is encouraged or enabled will have great impact on the relative performance of control subjects versus amnesic patients. The empirical outcomes, then, of testing preserved learning in amnesia with a given paradigm can easily differ among different investigators—either impairment or sparing can result. This is a point we have emphasized repeatedly in this book, and is the reason for our stressing the need to conduct probe tests to determine what representational strategies and which memory systems were actually used by subjects to drive performance. Unless this is understood, there are likely to be disagreements, "failures to replicate," and controversies in the field based solely on differences among tasks in the extent to which the two memory systems may jointly support task performance.

A particularly compelling example of a controversy about empirical outcome that turns on this issue concerns cognitive skill learning in amnesic patients on the Tower of Hanoi puzzle. In contrast to the claim of fully preserved learning on this task by amnesic patients (Cohen, 1985; Saint-Cyr et al., 1988), there are two other reports of less-than-normal learning (Butters et al., 1985; Gabrieli et al., 1988). As we shall see, this discrepancy in results becomes clear when we consider the relative use of procedural versus declarative memory by the subjects in the various experiments. On the Tower of Hanoi puzzle, explicit remembering of the outcomes of the training experiences can contribute significantly to performance in subjects who have—and make use of—declarative memory unless considerable care is taken in designing the testing conditions.

We noted earlier that there are a number of possible solution strategies and that subjects differ in the strategies they choose. For some strategies, the ability to remember specific moves and the outcome of having made those particular moves (e.g., moving the smallest block from the leftmost to the rightmost peg on the opening move leads to a good outcome) would help performance. But, for at least one strategy—the high-level strategy that Simon (1975) calls the *subgoal recursive strategy*—such explicit remembering is unnecessary; the best move from any given point in solving the puzzle can always be *derived* from the information at hand. That is, given (1) the rules of the task, (2) the overall goal of rebuilding the five-disc tower onto the rightmost peg, and (3) the recursive subgoal strategy of building smaller "sub-towers" on the way to building the full five-disc tower, subjects can engage their problem-solving abilities to compute the best next move on a move-by-move basis, *without having to remember particular puzzle configurations or moves, and without having to remember the previous moves that led to the current configuration of the puzzle* (Cohen, 1981; Cohen et al., 1985).

It was the existence of such a solution strategy for this task that prompted us to challenge amnesic patients with the task in the first place (Cohen, 1981). We reasoned that if all subjects were to base their performance on this strategy, declarative memory for specific moves and their outcomes would *not* play a significant role in performance, and the deficit in declarative memory suffered by amnesic patients would *not* place them at a disadvantage compared to control subjects. (If, on the other hand, the use of strategies that depend significantly on explicit remembering are encouraged, control subjects would gain an advantage and amnesic patients would show less than fully intact performance.)

Accordingly, in our work with the Tower of Hanoi puzzle, we employed a training procedure that encouraged *all* subjects to use the recursive strategy that permits moves to be derived, and thus leaves little role for declarative memory to play. Then, after training was completed, we used a set of probe tasks to verify that their performance was based on the recursive subgoal strategy. The training procedure involved the examiner's repeatedly asking subjects a formalized set of questions about what they were trying to accomplish, how they were going to accomplish it, and what they would then do next (described in Cohen, 1981; Cohen, Gabrieli, & Corkin in preparation). The examiner did *not* answer the questions for the subjects, nor give feedback on the subjects' answers, nor offer any suggestions, nor cue subjects about where to move. The probe tasks administered at the end of the experiment presented subjects with the puzzle in various optimal and nonoptimal configurations or stages of completion, and asked them to complete the puzzle from each configuration. The ability to solve the puzzle from each of these configurations, including ones that were not on the optimal solution path and were not likely to have been experienced during training, *requires* that they can *derive* the correct completions, in the sense described above (Cohen et al., 1985). Using these procedures, normal learning was observed in amnesic patients, and amnesic patients and control subjects alike were able to derive correct completions from probe configurations of the puzzle.

In the Butters et al. (1985) and Gabrieli et al. (1988) studies, however, no such control over the use of strategies was employed, and the likelihood of explicit remembering playing a significant role in guiding performance was therefore greatly increased. Nor was there any probe of the solution strategies actually employed by subjects. Moreover, Butters et al. (1985) adopted a procedure that, although unintended, undoubtedly served to *dis*courage rather than encourage the use of the recursive strategy. In their attempt to simplify the task, they permitted subjects to solve the puzzle to any empty peg, instead of the standard procedure to solve to the rightmost peg, and subjects did not have to specify in advance which peg they would consider to be the goal peg (figure 8.5). The idea, apparently, was that it is difficult to "see" or plan far enough ahead to anticipate what the initial moves should be in order to get the whole tower directly onto the rightmost peg. If subjects did not have to decide in advance which peg would constitute the goal peg, the investigators reasoned, then subjects could just start moving discs and later pick whichever peg seemed within reach given the way their solution was working out.

There is an unintended consequence of this manipulation, however, that undermines the ability of subjects to use the strategy we have argued is so important. That is, the manipulation serves to

THE TOWER OF HANOI PUZZLE

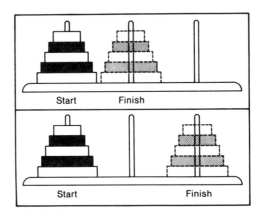

Figure 8.5
Schematic of the Tower of Hanoi puzzle as used in Butters et al. (1985). Subjects could use either the middle peg or the rightmost peg as the finish position on any given trial.

obscure the recursiveness of the problem, which depends on the
subject seeing the repeated stacking and unstacking of sub-towers
on particular pegs. One way to understand this point is to consider
the following way of viewing the recursive subgoal strategy in moving optimally (figure 8.6):

1. In order to get the whole 5-disk tower onto the rightmost peg,
there must be an earlier time when the 4-disk sub-tower (the topmost 4 disks) has been stacked on the middle peg, and the #5 disk
(the largest disk) is freed up to move to the rightmost peg.

2. In order to get the 4-disk sub-tower onto the middle peg, there
must be an earlier time when the 3-disk sub-tower has been stacked
on the rightmost peg, and the #4 disk is freed up to move to the
middle peg.

3. In order to get the 3-disk sub-tower onto the rightmost peg, there
must be an earlier time when the 2-disk sub-tower has been stacked
on the middle peg, and the #3 disk is freed up to move to the
rightmost peg.

4. In order to get the 2-disk sub-tower onto the middle peg, there
must be an earlier time when the #1 disk is placed on the rightmost
peg and then the #2 disk is freed to move to the middle peg.

Thinking of the puzzle in this way permits one to *derive* the
solution, move by move, seeing and taking advantage of the recursiveness. If, however, subjects are to just start moving without
specifying the goal peg in advance, reaching different solutions to
different pegs on different trials, there is no way to engage this type
of reasoning and no way to appreciate across trials the recursiveness
of the optimal solution.

A full consideration of the Tower of Hanoi work is beyond the
scope of the current discussion (but can be found elsewhere; see
Cohen, Gabrieli, & Corkin, in preparation). For the present purposes, let us emphasize that in obscuring the recursiveness of the
puzzle, these investigators reduced the likelihood of subjects being
able to use the recursive subgoal strategy that would permit them
to derive correct completions. Therefore, it reduced the possibility
of performance relying exclusively on procedural memory mechanisms, increasing the potential contribution that could be made by
declarative memory. The fact that amnesic patients would have

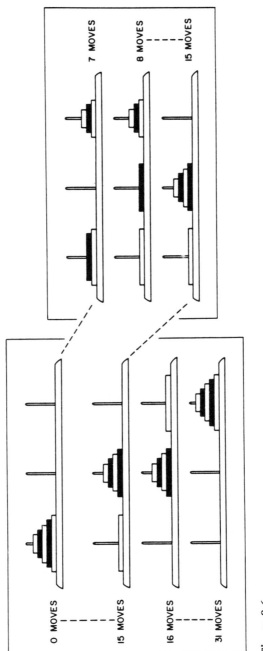

Figure 8.6
Schematic of the goal-recursion strategy in action, in which the overall (5-disc) problem is decomposed into a recursive set of smaller problems, i.e., with recursive subgoals. Using such a strategy, subjects can *derive* a solution to the puzzle from any given configuration of the discs. (From Cohen, 1981.)

more difficulty when tested under these circumstances—circumstances that are *not* a replication of the original testing procedures—becomes easy to understand.

The nature of our theory requires that strict attention be paid to the representational demands of various tasks and to the representational strategies employed by subjects in their performances. Assessments of the adequacy of our theory should do more than simply generate tasks and then assess whether the performance of amnesic patients is impaired or spared versus control subjects; they must also probe and verify the representational systems used by subjects in the tasks (see chapters 9 and 10). We employed just this strategy in our work with the Tower of Hanoi puzzle. A somewhat similar effort was made in the serial reaction time work by Nissen and colleagues, discussed above, who assessed whether individual control subjects had declarative memory for the repeating sequences that could affect their performance, and then excluded any such subjects from subsequent comparisons with the amnesic patients. This strategy is not used by the Butters et al. (1985) and Gabrieli et al. (1988) work.

Finally, the Butters et al. (1985) work was based largely on patients with Korsakoff's disease. Their problem-solving and planning deficits resulting from frontal-lobe pathology make them poor candidates for such an experiment. In the absence of intact problem-solving abilities, such patients would not be expected to show normal performance, even if they showed all of the normal procedural memory based tunings and modifications through experience. As we noted in our 1985 report (Cohen et al., 1985), frontal-lobe damage of the sort seen in patients with Korsakoff's disease causes severe impairment on a task called the Tower of London, a related task that directly assesses the number of moves ahead that subjects can plan in their heads (Shallice, 1982). Because of the problem-solving deficits of such patients, they would not be expected to be able to derive solutions to this or other problems as well as could control subjects, and hence are poor subjects on which to look for normal acquisition of problem-solving skill with practice.

In our treatment here of the Tower of Hanoi work, we have gone into considerable detail because the work illustrates so well one of the major themes we have articulated in this book. The Tower of Hanoi puzzle behaves in just the same way as all of the other paradigms we have considered, in revealing either spared or impaired performance in amnesic patients depending on the specific details of the testing circumstances: If it is administered in such a way as to encourage the use of strategies dependent on procedural memory, and if the basic processing machinery is intact to permit procedural-memory based tuning and modifications to occur as a result of experience, then amnesic patients can show fully preserved learning. If, however, these conditions are not met, both procedural and declarative memory will be enabled to make useful contributions to performance, and amnesic patients will be at a disadvantage relative to control subjects. The possibility that both procedural and declarative memory systems will contribute to any given behavioral performance is increased greatly with cognitive tasks, in which there are almost always multiple strategies that could be, and most likely will be, employed by different subjects. This is why *all* of the cognitive skill learning tasks that have been explored with amnesic patients, including the learning of simple numerical rules and of computer interaction situations (the sugar production and computer person tasks) discussed above, have now shown conflicting results and/or only partially spared learning. These apparent discrepancies in the data can be understood within the procedural-declarative framework.

REPETITION PRIMING

In this class of tasks, the phenomenon of interest is the facilitatory or biasing effect of previous exposure to the to-be-tested stimuli on the subsequent processing of those same materials. There is typically a study phase in which subjects are presented with some set of stimulus materials (e.g., words or line drawings of objects). Then, in a subsequent, unexpected test phase, those materials are re-presented along with new ones, often in fragmented or otherwise visually degraded form, and subjects are asked to name, identify, or otherwise categorize the stimuli. Subjects are *not* asked to recall their previous experiences or to judge whether or not the items had been presented previously. A facilitation in speed or accuracy of processing for the repeated items over items not previously presented, or a bias in responding toward the previously studied items, is taken to represent repetition priming. (There is a large literature on *semantic* priming effects, in which exposure to items can affect processing of *semantically associated* items if they are presented immediately after the priming stimulus. This type of priming is a different phenomenon, and will not be considered here. All subsequent uses of the term "priming" will therefore refer to *repetition* priming.)

Amnesic patients have shown robust priming effects in a large, and ever-growing, number of tasks. For example, upon studying or making some judgment about words on a list, amnesic patients have shown facilitation for those items over items not previously presented when subsequently asked to complete word stems (Cermak et al., 1988; Diamond & Rozin, 1984; Graf et al., 1984; Squire et al., 1987, Warrington & Weiskrantz, 1970; see figure 3.3) or word fragments (Squire et al., 1987); or when asked to identify briefly presented (Cermak et al., 1985, 1988) or visually degraded (Keane et al., 1988; Warrington & Weiskrantz, 1970) words.

Another set of examples of priming in amnesic patients involves the development of a bias toward previously studied items in spelling, category exemplar, drawing, or preference tests. The first of these examples involved pairs of homophonic words (e.g., *read* and *reed; bear* and *bare*). Patients with Korsakoff's disease were given questions presented auditorily that evoke one or another of each pair (e.g., Name a musical instrument that employs a *reed*), and were subsequently asked to participate in a spelling task. The prior exposure to one or another member of a homophonic pair "biased" the patients to give the spelling corresponding to that word (in our example—*reed*) with a higher probability than would have been the case without the prior exposure (Jacoby & Witherspoon, 1982). In the category exemplar task, there was an initial study phase in which patients read a word list that included randomly ordered exemplars of various categories. In a subsequent test phase, patients were asked to generate as many exemplars as they could for each of several categories. Generation of exemplars in this phase of the task was biased toward the items that were on the original study list (Graf et al., 1985). In the third example, the patient H.M. was shown a set of simple dot patterns in which the dots had been connected to produce a simple figure. He was subsequently shown the dot patterns again and was asked to connect the dots in any way he chose to produce a simple figure (figure 8.7). H.M. was biased

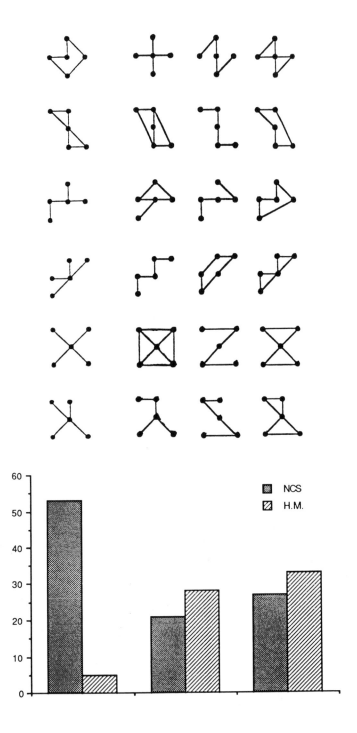

toward connecting the dots to produce the figures he had previously seen (Gabrieli et al., 1990). In the fourth example, patients with Korsakoff's disease exhibited preferences for novel melodies that they had heard earlier over ones that they had not heard earlier (Johnson, Kim, & Risse, 1985).

One last category of priming to be considered here concerns the priming effects seen in repeated trials of continuous perceptual processing tasks, in which processing performance measured on successive trials shows facilitation for repeated materials (without the usual study-phase then test-phase format). This effect has been seen in reading (Moscovitch et al., 1986; Musen et al., 1990), in identifying briefly presented words (Nissen, Cohen, & Corkin, 1981) or visually degraded words (Warrington & Weiskrantz, 1968) and line drawings (Milner et al., 1968; Warrington & Weiskrantz, 1968), in detecting hidden figures (Crovitz et al., 1981), in detecting anomalous features of pictures (Warrington & Weiskrantz, 1973), in making lexical decisions (word-nonword decisions) on letter strings (Gordon, 1988), and in detecting the axis of symmetry of checkerboard-based visual patterns (Cohen et al., 1986).

Dissociations

For some of the above examples of priming, the size of the effect in amnesic patients has not been systematically compared to that seen in normal subjects. For the great majority of these studies, however, the comparison has been made and most often shows priming effects to be fully intact (for reviews, see Schacter, 1987b; Shimamura, 1986; Tulving & Schacter, 1990). Fully in line with the

◀──

Figure 8.7
An example of pattern priming. (*Top*) Subjects see dot patterns such as those shown in the *pattern* column, and then for each pattern see one particular way of connecting the dots (of completing the patterns) to create the figures seen in the *target* column. They are subsequently tested either by being shown several alternative completions of each dot pattern and being asked to indicate which is the one they saw previously (recognition), or by being shown just the patterns and being asked to complete them in the first way that comes to mind (priming). (*Bottom*) Performance on these two tasks indicates that H.M. shows intact priming, i.e., he shows a normal tendency to complete the patterns to the figures that he had seen previously. But he is profoundly impaired in making recognition memory judgments. (From Gabrieli et al., 1990.)

phenomenon of preserved skill learning, discussed in the previous section, the preserved priming effects in amnesia occurred despite profoundly impaired recall and recognition of the materials that were primed and impaired recollection of the training experiences that served as the basis for the priming effects. That is, there is the same dissociation here between aspects of skilled performance and the explicit remembering of the materials whose previous presentation caused the learning effects.

The dissociation between priming of recently presented materials and recall or recognition of their previous occurrence also conforms with evidence from normal subjects indicating that these measures of memory are independent. First, experimental manipulations can influence *either* priming measures *or* measures of recall and recognition without affecting the other (e.g., Graf & Mandler, 1984; Graf & Schacter, 1987; Jacoby, 1983; Roediger & Blaxton, 1987a,b; Schacter & Graf, 1986; Sloman et al., 1988). Second, in experiments that assess both priming effects and recognition memory for the same items, performance on the two measures can be stochastically independent—that is, priming is *no* greater or more likely for items recognized as having occurred previously than for items not recognized (e.g., Jacoby & Witherspoon, 1982; Musen & Treismann, 1990; Tulving, Schacter, & Stark, 1982). This is *not* to say that the measures must be independent, or that priming effects and explicit remembering cannot interact in influencing certain behavioral performances. Indeed, as we shall see, some behavioral performances are clearly influenced by both classes of memory phenomena, just as some of the performances considered above were influenced by both skill learning and explicit remembering phenomena. However, the fact that these phenomena *can* be independent is critical for understanding their determinants and their implications concerning the organization of normal memory.

Less-than-Normal Performance

Some studies of priming in amnesic patients have reported the performance facilitation to be smaller than in normal subjects. First, several studies of identification of incomplete or fragmented line drawings of objects presented on multiple trials have found robust, but less-than-normal, facilitation upon the repetition of items in amnesic patients (Milner et al., 1968; Warrington & Weiskrantz,

1968). A second example comes from McAndrews, Glisky, and Schacter's (1987) work on priming for the solution of sentence puzzles—sentences whose meanings hinged on a key word or idea not provided with the sentence (e.g., the sentence "The haystack was important because the cloth ripped" becomes understandable when given the key word "parachute"). Amnesic patients showed facilitation in solving sentence puzzles that had been previously presented as much as one week earlier, but this priming effect was not as robust as that seen in normal subjects. A third example concerns priming for nonword letter strings in either word-stem completion (Diamond & Rozin, 1984) or perceptual identification (Cermak et al., 1985) tasks, in which amnesic patients showed less than the normal facilitation for repeated items.

An Area of Ambiguity: Priming of Relationships?

There is one class of experiments with considerable importance for which the current results remain ambiguous. As a means of addressing the question of whether amnesic patients can show normal priming for novel materials, namely, materials for which there is no prior stored representation of the stimulus item to be primed (the answer, by the way, is "yes"), several experiments looked at priming for arbitrarily paired words. Graf and Schacter (Graf & Schacter, 1985; Schacter & Graf, 1986) gave subjects pairs such as *window-reason* at study time and then looked at word-stem completion for items such as *window-rea____* at test time. Other test items included re-pairings of *window* and of *reason* with new items, plus brand new pairs. These investigators reported that priming was best for the studied pairings: Stems were completed best when paired at test time with the same item as appeared with it at study time (i.e., *rea____* was completed best at test time when the cue was *window-rea____*). Similar results were obtained in a task where the measure of priming came from reading speed (Moscovitch et al., 1986). Subjects read arbitrarily paired words, and then later read the same pairs together with re-pairings of the original words plus brand new pairs. The "old" word pairs were read faster than either re-pairings of the same words or brand new pairs.

However, subsequent work indicates that more severely amnesic patients show less than the normal magnitude of priming for word pairs. Several investigators have shown amnesic patients to be impaired on fragment completion for word pairs (Cermak et al., 1988; Mayes & Goodling, 1989; Shimamura & Squire, 1989). Musen and Squire (1990) failed to find superior priming for "old" word pairs over re-pairings of the original words in reading speed for either amnesic patients or normal subjects, unless they gave many repetitions of the same items, and even then the resulting effect was very small.

More recently, Musen and Squire (1991) found a pairing-specific reduction in Stroop interference that was of normal magnitude in amnesic patients, but only if the experiment was run in a specific way. In this task, subjects were shown color names (red, green, blue, etc.) displayed on a color monitor in colors that conflicted with those names (e.g., red displayed in green, blue displayed in red, etc.), and were asked to say the color in which each item was displayed (*green* for red displayed in green, *red* for blue displayed in red). The conflict (Stroop interference) between the color name and the color in which it was displayed makes it difficult to perform this task under speed pressure—a widely reported phenomenon. In this experiment, the particular conflict pairings were maintained across several trials, so that, for example, red was always displayed in green, blue was always displayed in red, and so forth. Across trials, subjects were able to speed up their responding (i.e., showed less and less effect of the interference). Then, after a series of trials, the conflict pairings were changed, such that, for example, red was now displayed in blue, green was now displayed in red, and so forth. On this trial, responses were slowed greatly; the reduction in Stroop interference that was learned over trials was lost, indicating that it was pairing-specific. Results were the same on this task for amnesic patients as for control subjects.

However, this result was only obtained when the conflicting information was conjoined in the same item; that is, when each individual stimulus item was both a color name and had a display color. When color names were displayed on patches of color or were surrounded by colored boxes (i.e., when the conflicts were between distinct physical objects), the above results did *not* obtain.

Explaining the Phenomena: Preserved Repetition Priming Effects

Priming effects entail the facilitation or biasing of (word recognition, object recognition, etc.) performance when previously exposed materials are re-presented; that is, when, from the point of view of a given processing module, there is a repetition of the original processing event and the original processing operations are again engaged. In such cases there is no need for the information acquired during training to be carried over to other domains or to novel situations outside of the original training context, and no need to gain access to the learning experiences that shaped the facilitated performance. Accordingly, there is no need of the representational flexibility and promiscuity mediated by declarative memory. On our account, priming effects can be supported fully by tuning or biasing of cortical processors and cognitive operations, mediated by procedural memory, expressed when the subject again engages these processors. Such tuning and modifications of the affected processors occur independently of the hippocampal system and hence can be fully intact in amnesic patients.

To understand how this can be realized, let us return to our discussion from earlier in the chapter about the way in which processing networks can continue to be shaped and molded by new experiences, making and keeping them maximally tuned to the inputs they actually receive most frequently and recently. The brain's various processing networks, having been organized by past experience, retain the ability to be tuned and modified in accordance with the particular regularities of their inputs. As modeled in current connectionist or neural network theory, such experience-induced tuning is accomplished by incremental modifications of the connection weights that capture the patterns present in the input. Recent exposure to a given stimulus item temporarily biases or exerts some "pull" in one or another direction in the "weight space" of the network, which will be detected for a time as an increased facility of the network for that item, until the pulls exerted in other directions of the network's weight space by subsequent presentations of other stimulus items obscures the earlier modification. Such effects are wholly within-network modifications, and can be mediated entirely independently of the hippocampal system.

Evidence supporting this view comes from positron emission tomography (PET) studies in normal subjects, in which the early stages (feature analysis) of visual word recognition are associated with increased metabolic activity in peristriate areas of cortex (secondary visual cortical areas) (Petersen et al., 1989, 1990), and these same areas show a significant change in activity (decreased activation) when subjects are performing a visual word priming task (Squire et al., 1992). A less direct piece of evidence comes from study of priming in patients with Alzheimer's disease, whose memory impairments are accompanied by other cognitive deficits (in language, attention, problem-solving, and visuospatial processing) and cortical pathology (frontal, temporal, and parietal association areas). Such patients exhibit normal repetition priming on tasks that seem to rely most heavily on *perceptual* processing and hence on the integrity of visual processing areas of the brain that are little affected in Alzheimer's disease (e.g., the peristriate cortex areas noted above in our discussion of the PET data); but they exhibit less-than-normal priming on tasks that seem to rely most heavily on *conceptual* processing and hence on the integrity of language-related and other association cortical areas greatly affected in Alzheimer's disease (Keane et al., 1991). We take the finding that different priming phenomena depend critically on specific cortical processing substrates as reflecting the dependence of these priming phenomena on tuning and modification of those specific cortical processing networks.

Explaining the Phenomena: Dissociations

The tuning and modification described above are dedicated to particular processors and are representationally *in*flexible. These procedural representations are accessible only when the processing networks that support skilled performance in reading, identifying objects, and so forth, are again engaged by re-presentation of the primed materials. When the performance requirements are changed to require recalling or recognizing the stimulus materials or recollection of the training experiences, the dedicated, inflexible representations supporting priming effects are not sufficient. Explicit remembering and recollection require that the information acquired during training be carried over to other domains or to novel situations outside of the original training context, and hence that it be accessible to other processors. This requires the representational flexibility and promiscuity that is uniquely characteristic of declarative memory and that is unavailable to amnesic patients in the absence of an intact hippocampal system.

Explaining the Phenomena: Less-than-Normal Priming Effects

As was the case with the skill learning phenomena, performance on repetition priming tasks can certainly be influenced by declarative memory—that is, by explicit remembering of the study materials. Repetition priming is defined only as a facilitation or other biasing of performance due to previous exposure to the test materials. However, facilitation can result from explicitly recalling the set of previously presented stimuli and then considering them as potential candidate answers in priming tasks such as identification or completion of visually degraded or rapidly presented items. The use of explicit remembering is encouraged in such tasks by making the set of study items small and the items particularly unusual or distinctive (thereby producing particularly robust declarative representations), or by making the identification or completion of the test items especially difficult (thereby making alternative sources of information particularly welcome). In such a case, facilitation of performance for repeated items over nonrepeated items would reflect an indirect measure of explicit remembering (i.e., of declarative memory). But this is not the situation that has attracted so much attention to priming phenomena; rather, it is the facilitatory or biasing effects of previous experience that can be shown to occur independently of explicit remembering. Perhaps the term *priming* should be reserved for just these instances of performance facilitation. Certainly, tests of priming in amnesia should be restricted to these instances; when explicit remembering does play a significant role, then the performance of amnesic patients would be expected to be impaired relative to control subjects.

Unfortunately, a number of the tasks employed with amnesic patients have permitted declarative memory to make a significant contribution, and it is just these tasks that have given rise to reports of less-than-normal facilitation in amnesia. Let us consider the examples noted above in light of this interpretation.

The tasks involving identification of incomplete or fragmented line drawings of objects (Milner et al., 1968; Warrington & Weiskrantz, 1968)—in which relatively short lists of visually distinctive items are presented under conditions in which identification is initially very difficult—have just the conditions noted above for encouraging an explicit-remembering contribution to performance, a point noted at the time by Milner et al. (1968) and by others subsequently (e.g., Schacter et al., 1990). Snodgrass (1989) has been carefully working out the multiple determinants of performance in this task. The point here is that the task is multidetermined and leaves considerable room for influences of declarative memory. Finding less-than-normal performance facilitation in amnesic patients on this task is easily understandable within the procedural-declarative framework.

The task involving priming for sentence puzzles (McAndrews, Glisky, and Schacter, 1987) leaves obvious opportunities for the influence of declarative memory on performance. The verbal nature of the materials and the ambiguity of the intended meaning requires on-line relational processing—the subject must process the materials for meaning, comparing and evaluating possible meanings with other stored information and evaluating the relationship of each sentence with the corresponding key word, in order to solve the sentence puzzles. Invoking relational processing necessarily leads to the opportunity for normal subjects to create new declarative representations that will be available the next time they try to solve the puzzles. Amnesic patients, without the luxury of being able to create new declarative representations during their initial exposure to the sentence puzzles, would be expected to be disadvantaged compared to normal subjects.

Finally, the failure to find normal priming in amnesic patients for nonword letter strings (Cermak et al., 1985; Diamond & Rozin, 1984) seems also to be attributable to the ability of normal subjects to make use of declarative memory to aid their performance. This conclusion is suggested by the fact that subsequent studies, in which either the tasks were changed to discourage the use of explicit remembering, or a patient with more profound amnesia (H.M.) was used, or both, found normal priming for these stimulus materials (Gabrieli et al., 1988; Haist et al., 1991).

Explaining the Phenomena: Priming of Relationships?

One of the key elements of the procedural-declarative theory as we have articulated it here is that building representations of the relationships among perceptually distinct cues is uniquely accomplished by declarative memory. Accordingly, any findings suggesting that amnesic patients could show normal learning of such relationships would provide a significant challenge to the theory. The initial work with word-pair priming suggested that amnesic patients might be able to accomplish such relational learning, at least when tested in the priming paradigm (Graf & Schacter, 1985; Moscovitch et al., 1986; Schacter & Graf, 1986). The subsequent work indicating that the performance of amnesic patients is *not* in fact intact when the potential contributions to performance of declarative memory are minimized (Cermak et al., 1988; Mayes & Goodling, 1989; Musen & Squire, 1990; Shimamura & Squire, 1989) suggests that declarative memory is indeed critical for relational learning, supporting our theoretical position. As to the work on pairing-specific reduction in Stroop interference (Musen & Squire, 1991), the critical finding with respect to the procedural-declarative theory is that the phenomenon only seems to obtain in amnesia when the learning is *not* of relationships among distinct physical objects but rather of different attributes of stimului conjoined in the same item. In this paradigm, as in the others we have considered throughout the book, learning relationships among perceptually distinct objects requires hippocampal-mediated declarative memory.

Explaining the Phenomena: Multiple Sources of Performance Facilitation and the Processing Loci of Priming Effects

We have discussed at length the fact that both procedural and declarative memory influences can be found on priming tasks, and have argued that the term "priming" should be reserved for those task situations in which declarative memory does *not* contribute to performance facilitation. However, limiting the scope of priming to only those examples of performance facilitation in which explicit remembering plays no role, although important in order to conduct meaningful analyses of preserved learning and memory phenomena in amnesia, cannot guarantee that priming reflects a unitary phenomenon. On the contrary, it seems prudent to recognize that there are various possible sources of facilitation in any given task. Thus, for example, in identifying visually degraded line drawings of objects on repeated occasions, performance facilitation might well reflect the contributions of each of the following: explicit remembering of the presented items, a temporary activation of the (logogen-like) representation of the names of the objects, a temporary activation of the (pictogen-like) representation of the perceptual forms of the objects,[1] and a procedural tuning or modification of the pattern-analyzing and object-recognition networks themselves. The point is, even after excluding the contribution to performance of explicit remembering, priming can be multidetermined, and various dissociations among priming effects are to be expected.

The procedural view of priming offered here is intended to be about one particular source of performance facilitation. Thus, at least one of the determinants of performance on tasks such as the one noted above is claimed to be based on procedural memory, and is characterized by the inflexibility and dedicatedness of that kind of representation system, as discussed at length. Indeed, we propose that the features of representational inflexibility and dedicatedness that we have attributed to procedural memory can be used diagnostically to discern which memory system is supporting a particular memory performance. Thus, Glisky and Schacter's (Glisky, Schacter, & Tulving, 1986; Glisky & Schacter, 1987) work on teaching an amnesic patient several computer terms is particularly germane. They were able to teach computer terms (e.g., *print*) through the method of vanishing cues, in which a set of terms was presented in the context of computer commands, and then over a series of trials, various letters were removed from the terms, with the task being to type the terms to complete the computer commands. Over training, the patient was able to type the appropriate terms to complete the commands with fewer and fewer letters of the terms present as cues, until it eventually became possible to type entire computer terms without letter cues. What is relevant here is the nature of what was learned by the patient. First, the learning was very gradual and incremental, taking much longer than was the case with control subjects. Second, and more to the point of the present discussion, the information was "hyperspecific"—the patient could use the terms only in the context of this particular computer task with the particular commands as completion cues.

A particularly compelling piece of evidence for the claim that at least certain aspects of priming reflect the use of inflexible or hyperspecific *procedural* representations, comes from work by Tulving, Hayman, and Macdonald (cited in Tulving & Schacter, 1990) on word fragment completion. Previous work had shown that if subjects are given a list of words to study (including items such as *pyramid, mosquito,* and *aardvark*) and then given a word-fragment completion task (for example, complete the fragment _y_a_id), subjects show a facilitation of completion performance for items that had been on the study list, independent of their recognition of the previous occurrence of those items. Tulving et al. have now found that completion performance given one possible fragmented version of an item is independent of completion performance given a different fragmented version of the same item (e.g., _o_q__to versus __s_ui_o or even _a_d__r_ versus _ard_ar_). The tuning and modifications of word recognition networks by recent exposure to individual words is apparently sufficiently specific to permit temporary changes in the weights of links between particular visual features, letters, and words. In this way, priming would be sensitive to the precise match between the particular letter combinations in the studied word fragments and the letter combinations of the fragments presented at test time.

Another point about the procedural memory view of repetition priming is that, in tying procedural memory to the particular processors engaged during a learning event, it becomes natural to think about the processing loci of the effects of experience. That is, if we return to the example of identifying visually degraded line drawings of objects on repeated occasions, we find ourselves asking, Where in the stream of processing of the materials do the effects of learning manifest themselves? Each of the different processing networks—from those supporting visual pattern analysis to those mediating visual object recognition to those concerned with lexical analysis—may well contribute to the priming effects, each being separately tuned and biased by experience (Cohen, 1981, 1984). Similarly, in the word-fragment completion work just discussed, we turned very naturally to discussion of priming effects as likely being due to changes between the visual feature, letter, and whole-word levels of processing; or there could be effects at all three levels.

The important point, we think, is that rather than asking, What is priming?, as though it were a unitary entity across all the tasks in which performance facilitation is seen, and as though data from any single task could fully illuminate its nature, it seems more productive to ask, Where is priming?, adopting the view that there are multiple sources of performance facilitation and multiple processing loci that are modified by experience.

ON THE RELATIONSHIP BETWEEN SKILL LEARNING AND REPETITION PRIMING

Nearly all of the examples of repetition priming considered here, and in the literature generally, are based on domains of processing in which subjects are already expert and no further generalized skill learning occurs, such as in reading and in word or picture identification. Conversely, studies of skill learning generally involve repeated practice on tasks for which subjects have little or no previous expertise. As a result, studies of these two phenomena have been conducted separately, and within largely separate theoretical frameworks. Many investigators treat these aspects of memory as functionally distinct phenomena based on separate mechanisms and have made almost no effort to try to accommodate both of them into a single theory of memory and amnesia.

One line of work that has considered the relationship between skill learning and repetition priming has made much of the fact that basal ganglia disease, as is seen in Parkinson's disease and Huntington's disease, produces impairment in (motor) skill learning but not in (verbal) priming (Heindel et al., 1988, 1989). Such a result strikes us as being open to many interpretations. Our work, by contrast, has attempted to look at these two aspects of memory within the same paradigm and within a single theoretical framework. In the work already discussed on reading mirror-reversed or otherwise transformed text, skill learning and repetition priming are seen together, in control subjects and amnesic patients alike. We have extended the combined study of generalized skill learning and item-specific repetition priming effects in a task involving detection of the axis of symmetry of repeating and unique checkerboard-based visual patterns (Cohen et al., 1987; figure 8.8). Subjects are presented with a series of visual patterns that are symmetric about one and only one axis—either the vertical, horizontal, left diagonal, or right diagonal. The patterns are presented very briefly (for less than 200 msec) and are masked by a true checkerboard (which is symmetric about all four axes). Subjects are to move a hand-held optical computer mouse in the direction of the perceived axis of symmetry of each pattern presented. In this work, we have shown that repetition priming occurs at all levels of skilled performance, both when subjects are novices in the domain and show robust skill learning, and when subjects have become "experts" and show asymptotic performance for unique items.

From the perspective of the procedural-declarative framework, we see skill learning and repetition priming as both arising from the same procedural mechanisms of tuning and modifying of the processors. Indeed, we propose that skill learning is the sum total of all of the individual item-specific repetition primings. The separate "pulls" exerted by the specifically trained items will provide the processing network(s) with some advantage or bias in processing for those items over novel items. Items that are presented most often and most frequently will have the largest bias or advantage. However, as long as training ensures that items are sampled fairly broadly within the domain, then the pulls exerted by the various trained items will also begin to confer some processing advantage for all those novel items that are consistent with the regularities already captured by the network(s). In this way, there would be both generalized skill learning and an additional facilitation for repeated items, just as is observed in behavior.

RECALL AND RECOGNITION

A huge body of work has documented the impairment of amnesic patients such as H.M. on a variety of recall and recognition memory tasks (Corkin, 1984; Milner, 1966; Milner, Corkin & Teuber, 1968; Milner & Teuber, 1968). When given a quantity of information that exceeds the patients' span and when asked to bridge any significant (particularly if interference-filled) delay, amnesic patients are markedly impaired in recalling and recognizing (or even relearning) the materials. Indeed, profound deficits on recall and recognition tests are diagnostic of amnesia, and will have had to be documented in screening tests (such as the Wechsler Memory Scale–Revised [WMS-R], in which recall across interference-filled delay is critical, and the Warrington Recognition Test) in order to identify patients as being amnesic.

This is not to say that the extent of the deficit in amnesia is, or needs to be, identical for recall and recognition. Work by Hirst and

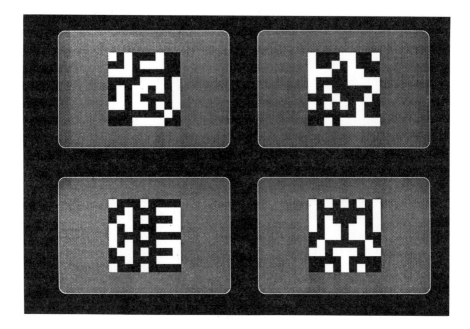

SYMMETRY DETECTION

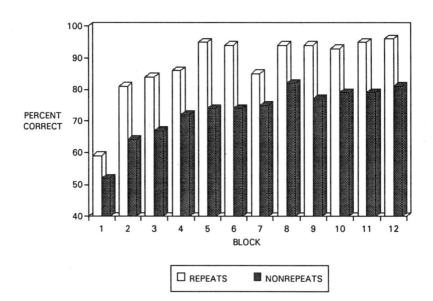

colleagues (Hirst et al., 1986, 1988) has suggested that recall may be disproportionately more impaired than recognition in at least some examples of amnesia, compared to the respective performances of control subjects. On the other hand, H.M.'s amnesia is so profound that his recognition memory performance is almost always at chance levels and hence is as impaired as it is possible to be. Squire (1992) has taken issue with the idea that recall is disproportionately impaired in amnesia, suggesting that this may be true only for patients with additional deficits attributable to frontal-lobe involvement. Still, there is some reason to expect recognition memory performance to be less severely impaired in amnesia than recall if, as suggested by several investigators (see below), phenomena related to priming effects (intact in amnesia) may sometimes contribute to recognition task performance. Regardless of which way this issue turns out, what is important for our purposes here is that hippocampal system damage causes deficits of both recall and recognition.

Impairment of recall and recognition memory performances occurs for the very materials on which amnesic patients demonstrate normal repetition priming and skill learning. Accordingly, just as with the animal amnesia data, either impairment or sparing is seen for the very same materials depending on the nature of the processing demanded, and hence on the representations needed to support performance. As discussed at some length earlier, recall and recognition inevitably depend on stored information about the outcomes of specific processing events and on the relational flexibility and promiscuity of the resulting declarative memory representations. The dependence of such performances on declarative representations results in amnesic patients being impaired.

◄————————————————————————————————

Figure 8.8
Skill learning and priming in detection of the axis of symmetry in checkerboard-based visual patterns. (*top*) Examples of stimulus materials, each of which is symmetric about one and only one axis (in these examples: left diagonal, right diagonal, vertical, and horizontal, starting in the upper left-hand corner and moving clockwise). (*bottom*) Increases in percent correct detection of the axis of symmetry for both novel stimuli (dark bars) and repeating stimuli (white bars), documenting both skill learning and repetition priming.

MULTIPLE DETERMINANTS OF RECOGNITION MEMORY PERFORMANCE?: AN ASIDE

Paralleling the issue of there being multiple sources of performance facilitation in priming tasks, there may also be multiple determinants of recognition memory performance. Several investigators, most notably Mandler (1980) and Jacoby (1983, 1991) have suggested that recognition memory includes not only the conscious *recollection* component that is usually discussed, but also a *familiarity* component that may include the increase in perceptual *fluency* caused by being (procedurally) primed. This two-factor view of recognition memory becomes more interesting for our present purposes with the possibility that amnesic patients may be able to demonstrate some significant measure of familiarity (Jacoby, 1992). If there is indeed a familiarity component of recognition memory that is not completely dependent on declarative processes, then to the extent that amnesic patients' recognition memory judgments are capable of making use of familiarity their recognition memory performance would be expected to be superior to what would be predicted on the basis of their recall performance, just as claimed by Hirst et al. (1986, 1988).

DISSOCIATIONS AMONG PERFORMANCES IN NORMAL SUBJECTS

As was noted earlier in this chapter, dissociations between skill learning and repetition priming effects, on the one hand, and recall and recognition memory performance, on the other, have been noted in the performances of normal subjects: Skill learning and repetition priming are not dependent on, nor are they influenced by the same variables as, recall and recognition. The observation of this dissociation in normal subjects is heartening; after all, one would hope that inferences about multiple memory systems in normal memory drawn from studies of amnesic patients with selective memory impairments could actually be confirmed in normal subjects.

Another dissociation in normal subjects that parallels the amnesia phenomena concerns the relationship between skilled performance and the ability to introspect about its determinants. For amnesic patients, this dissociation is remarkably profound: Improvements in skilled performances occur in the absence of any awareness of the determinants of the newly skilled performance, or even of knowledge that improvement occurs. Any such dissociation in normal subjects is necessarily less marked. Nonetheless, strong claims have been made by investigators such as Broadbent (Broadbent et al., 1986), Reber (1967, 1976, 1989), and Lewicki (Lewicki, 1986; Lewicki et al., 1988), among others, suggesting that normal subjects exhibit robust "implicit learning" about the regularities of their input without being able to articulate those regularities in their verbal reports. That is, there seems to be the same dissociation between increasingly "skilled" performance and inadequate verbal reports as is seen in amnesic patients. However, it must be said that this area of research has received much criticism, and the extent to which it really parallels the amnesia phenomena is not entirely clear. Thus, investigators such as Dulany et al. (1984), Perruchet and Pacteau (1990), and Sanderson (1989) have been critical of the methodologies employed and have suggested that subjects' verbal reports match the information guiding their skilled performance rather better than had been claimed.

We continue to be impressed, however, with examples such as the one offered by Posner (1973) about the dissociation in normal skilled typists between ability to perform with skill and their inability to introspect about their skilled performance. Thus, such subjects are much more proficient at typing the alphabet from a to z than at indicating on a schematic keyboard where each of the 26 letters is located spatially, even though they must "know" the location of each letter in order to type it (Cohen et al., 1985). This dissociation is very much like the SHRDLU example that we discussed earlier.

This dissociation, along with the others discussed earlier, are understood within the procedural-declarative framework as reflecting the fact that skilled performance is mediated by procedural memory, whose representations are dedicated and inflexible, inaccessible to the processes that mediate conscious introspection. The representations driving skilled performance can only be expressed in the context of performing the learned task. The ability to consciously recollect one's training experiences and to introspect about the contents of one's memory requires the flexible, relational representations mediated by declarative memory. Although normal subjects have both of these memory systems, and although these memory systems can interact in mutually supporting certain task performances, they are functionally distinct systems with different capabilities and are manifested in different types of memory performances.

OTHER PHENOMENA

There are a few other demonstrations of previous experience exerting an influence on the performance of amnesic patients despite their impaired memory for the relevant learning events. These include eyeblink conditioning (Daum et al., 1989; Weiskrantz & Warrington, 1979) and longlasting perceptual aftereffects (Benzing & Squire, 1989; Savoy & Gabrieli, 1988; Weiskrantz, 1978). These performances would appear to reflect the ability of basic cortical processors and subcortical brain circuits (e.g., cerebellum) to exhibit incremental tuning and modification of processing networks in the manner we have described for procedural memory. Being tied inflexibly to particular processing networks, these (procedural) representations give rise to the observed dissociation between the experience-induced modifications of performance and the inability to recollect the learning events, just as we have described for skill learning and repetition priming.

Summarizing the Fit of the Theory to Data

We have endeavored to show how the procedural-declarative framework articulated here provides a comprehensive account not only
of the human amnesia data but also of the animal model work; and
not only of the behavioral findings but also of the anatomical and
physiological data. With regard to the behavioral data, we conclude
that the procedural-declarative account offers an explanation of the
pattern of impairment and sparing following hippocampal system
damage in each of the major behavioral paradigms used in work
with rats, monkeys, and humans. With regard to the anatomical
and physiological data, we conclude that the hippocampal system
has the anatomical connections and physiological characteristics
necessary to perform the functional role ascribed to it by the procedural-declarative account. These conclusions are explicated
below.

BEHAVIORAL DATA

In evaluating the fit of our account to the behavioral data, five
summarizing conclusions emerge about the relationship of declarative and procedural memory systems to task performances. They
are as follows:

1. *Particular paradigms give rise to either impaired or intact
performance in amnesic subjects, even for the same to-be-learned
materials.* Different variants of the water maze, radial-arm maze,
and conditional discrimination tasks considered above have produced either impairment or intact performance in animals with
hippocampal system damage. On sensory discrimination tasks, the
performance of animals with hippocampal system damage was
shown to be impaired, intact, or even facilitated depending on the
specific task variant. In humans, testing with a single set of mate-

rials produced either impairment or sparing depending on whether it was skill learning and repetition priming or recall and recognition that was assessed.

2. *The nature of the representations required by the task determines whether impaired or intact performance is seen in amnesic subjects on any given task variant.* The behavioral outcome of damage to the hippocampal system was shown to depend on the extent to which performance on each task variant required the use of declarative memory or could derive benefit from making use of declarative memory. Subjects with hippocampal system damage were impaired whenever declarative representations of experience were necessary for, or contributed significantly to, the successful performance of intact subjects. That is, impairment was seen in tasks that emphasized learning of the relationships among multiple perceptually distinct stimuli and/or required that memory be used flexibly in novel testing situations. Sparing was observed in amnesic subjects whenever successful performance could be mediated in the absence of the hippocampal-dependent declarative system; that is, when performance could be mediated by an inflexible, dedicated representation supported by the tuning and modification of specific processing modules, and when the consequent biasing or adaptation of processing needed only to be expressed in a repetition of the original learning situation.

Sometimes differences in performance on the same learning materials could be attributed largely or even wholly to quantitative differences in the strength and persistence of contributing representations from separate memory systems rather than to distinctions in the qualitative nature of representation in separate memory systems.

3. *Even for those task variants on which amnesic subjects exhibit impaired performance, there is some preserved procedural memory.* Even when animals with hippocampal system damage were profoundly impaired on various task variants of DNMS, of the water maze and radial-arm maze, and of conditional discriminations, elements of their performance revealed a preservation of procedural memory. They had no impairment in learning to search for food by choosing objects to displace or by choosing maze arms to run down, and in learning to escape from the water by swimming to and climbing onto a submerged platform. That is, they were intact as

long as they were *not* asked to learn and remember about the particular objects that had been presented previously in DNMS, the particular arms that had been baited and had not been visited recently in the radial-arm maze, the specific location of the escape platform in the water maze, and the particular contingencies that predicted reward in conditional discrimination. Their impairments on these tasks were manifested only for attempting to use past experience to permit a determination of *which* objects and maze arms to choose, and *which* locations to search first, expressions of representations of past experience that require more than what the intact procedural memory system can deliver.

Likewise, human amnesic patients were able to keep track of the task procedures in tasks such as recall or recognition memory, demonstrating the ability to learn the response requirements; unfortunately, in the absence of declarative memory–mediated remembering of specific objects and events and the relations among them, they failed to come up with the substantive content required for correct responding. More fundamentally, even while unable to explicitly remember their learning experiences and the materials to which they were exposed during training sessions, they were able to show increasing skill in processing such materials, both when the very same materials were subsequently re-presented (in repetition priming conditions) and when further materials of the same class were subsequently presented (in skill learning conditions).

4. *Even for those task variants on which the performance of amnesic subjects is intact, the ability to express learning flexibly is impaired relative to normal subjects.* Findings of spared performances in subjects with hippocampal system damage did not guarantee that the same information was acquired and stored by such subjects as was acquired and stored by normal subjects. Rather, the equivalence of performance between amnesic and normal subjects on some tasks was accompanied by performance discrepancies in subsequent probe tasks. Rats with hippocampal system damage could eventually learn several olfactory discriminations in the simultaneous-cue task, but were impaired with respect to controls in subsequent probe tasks involving novel pairings of the trained odors. Similarly, monkeys with hippocampal system damage who showed intact learning of object-pair discriminations containing common elements were impaired with respect to controls in sub-

sequent probe tests in which the originally learned pairs were segregated. For human amnesic patients, the intact facilitation of
performance in priming and skill learning tasks did *not* carry over
to other tasks or other test contexts involving different processing
operations, such as those required for success on recall and recognition tasks, whereas normal subjects were able to access their
stored representations and express them flexibly in many different
test contexts or task environments. In short, although fully spared
learning by amnesic subjects could be seen on those tasks for which
their inflexible procedural representations sufficed for successful
performance, their lack of an intact declarative system hindered
their performance whenever additional probe tests required the flexible use of the knowledge acquired during training.

   5. *For many paradigms, and certainly for most real-world problems, the performance of amnesic subjects will be neither fully
intact nor systematically impaired; rather, there will be both
spared and impaired components.* In several variants of the priming
and skill learning tasks considered above, explicit remembering of
Evaluating the form of the representation is based on the criteria of
processing operations performed during training was able to contribute to the performance of normal subjects; on those variants,
amnesic patients with only a procedural system to draw on demonstrated less-than-normal learning. The priming tasks on which
amnesic subjects showed fully spared performance were those carefully (or fortuitously) constructed to eliminate the possible contribution of explicit remembering. Similarly, the performance of
amnesic subjects on cognitive skill learning tasks depended on the
extent to which the procedural system alone was capable of supporting successful performance; on those task variants in which
both procedural and declarative systems ordinarily contribute, amnesic patients showed intact learning of some but not all components of the skill. It was only when the task was carefully
constructed to rule out any benefit from declarative representations
that amnesic patients demonstrated fully intact performance.

Summary and Implications

The above conclusions indicate the scope of the procedural-declarative account, explaining the range of fully and partially spared and
impaired performances following hippocampal system damage in

humans and animals. It also permits us to offer the admonition that real-world performance depends on the coordinated activity of various brain systems or processing modules. Normal memory, like other cognitive capacities, reflects the seamless operation of its component systems and processes. It is only when damage is restricted to one or another of the components—as is the case in amnesia, where damage selectively affects the declarative system— that the separate contributions of the different components can be ascertained. And it is only in carefully constructed and selected tests that the separate contributions of the various components can be assessed.

The implications of this point for testing the theory offered here, and, more generally, for understanding the nature and organization of normal memory, are very significant. A fair and legitimate test of this theory, or of its competitors, will require more than has been the standard of the past. We will need to have information about, or else strict control over, the nature of representation used by subjects in solving the tasks with which we challenge them in testing the theory. We propose, and have here illustrated the use of, a two-stage testing process, in which probe tests are used to determine the form of representation actually employed by subjects. Evaluating the form of the representation is based on the criteria of representational flexibility and relationality articulated in our theory. This issue is tackled more fully in the next chapter.

ANATOMICAL AND PHYSIOLOGICAL DATA

Anatomical and physiological data about the hippocampal system provide a further test of the adequacy and explanatory power of the procedural-declarative account. Three summarizing conclusions can be offered to describe the fit of our theory to findings about the anatomical connections and physiological properties of the hippocampal system:

1. *The anatomical connections of the hippocampal system place it in a position to receive, and to compute the relationships among, converging inputs from multiple higher-order associational areas that convey information about the functional characteristics of "objects," "events," and "actions."* The hippocampus receives as input the outcomes of processing of the brain's various processing

modules. The inputs to hippocampus are intermixed in topographic gradients, providing weighted partial overlaps of input. This places the hippocampal network in a position to process the conjunctions or associations of objects and events, and of their relative behavioral significance or task relevance, as required and explained by our theory. Information processing by the hippocampal system entails the convergence of representations generated by two different pathways within the hippocampus proper.

2. *Hippocampal neurons are activated by and seem to participate in the encoding or representation of all manner of relationships and conjunctions of significant events or objects.* The activity of hippocampal CA1 neurons is sensitive to a variety of different relationships. The relationships thus coded by hippocampal activity may be quite abstract and multidetermined. Hippocampal neural activity reflects the processing of relationships among spatial cues, among objects and their spatial locations, and among objects or events and the task-defined relevance or significance of those objects or events. Confronted with different task environments on different occasions, the same hippocampal networks process different relationships among the events and objects they receive as inputs. Thus, the firing properties of hippocampal neurons parallel aspects of relational processing and flexible representation that characterize the deficits seen after damage to the hippocampal system, thereby bringing the behavioral and physiological findings into strong correspondence.

3. *The hippocampal system supports a powerful associative learning mechanism (LTP) capable of mediating the representation of relationships.* The physiological characteristics of hippocampus include the presence of a form of synaptic plasticity, called LTP, that exhibits many of the properties of behavioral memory. LTP is best elicited by activation of multiple inputs arriving in close temporal proximity—just the conditions required to support the relational processing that we propose is characteristic of hippocampal-mediated declarative memory. More generally, LTP is preferentially induced by patterns of conjunctive neural activity that occur naturally during hippocampal-dependent declarative learning.

Summary and Implications

The data indicate that the hippocampal system possessed the requisite connections and physiological machinery to perform the relational processing and support the declarative representations proposed in our theory. Said the other way around, the procedural-declarative theory provides an account of the specific anatomical and physiological properties of the hippocampal system; these properties correspond directly to the characteristics of declarative memory inferred from the behavioral data, bringing the two sets of data into register. This is not to say that the anatomical and physiologically data prove or even uniquely support the procedural-declarative framework; rather, they conform with what must be the case in order for the theory to make sense, and hence provide support for it. These data, and the theory we offer, also permit some speculation about the particular functional role played by the hippocampal system in declarative memory. This will be the subject of the final chapter of the book.

10 What Constitutes a Test of This Theory?

Continuing the theme sounded in the previous chapter, testing this theory will require rather more than has been the standard in the past. Indeed, there needs to be a re-thinking of how experiments are to be designed to test such theories of the role of the hippocampal system in memory. We hypothesize here that the hippocampal system automatically and obligatorily creates a declarative representation of every learning event, whether or not it is required for successful performance on the task at hand, and whether or not the specific experimental design is equipped to assess its presence. Such representations may or may not contribute to task performance, depending on their utility to or necessity for successful performance, on idiosyncratic preferences of the individual subject or species, and on the structure of the task environment as manipulated and controlled by the experimenter.

Likewise, in any learning event, the plasticities inherent in the brain's various processors will cause some tuning or biasing of the engaged systems in the direction of the particular materials available for processing—that is, procedural memory. This will affect subsequent performance whenever the biasing or weighting of perceptual processing or response tendencies, caused by prior learning events, can make a significant impact on behavior.

Behavioral paradigms cannot be simply categorized into "impaired in amnesia" versus "spared in amnesia" with complete assurance, without knowing about the specific representational demands of each of the different paradigms and their many variants. As we have documented in considerable detail, different variants of nearly every paradigm can end up in either the "impaired" or the "spared" category for the very same stimulus materials, depending on the extent to which the given variant requires declarative memory for successful performance or confers an advantage on performances based on declarative memory. Thus, the issue of "replication" from study to study is more complicated that it has appeared. Moreover, tasks can have distinct components with different representational demands, such that some aspects of task performance can be intact despite an overall impaired performance level while others can be impaired despite an overall normal performance level. The differences in strength and persistence between hippocampal-dependent and hippocampal-independent respresentations further complicate an assessment of any particular task; the existence of these differences in operating characteristics requires that parameteric studies on learning and forgetting rates be done to distinguish dissociations based on these characteristics versus differences in the qualitative nature of memory representation demanded by the task.

Returning for a moment to the issue of automatic and obligatory encoding of declarative memories, as outlined in detail elsewhere in this book, the hippocampal system forms a representation of learning events even in such non-hippocampal-dependent tasks as simple classical conditioning. The existence of a declarative representation in classical conditioning of the nictitating membrane response in rabbits can be revealed by a probe test—as has been done by testing reversal learning; and it can be revealed by changing subtle variables in training—as has been done by interposing a brief delay between the CS and UCS. Furthermore, the existence of the hippocampal representation is reflected in the activation of hippocampal neurons during performance of such tasks, both those tasks (and task variants) for which performance requires hippocampal-system participation and those tasks (or variants) that do not.

This latter point suggests that great care must be taken in drawing inferences from physiological work about the role of the hippocampal system in any particular memory task. Neither the single-unit recording data, nor metabolic or activation measures of brain areas in humans (PET, EEG, MEG, MRS), will be particularly useful in determining which tasks *require* the participation of the hippocampal system—it should be activated to some extent by all learning events. It may be possible to show, however, that tasks that put a greater demand on declarative processing result in a quantitatively larger or more persistent degree of hippocampal system activation.

Similarly, electrophysiological or metabolic data indicating changes in particular processing systems that might be the substrate of procedural memory cannot tell us much about what role such changes play in guiding the learning and memory performance.

This perspective leads us to propose the following alternative experimental design in investigations of the hippocampal-system's role in learning and memory. Experiments seeking to further elaborate, or to test our theory's assertions about, the role of the hippocampal system in any single learning paradigm should proceed in two stages:

First, challenge subjects on a set of closely related tasks or task variants that differ in their dependence on declarative representations and the relational processing supported by the declarative system. The more that performance depends on (1) memory for the relationships among multiple perceptually distinct items, (2) the ability to make comparisons or relative judgments among, or to otherwise manipulate, stored representations, and (3) the ability to flexibly use memory in new test environments or novel contexts, the greater the requirement for declarative memory, and hence the greater the impairment that should occur in subjects with damage to the hippocampal system. For task variants that absolutely require declarative memory, the performance of amnesic subjects should be grossly impaired; subjects with severe enough amnesias should be incapable of performing successfully on such tasks.

Second, employ probe tasks that assess the extent to which the performances actually produced by subjects in the various tasks exhibit the representational flexibility and promiscuity characteristic of declarative memory, as opposed to the dedicated and inflexible nature of the representations characteristic of procedural memory. The specific design of these probe tests will vary widely, depending on the nature of the behavioral paradigm (see examples above). However, common in the procedures for all such probe tests should be that the context or the specific examples presented are altered from what was used in training in order to produce novel testing circumstances to permit assessment of the relational character and of the representational flexibility of the learned information. That is, the probe tasks should be capable of asking: Does the knowledge acquired by subjects transfer to new test environments?

Can it be manipulated and used flexibly by various processors? The representations of experience actually acquired, stored, and used by amnesic subjects should differ qualitatively from those available to intact subjects, in the extent to which they possess representational flexibility and promiscuity.

11 Comparing the Theory to Other Accounts: Animal Models

In this and the following chapter, we compare our account to and distinguish it from others in the animal model and human amnesia literatures, providing us with one final way in which to communicate the critical features of our theory. This comparative discussion of alternative accounts cannot, of course, be fully exhaustive, but it will include the proposals with the greatest currency and impact in the two literatures. In the course of this discussion, we shall point out the commonalities between our account and others, taking the opportunity to point out some intellectual debts we owe. We shall also point out the areas in which our account diverges from others. The scope of various alternative accounts will emerge importantly in this discussion, because many of the alternative proposals turn out to be limited-domain accounts whose ability to explain the pattern of sparing and loss in amnesia is limited to particular paradigms and particular species and whose coverage of the data is limited to only the behavioral findings, as we had warned in chapter 2. In such cases, our procedural-declarative account provides coverage of phenomena for which others have no explanation. This is shown by challenging each of the alternative accounts with the entire range of human and animal (behavioral, anatomical, and physiological) data with which we evaluated our own theory.

COGNITIVE MAPPING VERSUS TAXON LEARNING

O'Keefe and Nadel (1978) distinguished between a hippocampal-based cognitive mapping system, necessary for representing and using spatial maps of the environment, and a hippocampal-independent taxon learning system, which mediates behaviors cued by "taxons" (or "guidance" stimuli) contiguous with reward. They argued that the deficits of animals with hippocampal system damage are of "place" learning and can be attributed to their inability to construct, maintain, and/or make use of spatial maps. Preserved memory performances, on this view, occur in situations in which (even spatial) responses can be guided by specific taxon cues.

The nature of this proposal can be appreciated by considering the way in which it would explain the results of the O'Keefe and Conway (1980) maze-learning study (see chapters 3 and 6). Performance in the distributed cues condition, in which orienting stimuli were distributed around the environment, places demands on the hippocampal system because of the need to represent the relationships among the multiple spatially separate cues in order to learn the goal "place." When the cues were concentrated at the goal site performance could be supported without hippocampal-mediated place learning, because animals could directly associate the goal with contiguous taxons guiding them to reward; they need only orient in the direction of the collection of cues on each trial and would therefore not need the cognitive mapping capacity of the hippocampal system.

In support of this view is the enormous number of reports of profound impairment following hippocampal system damage on various spatial learning tasks, including the water maze and radial-arm maze tasks discussed in chapter 7; and numerous reports of preserved learning on various nonspatial tasks, such as sensory discrimination learning (see chapter 7). Further support for this account comes from the striking and well-documented finding of spatially determined firing of hippocampal neurons—the phenomenon of cells with place fields discussed in chapter 5 (see figures 5.1–5.5).

This account has been enormously influential, and justifiably so, for a number of reasons. It provided a powerful framework for understanding the discrepancy between impaired performance on some learning tasks and intact performance on others in rats with hippocampal system damage, at a time in the history of the field when the alternative theories of animal amnesia were framed in terms of "response inhibition" or other *non-memory* functions that had little chance of making connections to theories of human amnesia (see chapter 2). Moreover, the cognitive mapping account successfully emphasized the importance of inquiring below the performance level of analysis, helping to point out that the strategies actually used by animals in performing a given task and the nature of the stored information driving their performance play a determining role in preservation versus sparing. Finally, the account certainly captures a large portion of the variance in the rat amnesia data: Spatial learning is an enormously significant aspect of the rat's behavioral repertoire, and there is now little doubt that the hippocampal system plays a critical role in much spatial learning.

However, the O'Keefe and Nadel proposal can only be considered a limited-domain account. The claim they have championed for years, for example as stated in Nadel's (1991) recent "revisiting" of the issue, is that "it is the spatial nature of a given task that determines whether or not hippocampal disruption will influence learning." Yet the evidence we have reviewed here indicates that spatial learning is *not* the only type of learning impaired after hippocampal system damage; and spatial relationships are *not* the only type of relationships for which the hippocampal system plays a critical role. Accordingly, their theory can only apply to a subset of the phenomena to be explained, failing to generalize or to provide an account of the findings across species across the full set of paradigms against which we earlier tested our own account.

We have shown, instead, that the critical variables across paradigms that determine which task variants will be impaired and which will be spared following hippocampal system damage have to do with representational flexibility and relationality no matter whether the to-be-learned materials are spatial—variables that are just not accommodated by the O'Keefe and Nadel account. Moreover, their account fails to accommodate the full scope of anatomical and physiological data against which we tested the procedural-declarative theory offered here. Let us now consider some of the behavioral and anatomical/physiological data that illustrate these points. We will spend a good deal of time on this particular alternative account—more than on the others—because its claims have been spelled out particularly clearly and because it has been the subject of so much discussion.

DNMS Task Performance

In the DNMS task (see figure 7.1), the dependence of performance on remembering the identity of previously presented objects and responding to novel objects (rather than to those already represented in memory) in the match-phase display occurs irrespective of spatial locations or spatial strategies. That is, the critical processing demands made by this task seem to require the ability to perform comparisons between stored representations of the sample-phase objects and the objects present in the match-phase displays, and the ability to use the stored representations of the studied objects when tested with *new* stimulus arrays. The more objects that have to be stored, the more comparisons that have to be made, and the longer the delay interval over which the comparisons must be made, the more sensitive performance is to hippocampal system damage. Accordingly, the critical variables that determine sparing versus loss in this task are *not* spatial ones. Exactly the same state of affairs obtains for recognition memory performance in humans.

Radial-Arm Maze Task Performance

In many or most experimental situations, the radial-arm maze task (see figure 7.4) certainly requires spatial processing, and the cognitive mapping account predicts the observed sensitivity of performance on this task to hippocampal system damage. However, as we have discussed, at least one nonspatial variable is critical in determining whether impaired or intact performance will be observed in amnesic rats, namely, whether the maze arms are baited once on each trial versus never baited across trials. Intact animals are able to learn across trials to avoid entering the never-baited arms, and to enter the once-(per-trial)baited arms only one time per trial. In some experimental environments, animals with hippocampal system damage are able to learn to avoid the never-baited arms, but *not* able to learn to avoid multiple entries into the once-baited arms. The spatial demands of these two conditions are the same. What differs seems to be whether or not animals have to support a continual updating of their representation of which arms were and were not visited earlier in the trial and across trials (i.e., maintaining representations of visited arms for some period, plus computing temporal relationships—comparisons across time), plus whether their representations of the arms are to guide later choices toward or *away* from those arms (i.e., representation flexibility).

Accordingly, while one critical variable in determining the consequences of hippocampal system damage on radial-arm maze performance is indeed the requirement for spatial processing, there are other *nonspatial* variables that determine the full pattern of sparing and loss on this task. Even within some of what are formally categorized as among the spatial learning paradigms under consideration here, then, the spatial mapping hypothesis offers only a limited-domain account.

Conditional and Contextual Discrimination Task Performance

The conditional discrimination work is similarly problematic for the spatial mapping hypothesis. There are deficits on variants of conditional discrimination involving spatial processing (i.e., where discriminative responding is conditional on spatial location) as predicted by the O'Keefe and Nadel account. But there are numerous examples of deficits on other task variants in which discriminative responding is conditional on nonspatial (e.g., *temporal*) contingencies. Two examples documented in chapter 7 are serial feature–positive conditioning, in which animals have to learn that presentation of a specific tone stimulus is followed by food delivery conditional on the tone being preceded by the visual stimulus, and the negative patterning problem, in which a tone or light signifies the availability of reward but the combination of tone plus light signifies the absence of reward (see figure 7.5).

Even in conditional discrimination tasks for which spatial processing is a factor, either impaired or spared learning may result depending on how spatial variables are used. For example, Gaffan and Harrison (1989b) looked at different forms of conditional place-object discrimination in monkeys with fornix lesions and found that the monkeys were impaired in their object discriminations when their choices were conditional on the "place" in which the set of cues were presented within the same background "scene." By contrast, they performed normally when their choices were conditional on the "place" of the monkey in the test area, resulting in different background "scenes" behind cues presented in the same location on each trial (see chapter 7). Again, the spatial mapping hypothesis fails to capture the full pattern of sparing and loss.

Odor Discrimination Learning Performance

The results from our olfactory work are clearly outside the scope of the cognitive mapping hypothesis. The major variable determining impaired versus spared performance following hippocampal system damage is whether the odor cues are presented simultaneously or successively. In the successive odor discrimination task, where the single spatial location for cue presentation and responses precludes any significant spatial processing component, the representations generated during performance by animals with damage to the hippocampal system differed from those generated by intact animals, and hippocampal neurons recorded during performance revealed preferences for nonspatial, temporally defined configurations of stimuli (e.g., S+ preceded by S−). In the simultaneous odor discrimination task, moreover, the representations generated by animals with damage to the hippocampal system differed from normal animals in the extent to which they could be flexibly expressed when presented in novel pairings, despite identical spatial demands for trials involving the standard versus novel pairings. Impairment on simultaneous discrimination in this paradigm and others cannot be attributed to a spatial mapping deficit, because the spatial component of these tasks involves simple left-right positional judgments (as opposed to spatial mapping), and because predictive taxon cues are readily available.

Human Amnesia Work

As has been pointed out by various authors in response to O'Keefe and Nadel's proposal, the pattern of preserved and impaired learning capacities in human amnesia just cannot be accounted for by the spatial mapping account. The critical variables determining why, for a given set of study materials, amnesic patients will show normal performance when tested via repetition priming or skill learning but impaired performance when tested via recall or recognition (see chapter 8) have nothing to do with spatial mapping. Rather, the issue is whether the materials need to be explicitly remembered in a flexible way, or whether instead they need only be expressed in performances that constitute repetitions of the original learning events.

The Graf et al. (1984) example is illustrative once more here. Amnesic patients show either impairment or sparing for the very same words studied in the same way and then tested with the same word-stem cues, depending on whether they are asked to *use* the word-stem cues to help them recall words from the study list or are instead asked to generate the first word that comes to mind completing each word-stem (see chapters 3 and 6). The spatial mapping hypothesis has nothing to say about these findings or, more generally, about the bulk of the enormous body of related work on repetition priming effects (see chapter 8).

Physiological and Anatomical Work

Paralleling the inability of the spatial mapping account to handle the full set of behavioral findings against which we have tested our procedural-declarative theory, the anatomical and physiological data discussed in chapters 4 and 5 require a more comprehensive account than is provided by the O'Keefe and Nadel theory. We have discussed that the anatomical connections of the hippocampal system include the higher-order processing areas for each sensory modality, as well as action and limbic associations areas. Thus, the hippocampal system receives converging inputs representing the outcomes not just of spatial processing—to which the O'Keefe and Nadel account is limited—but of the processing of objects and events of all sorts.

Likewise, the O'Keefe and Nadel account of the physiological data is too restrictive. The discovery that hippocampal neurons have place fields when animals were engaged in spatial exploration was the initial impetus for, and provided strong evidence supporting, the spatial mapping hypothesis (see above and chapter 5). Indeed, these cells were thought to exclusively provide the physiological substrate for representing space. The problem is that, as shown in chapter 5, the same neurons that are activated by animals exploring one or another specific place in the environment are also activated by a variety of nonspatial, task-relevant contingencies and relationships (see figures 5.5 and 5.6). Thus, these neurons are *not* place cells, but rather relational cells that are capable of representing spatial relationships as well as all manner of temporal and configurational relationships among objects, events, and their functional significance.

Disproportionate Involvement in Spatial Learning

The mixture of results on spatial and nonspatial learning described above has led some to ask whether the hippocampal system is only *disproportionately or preferentially*, but not exclusively, involved in spatial learning (Morris, 1991; Nadel et al., 1991; Squire Mishkin, and Shimamura, 1990). While this view is less restrictive and so incorporates all findings, it unfortunately provides little insight about the processing functions or nature of memory representation of the hippocampal system. Taking a view that focuses on "proportionate" involvement in different types of learning necessarily leads one to view processing by the hippocampal system as, for example, 40% "spatial learning" plus 20% "recognition memory" (DNMS) plus 10% "conditional and contextual learning" plus 10% "sensory discrimination," and so on, eventually leading to 3% "timing" (e.g., DRL) and 1% "classical conditioning" (trace conditioning only). Once elaborated this way, it becomes apparent that a characterization based on proportionate involvement is not a theoretical account but merely a numeric summary of the current "spreadsheet" on different categories of findings. It is not a meaningful explanation of hippocampal function in memory.

Our account of the robust and largely consistent findings of deficits in spatial learning after hippocampal system damage is that place learning usually puts a heavy emphasis on relational processing (see chapter 7). The use of Morris water maze, the radial-arm maze, and similar paradigms to compare "spatial" versus "visually cued" learning is deceptive; it is not equivalent to a comparison between, for example, learning guided by visual versus auditory cues. Rather, what is compared in such analyses is learning guided by visual (or other) cues versus learning guided by spatial *relationships* among cues. Consistent with our account, place learning is a powerful example of relational representation in just the way described for the example of water maze learning given above. Thus we have no argument with the cognitive mapping theory of hippocampal function except that, as proposed by O'Keefe and Nadel, this view is limited to the domain of spatial memory. On this point our account of the hippocampal system as supporting a "memory space" (see chapter 3) differs from their view of this system as mediating "spatial memory."

Summary

Consideration of the behavioral, anatomical, and physiological data indicate that the hippocampal system is critically involved in place learning but the spatial mapping theory is a limited-domain account. The behavioral impairment following hippocampal system damage extends well beyond spatial learning; anatomical projections to the hippocampal system provide information from many processing systems in addition to spatial systems; and hippocampal neurons are activated by all manner of relationships among objects and events. Thus, as we have noted elsewhere (Cohen & Eichenbaum, 1991) in considering the O'Keefe and Nadel hypothesis, the hippocampal system "processes whatever critical relations among cues and events it finds in the environment." This is just as required by the procedural-declarative account we have offered, but clearly inconsistent with the spatial mapping hypothesis.

WORKING MEMORY VERSUS REFERENCE MEMORY

Olton and colleagues (1979) have offered an account based on Honig's distinction between working memory, namely the storage of information relevant only for the current trial (and contradictory on others), and reference memory, namely, the storage of information that is consistent across trials and presented repeatedly with the same (reward) contingencies. Performance on tasks depending on reference memory are said to remain intact, while performance on tasks requiring working memory are said to be selectively impaired.

The primary evidence offered in support of this account is the dissociation between performance on once-baited versus never-baited arms in the radial-arm maze task (see figure 7.4). To explain, performance on once-baited arms is dependent on the ability to continually update memory for the arms already visited and the arms not yet visited *on that trial*, and thus is taken to require working memory. Performance on the never-baited arms, by contrast, is dependent on memory for the constant-across-trials contingencies, that is, learning which arms are *always* baited and which *never* baited, and thus is taken to require reference memory. Numerous reports indicating that rats with hippocampal system damage cannot learn to avoid multiple entries into the once-baited arms while nonetheless learning to avoid making entries into the never-baited arms (see chapter 7), has been taken as providing strong support for the working memory–reference memory distinction.

This proposal has provided a powerful account of an increasingly large set of findings with the radial-arm maze task in rats, explaining phenomena that cannot be accommodated by the cognitive mapping hypothesis, against which it has frequently been pitted in empirical tests. The proposal may also be used to understand the impairment caused by hippocampal system damage on the DNMS task in monkeys and recognition memory in humans; both of these tasks could be construed as tapping working memory, in that they too require memory only for a given trial's items on a changing trial-by-trial basis.

However, the proposal has problems with respect to its ability to handle the data from different variants of the radial-arm maze paradigm and in its ability to be extended beyond this paradigm to the others under consideration here. With respect to the radial-arm maze data, we have already noted findings from other investigators that are at odds with the claim of dissociation in performance between once-baited and never-baited arms (see chapter 7). In variants in which perceptually distinctive guidance cues on the maze arms were eliminated, leaving only distal spatial cues to guide performance, both Jarrard et al. (1984) and Leis et al. (1984) found impairment on *both* types of arms. Using Olton's framework, these results suggest impairment of *both* working and reference memory, clearly incompatible with his proposal.

Attempting to extend the proposal outside of the radial-arm maze paradigm proves to be even more problematic. Nearly all of the paradigms we have considered in this book would fit the definition of reference memory according to Olton's framework, and should therefore be spared following hippocampal system damage; yet, as we have discussed at length, they actually show either impairment or sparing depending on the specific task variants chosen. Accordingly, the variables that determine whether impairment or sparing will be seen across this set of task variants are outside the scope of the working memory–reference memory proposal. Several examples are offered to illustrate this conclusion.

Water Maze Task Performance

In the water maze task, the location of the escape platform remains constant across trials. It should therefore be learned through the use of reference memory and should be intact in the face of hippocampal system damage. Yet, on the standard variant of this task, a severe impairment results from hippocampal system damage. We did discuss a variant of the task in which learning does occur, but this variant too is a reference memory task. This pattern of sparing and loss cannot offer any support for the Olton theory because it is clearly determined by variables (whether or not the escape platform is visible to the swimming animal, and whether a constant start location or variable start location was used during training) that are outside the scope of the working memory–reference memory distinction.

Odor Discrimination Learning Performance

In our olfactory discrimination learning work, all of the paradigms would be considered reference memory tasks because the contingencies and relationships to be learned are all held constant across trials: A particular odor or odor-location pairing is always "positive" and another is always "negative." According to the Olton framework, then, they should all be learned normally in animals with hippocampal system damage. Yet we have shown that performance can be either impaired or preserved following hippocampal system damage depending on whether the same odors are presented simultaneously or successively. The variables that determine sparing or loss here are not within the scope of the working memory/reference memory account.

Conditional and Contextual Discrimination Task Performance

The conditional discrimination tasks we have considered involve learning particular conditional relations and their association with reward that remain constant across trials. According to the Olton framework, then, they would be considered reference memory tasks, and would be expected to survive hippocampal system damage. However, we have seen that performance in this paradigm can be markedly impaired following hippocampal system damage and that different variants can produce impairment or sparing depending on the specifics of the task variant chosen. The variables that determine the behavioral outcome, such as the relationship between the discriminative objects and the background stimuli as varied by Gaffan and Harrison (1989b), are clearly beyond the scope of the working memory–reference memory account.

Human Amnesia Work

In human amnesia, too, there are numerous examples of deficits on what would have to be considered reference memory tasks, contrary to the predictions of the working memory–reference distinction. Amnesic patients *cannot* learn the constants in their lives in a normal fashion; patients such as H.M. require an inordinate amount of repetition in order to gain some familiarity with their doctors or caregivers, or to begin to learn their way around a new home or health facility, if they are able to do so at all. Objective testing clearly shows that amnesic patients have profound learning impairments despite constant repetition of the same materials and the same relations across multiple trials.

Consider, for example, Drachman and Arbit's (1966) study of extended digit span. What they did was the following: First they ascertained each subject's digit span. This was accomplished by the standard method of presenting a series of digit strings of increasing length, one at a time, at the rate of one digit per second, with the subject being required to recall the digits in a string in precisely the order as presented. The largest string length that could be reliably recalled was considered the digit span. Then, for each subject, strings were presented that exceeded the digit span, each string being repeated as many times as necessary (up to 25 repetitions) to permit recall. Each time a subject succeeded in recalling a string of a certain length, a new string was presented that was longer by one digit. Using this procedure, with as many as 25 consecutive repetitions of the same string being permitted, normal control subjects could recall strings as long as 20 digits. Yet, H.M. was not able to recall a string of digits even one longer than his 6-digit span, even with 25 consecutive repetitions.

The same conclusion obtains from work with a very similar task in which subjects are again presented with digit strings, each string one digit longer than each individual subject's digit span, and asked to repeat each string exactly as presented. Unbeknownst to the subject, one particular string appears on every third trial. Hebb (1961) had shown that normal subjects exhibited an increase across trials in the likelihood of recalling the recurrent digit string, but no increase over trials in the ability to recall the nonrecurring strings. Using this same method, Corsi (1972) showed that H.M. differed from normal subjects by being unable to take advantage of the repetitions, failing to show an improvement across trials on the recurring string.

Cohen (1981) confirmed this impairment in the same amnesic patients who showed intact acquisition of skilled performance across trials in mirror reading. This contrast between impaired performance on the recurring digits task and intact performance on the mirror reading task was part of what led to proposing the procedural-declarative distinction; it seemed apparent that what was important for determining which aspects of learning would be preserved in amnesia was *not* the repetition or constancy across trials of the same materials but rather what must be remembered and how that material must be represented. No matter how many repetitions are provided or how constant the relations, if what must be remembered are facts and events that reflect the outcomes of processing experiences, then there will be impairment after damage to the hippocampal memory system; yet, normal learning can be achieved by amnesic patients across trials as long as it is based on tuning and shaping of the processors themselves.

One final demonstration of this point that we shall consider here comes from Gabrieli, Cohen, and Corkin's (1988) testing of vocabulary in H.M. They found that H.M. was unable to learn the meanings of a set of 8 unfamiliar words, despite days of repeated testing. Because these results will prove to be important for several issues under discussion in this book, we will describe the experiment and results in some detail. Subjects were trained and tested in the following way: In the initial study phase, they were presented with a list of the 8 words, each with a one-line definition, on a computer display (figure 11.1, top panel). After studying the words and definitions, they were tested with the displays such as the one illustrated in figure 11.2 (left panel). The definitions were presented in a list in random order, with each of the to-be-learned words appearing at the bottom of the screen, one at a time. Subjects were asked for each word, "Which of the definitions in the list goes best with the word at the bottom of the screen?" When correct, the word was replaced with another of the 8 to-be-learned words, and the definition was removed from the list, the list of possible choices thereby being reduced. When incorrect, subjects were told the correct answer, the word was replaced with another, and the definition was removed from the list. This was done for all 8 words. When

LEARN DEFINITIONS

tyro	a beginner in learning
cupidity	inordinate desire for wealth
manumit	to release from slavery
anchorite	one who lives in seclusion
.	.
.	.
.	.
.	.

LEARN SYNONYMS

tyro	novice
cupidity	greed
manumit	emancipate
anchorite	hermit
.	.
.	.
.	.
.	.

Figure 11.1
Items from the definition learning (*top*) and synonym learning (*bottom*) phases of the Gabrieli et al. (1988) vocabulary learning experiment.

correct responses were given to all 8 words on a single trial, the next phase of testing was introduced. For trials on which any errors occurred, however, the testing procedure was repeated with a different random-order listing of the definitions and a new random order of presentation of the words. This procedure was repeated until a fully correct trial was accomplished.

Subjects were then presented with the same 8 words, this time paired with synonyms, as shown in figure 11.1 (bottom panel). After studying the words and synonyms, the next testing phase began. A random-order listing of synonyms, such as that in figure 11.2 (mid-

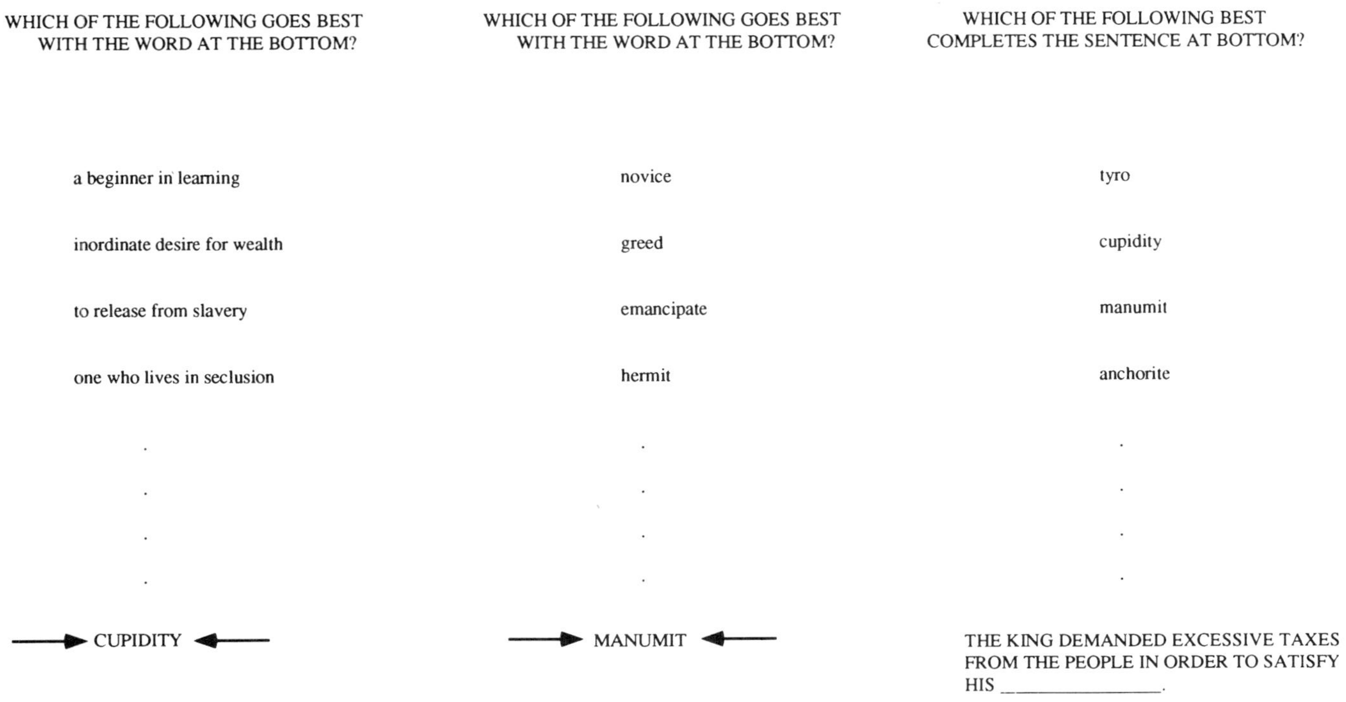

WHICH OF THE FOLLOWING GOES BEST WITH THE WORD AT THE BOTTOM?

a beginner in learning

inordinate desire for wealth

to release from slavery

one who lives in seclusion

. . .

CUPIDITY →

WHICH OF THE FOLLOWING GOES BEST WITH THE WORD AT THE BOTTOM?

novice

greed

emancipate

hermit

. . .

← MANUMIT →

WHICH OF THE FOLLOWING BEST COMPLETES THE SENTENCE AT BOTTOM?

tyro

cupidity

manumit

anchorite

. . .

THE KING DEMANDED EXCESSIVE TAXES FROM THE PEOPLE IN ORDER TO SATISFY HIS _____

Figure 11.2
Testing of vocabulary learning using indirect or implicit methods in the Gabrieli et al. (1988) experiment. (*Left*) Items from definitions test phase. (*Middle*) Items from synonyms test phase. (*Right*) Items from sentence frames test phase.

dle panel), was presented in the center of the computer display, with each of the 8 words appearing one at a time at the bottom of the display. The instructions were parallel to the definition test, this time requesting that subjects indicate which of the listed synonyms "goes best with" the word at the bottom of the display. The procedure was identical to that used in the definition test, involving the presentation of as many trials as necessary for subjects to attain errorless performance.

There was one final test, illustrated in the right panel of figure 11.2, in which the 8 words now appeared in a random-order listing in the center of the display, and sentence frames appeared one at a time at the bottom of the display. Subjects were asked to indicate "which of the words on the list best completes the sentence." The procedure was identical to that used in the definition and synonym tests, involving the presentation of as many trials as necessary for subjects to attain errorless performance.

The results are shown in figure 11.3. Normal subjects learned the new vocabulary words readily, producing errorless choices of definitions within an average of 2.2 trials, of synonyms within 1.9 trials, and of sentence frame completions within 2.3 trials. By contrast, H.M. received 20 trials of definition testing, producing over 200 errors, without showing improvement; then 20 trials of synonym testing, producing over 200 errors, without showing improvement; and then 20 trials of the sentence completion test, again without showing improvement. He just could not learn these words, despite the multiple repetitions of the same materials, with meaning and task contingencies held constant, trial after trial.

This task, like the others we have discussed in this section, clearly falls within the category of reference memory in the Olton framework, and thus should be spared in amnesia; yet, as we have seen, there is profound impairment. Simply providing repeated presentations of the same materials with the same contingencies will not suffice to permit preserved learning in human amnesia if the task requires memory for the relationships among words, definitions, and synonyms, and if it requires the ability to use that knowledge flexibly in the context of unfamiliar sentences. Indeed, in many ways this is a prototypical declarative-memory situation. What must be learned are the arbitrary associations between words and their meanings and synonyms. That is, there is no way to *derive*

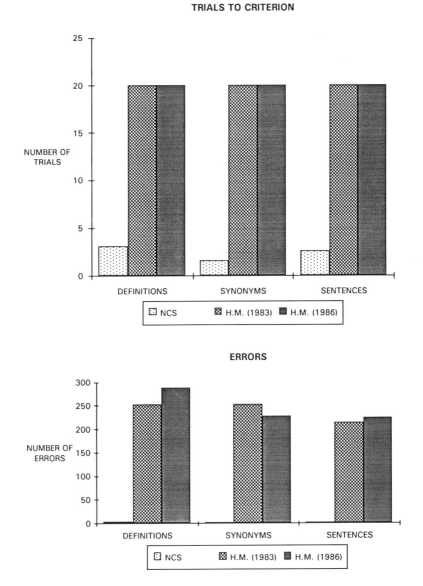

Figure 11.3
Performance of H.M. as compared to control subjects on the tests in figure
11.2, depicted in terms of number of trials to meet the learning criterion
(*top*) and in terms of the number of errors produced (*bottom*). H.M. was
profoundly impaired on both measures for all testing phases. (Data from
Gabrieli et al., 1988.)

that the word that means "a beginner in learning" and that is synonymous with "novice" is *tyro;* there is nothing to do but learn the relationship declaratively. Moreover, using knowledge about words to complete sentence frames requires the representational flexibility of declarative memory.

At the same time, a *single* presentation of material is sufficient to produce normal learning effects under the conditions that obtain for repetition priming effects, that is, when learning can be revealed through a facilitation of performance supported by tuning or biasing of particular processors. The repetition priming effects cannot be considered phenomena of the Olton account's working memory; contrary to its definition as being the storage of information relevant only for the current trial, the priming effects occur across trials within a task and even across tasks (e.g., when the item is seen once in a letter detection task that acts as the study phase and is then repeated some time later in a word-stem completion task that serves as the testing phase). Thus, the sparing of repetition priming in amnesia is not accommodated within the working memory–reference memory hypothesis.

Physiological Work

The activity of hippocampal neurons during behavioral performance does not seem to be consistent with the working memory–reference memory account. Hippocampal cells seem to participate critically in representing all manner of temporal and configurational relationships among objects, events, and their functional significance that remain constant across trials. That is, contrary to the view that the hippocampus is critical for mediating memory necessary only for the current trial and (potentially) contradictory on others, hippocampal neurons manifest stable place fields during and throughout spatial navigation tasks, and exhibit stable encodings of various other relationships that remain unchanged during the course of the other tasks we have considered here.

Summary

The working memory–reference memory distinction is clearly a limited-domain account. Although it does capture much (but not all) of the performance data from rats in the radial-arm maze paradigm, and while it is important in emphasizing the temporal factors that can find no account within the spatial mapping hypothesis, it cannot provide an account of the impaired versus spared performances for the other paradigms with which we have challenged our procedural-declarative theory. This is particularly true for the human amnesia data. Moreover, this account offers no explanation of the growing body of findings from electrophysiological recording studies indicating the stable relational properties of hippocampal neurons.

TEMPORAL BUFFER HYPOTHESIS

Rawlins (1985) has argued that the hippocampal system is a restricted-term ("short-term" or "intermediate-term") memory storage device. It serves to hold information temporarily in a representation that can bridge temporal discontinuities so that the information can be referenced in a subsequent test trial.

Offered as evidence for this view are the deficits seen following hippocampal system damage in: DNMS, where information about the object presented during the sample phase would have to be maintained over the delay interposed before the match phase (and where larger delays cause larger impairment); working memory tasks, where information would have to be maintained across arm entries for the duration of the trial; delayed alternation tasks, in which memory of the previous arm visited has to be maintained during the delay while waiting to visit the alternate arm; and recognition memory tasks in humans, where information presented during a study phase must be maintained over the delay interposed prior to the test phase (and where, again, the size of the deficit is proportional to the length of the delay to be bridged). Rawlins also cited the deficits that follow hippocampal system damage in a variety of timing tasks, such as DRL, where some sort of temporal buffer or "timer" would seem to be required. By contrast, tasks that have no requirement to bridge a lengthy delay interval are performed well by human and animal amnesics.

The temporal component of amnesia is clearly important, and the difference in performance between tasks requiring long-term retention and short-term retention is both well documented and an important part of any serious account of amnesia. Indeed, differences in the persistence of hippocampal-dependent and hippocampal-independent memories is often the primary if not sole source of the dissociation in performance between normal and amnesic subjects. However, this proposal can only be construed as a limited-domain account. The findings we have discussed in earlier sections should make evident the fact that only some types of long-term retention are impaired while others remain preserved, a distinction that has no explanation in the temporal buffer account. That is, the temporal buffer proposal has no account for the variables that determine whether sparing or loss will be seen among the tests requiring long-term retention. Several illustrative examples are provided.

Sensory Discrimination Task Performance

Sensory discriminations are learned gradually across trials, requiring maintenance of stored representations from each trial to the next, thus placing demands on a temporal buffer. Yet different variants of sensory discrimination learning that place identical demands on such a buffer can be either impaired or spared following hippocampal system damage depending on such variables as whether the discriminative stimuli are presented simultaneously or successively, as was seen in our olfactory discrimination work, or the type of pretraining given prior to the start of discrimination learning, as in the reversal learning experiments (see chapter 7).

Radial-Arm Maze Task Performance

In the radial-arm maze work, performance on both the once-baited arms and on the never-baited arms require bridging temporal discontinuities and the maintenance of representations across arm entries. Furthermore, the magnitude of the temporal gap to be bridged is of the same magnitude for both types of arms. Yet the effects of hippocampal system damage are different on these two components of radial-arm maze performance (see chapter 7).

Water Maze Task Performance

Similar issues arise in the water maze work. Different variants of the water maze task, involving the use of a visible escape platform rather than the standard submerged one, and use of a constant start location rather than the standard use of multiple start locations, determine whether hippocampal system damage will result in impaired or intact performance. Yet these variants place identical demands on a temporal buffer.

Human Amnesia Work

Finally, the variables that determine sparing or loss on tests of long-term memory in human amnesic patients cannot be accounted for by the temporal buffer hypothesis. We have shown that performance at a given delay after learning will be either impaired or intact depending on whether the learned material is to be explicitly remembered in a flexible way—as in recall or recognition memory tests, in which case there will be impairment—or whether the material can be expressed in situations that constitute repetitions of the original learning events—as in repetition priming effects and skill learning, in which case there will be intact performance. These two classes of performance must bridge the same delays and would place the same demands on a temporal buffer, yet fare differently after hippocampal system damage.

Physiological Work

The phenomenon of LTP might be taken as supportive of the temporal buffer account, providing evidence that the hippocampus has a mechanism for maintaining information over a temporary period. However, the activity of hippocampal neurons during behavioral performance is not consistent with the temporal buffer account. Hippocampal neurons clearly develop and maintain stable place fields during and throughout spatial navigation tasks, and exhibit stable encodings of various other relationships that remain unchanged throughout the course of the other tasks we have considered here, well beyond the time span of the proposed temporal buffer. The relationships and contingencies coded by the activity of hippocampal neurons reflect the participation of the hippocampal system in building representations from the accumulation of various processing events, and permitting the use of these representations in flexible ways, a view that has no place within the temporal buffer hypothesis.

Summary

Notwithstanding the importance of temporal parameters in characterizing amnesia *within the domain of memory that is impaired,* in order to understand and predict which behavioral performances will be impaired and which spared after hippocampal system damage, we need more than description of temporal parameters and temporal limitations (see Cohen & Shapiro, 1985). Rawlins, too, has recently moved in this direction (Gray & Rawlins, 1986). What is required is an explanation of how "memory" is capable of bridging temporal gaps in some circumstances but not in others, or, said differently, why some tasks or performances place large demands on a temporal-buffer capacity while others do not. Such an account must inevitably turn to issues of representation—what is the nature of the representations that permit the bridging of temporal gaps, and how does it differ from the representations that apparently degrade so rapidly in amnesic patients? This is what the procedural-declarative account offers.

CONFIGURAL, CONDITIONAL, AND CONTEXTUAL HYPOTHESES

Three related proposals about hippocampal-dependent memory speak to the involvement of the hippocampal system in the processing of and memory for specific types of relationship among the test stimuli or between those stimuli and the context in which they appear. In the *configural association theory*, Sutherland and Rudy (1989) posited that perceptually distinct stimuli are combined by the hippocampal system into "configural" stimuli; the association of these stimuli with reinforcement is used to support performances that cannot be mediated by unambiguous association with individual stimulus elements. Hirsh (1974, 1980) argued that the hippocampal system supports conditional logic operations by mediating the learning of *conditional cues*—cues whose significance is determined by the presence of additional "contextual" stimuli. Winocur's (1980) *stimulus selection theory* (or *contextual hypothesis*) held that the hippocampal system is critical in learning situations requiring the disambiguation of behaviorally relevant stimuli from background contextual cues. These ideas are considered in turn.

Configural Association Theory

This account was offered by Sutherland and Rudy (1989) to explain their results on the negative patterning problem, in which rats were trained to treat the presence of a tone alone or a light alone as a positive stimulus, but of a tone and light together as a negative stimulus (see middle panel of figure 7.5). Rats with hippocampal system damage were unable to learn this conditional discrimination task. Sutherland and Rudy's interpretation was that an intact hippocampal system is required to create a configural representation of the two stimuli, permitting the joint presentation of the two stimuli to be treated as a unique stimulus distinct from either of the two stimuli presented separately. In the absence of this configural system, animals for whom each of the individual stimuli had acquired strong rewarding value would be unable to withhold responses to the joint presentation of the stimuli.

This account can be extended to the other examples of conditional discrimination learning discussed earlier. Thus, in the serial feature—positive conditioning task (Ross et al., 1984; see top panel of figure 7.5), the finding that animals with hippocampal system damage could not learn to associate a tone CS to a food US *conditional* on the tone being preceded by a visual stimulus could be explained by assuming that such animals were unable to form a configural of the visual-stimulus-plus-tone and thus unable to separate conditioning to the tone alone from conditioning to the tone preceded by the visual stimulus. Similarly, in Gaffan and Harrison's (1989b) place-object discrimination (an example of the contextual discriminations discussed in chapter 7; see bottom panel of figure 7.5), the failure of monkeys to learn to make their discriminative responding conditional on the spatial location of the stimulus objects relative to their own position could be attributed to an inability to form configurals of the objects in one spatial position versus the objects in the other spatial position. In both cases, an ability to create configurals that literally combine the discriminanda and conditional cues would serve to remove the need for performing conditional logic operations (see discussion of representational and processing demands of conditional discrimination learning in chapter 7). To the extent that such a strategy is advantageous to performance and is mediated by the hippocampal system, animals with hippocampal system damage would be impaired relative to controls.

There are two serious problems with this account. The first problem is that although Sutherland and Rudy have attempted to extend the proposal beyond the initial paradigms of interest to them, it remains a limited-domain account. For example, Sutherland and

Rudy attempted to extend their account by arguing that the hippocampal system mediates place learning by constructing distinct
configural cues out of combinations of visual cues that are seen
from specific locations and orientations in the environment. According to this account, intact animals learn a specific and unambiguous approach response for each of the views it has previously
associated with reinforcement or nonreinforcement. However, the
configural association theory remains limited in the scope of the
coverage it can provide. In particular, it can offer no explanation of
the representational flexibility exhibited by hippocampal-dependent
memory but not by hippocampal-independent memory in novel
testing situations, including, for example, those commonly experienced in spatial learning. The ability of normal animals, but not
animals with hippocampal system damage, to find the escape platform from novel starting positions after training in Eichenbaum
et al.'s (1990) constant-start-location variant of the water maze has
no explanation within the configural association theory. Likewise,
the fact that, after being presented with a list of study items, normal
human subjects can express their learning in a variety of novel
testing situations (e.g., recalling or recognizing the items, making
judgments based on the studied items, and recollecting the training experiences) but amnesic patients can only express their learning or memory of the materials in a repetition of the initial learning
situation (as in repetition priming) has no explanation within the
configural association theory. The same conclusion follows from
consideration of the other paradigms discussed here, as well.

The second problem is that, contrary to Sutherland and Rudy's
proposal, it is in the *absence* of the hippocampal system that animals fuse perceptual distinct stimuli into configurals, at least in
some circumstances. As noted in chapter 7, animals with hippocampal system damage seem to "fuse" multiple cues into compounds, or configurals, at times when intact animals do not. Thus,
the context-shift experiments of Winocur and colleagues (Winocur
& Gilbert, 1984; Winocur & Mills, 1970; Winocur & Olds, 1978)
suggest that animals with hippocampal system damage fuse contextual cues with the differentially rewarded stimuli in discrimination learning. Such animals show increased conditioning to the
background (contextual) cues and are abnormally sensitive to context shifts. Similarly, our own work on olfactory discrimination

learning in rats (e.g., Eichenbaum et al., 1989) and Saunders and Weiskrantz's (1989) study of object discrimination learning in monkeys suggest the fusing of the discriminative stimuli into compound (or configural) cues following hippocampal system damage: These animals were impaired when the stimuli were unpaired or re-paired. Thus, contrary to the Sutherland and Rudy account, the hippocampal system is required in order to treat the learned materials as anything *other than* configurals.

The ability of the hippocampal system to support the flexible use of representations of the originally studied cues and the relationships among them, required for the probe-test performances of normal animals in the Eichenbaum et al. and Saunders and Weiskrantz studies, follows from the *compositionality* of declarative representation. As discussed in chapter 3, the relational quality of declarative memory permits representation simultaneously of both the individual cues that were constituent elements of the original event or scene and the across-cues relationships that characterize the scene or event. Such ideas have no counterpart in the configural association theory.

Learning of Conditional Cues or Contextual Labels

Hirsh's (1974, 1980) view of hippocampal-dependent memory, like that of Sutherland and Rudy, started with findings of impairment on conditional discrimination tasks following hippocampal system damage. His claim, however, was that the hippocampal system actually supports conditional logic operations rather than the reduction of such problems through storage of configurals. The hippocampal system was said to be responsible for learning and storage of conditional cues or contextual labels. On this view, the conditional-discrimination deficit of animals with hippocampal system damage follows from their inability to form and store representations of the critical conditional relationships—the conditionalizing of the tone-food association in the serial feature–positive task on the tone being preceded by a visual stimulus; the conditionalizing of reward to the tone or light in the negative patterning task on the stimuli being presented individually rather than jointly. Hirsh cited the failure of rats with hippocampal system damage to learn to "go left" to get food when hungry and "go right" to drink when thirsty (Hirsh et al., 1979; Hsiao & Isaacson, 1971) as an example of the failure to represent the conditional relationship between motivational context and responses leading to reward.

In attempting to extend this account beyond the conditional discrimination task, Hirsh (1974) applied it to the common finding of reversal-learning deficits in animals with hippocampal system damage. On his account, the acquisition of the initial discrimination can be mediated by a stimulus-response system operating independently of the hippocampal system, but learning to reverse the just-learned associations requires the application of contextual labels to *old* versus *current* cue-valences, a capacity provided only by an intact hippocampal system. Animals with hippocampal system damage cannot use such contextual labels and can acquire the reversal only by first extinguishing the old associations and then learning the new ones through the intact stimulus-response system. This two-stage process would require many more trials than learning based on contextual labeling, thus accounting for the slower reversal learning of animals with hippocampal system damage.

Unfortunately, such an account cannot be extended to the other paradigms with which we have challenged our own view and the others. That is, while the emphasis placed by this account on the representation of conditional and cue-context relationships mirrors the stress our own account places on relational representation, it is limited to just that set of relationships. Accordingly, it is difficult to see how a proposed deficit in representing conditional cues or storing contextual labels would account for the full range of sparing and loss following hippocampal system damage in the DNMS, radial-arm maze, and water maze tasks, or in the tasks used with human amnesic patients, in which the critical variables have little if anything to do with conditional relationships. For example, the critical variables determining sparing or loss following hippocampal system damage in DNMS are the importance of the non-match requirement, the number of to-be-remembered objects, and the length of the delay period; in our olfactory learning work, it is whether the very same odor stimuli are presented successively or simultaneously; on the radial-arm maze, it is whether performance is being assessed on the once-baited or never-baited arms. None of these receive an explanation within Hirsh's theory.

More generally, we have shown that across the different paradigms, a critical variable determining whether hippocampal system damage will produce sparing or loss is whether the information must be represented in a flexible way to permit its expression in novel testing situations or whether, instead, the representation need only support performance in repetitions of the original learning situation. This variable—central to our procedural-declarative account—has no explanation in the conditional cue account.

Stimulus Selection Theory or Contextual Hypothesis

Winocur (1980) has posited a critical role for the hippocampal system in disambiguating behaviorally relevant stimuli from background contextual cues. Three major findings about the performance of rats with hippocampal system damage have been cited in support of this idea: Such animals showed normal learning of an instrumental visual discrimination but were impaired in relearning the discrimination in an environmental context different from that of original acquisition; demonstrated abnormal negative transfer when the same discrimination problem was presented in a new environment; and outperformed normal animals in reversing a discrimination learned in a different context while impaired at the same reversal when learned in the same context as the original discrimination. Each of these findings was taken to indicate that rats with hippocampal system damage give too much weight to salient but unimportant cues that distract behavior away from correct performance. It would seem that animals with hippocampal system damage show conditioning to the entire cue-context compound.

Extending this account, Winocur cited demonstrations of deficient latent inhibition, overshadowing, and blocking by animals with hippocampal damage in classical conditioning paradigms (cf. Solomon et al., 1986). In the latent inhibition paradigm, animals are repeatedly pre-exposed to a stimulus without reinforcement before training with the same stimulus as the conditioned stimulus. Acquisition of training in normal but not hippocampal-damaged animals is retarded by CS pre-exposure (Solomon & Moore, 1975). Blocking and overshadowing are related paradigms in which certain stimuli normally come to predominate over others owing to prior exposure. In blocking, animals are trained in two stages, initially with a single CS and later with a compound stimulus including the original CS. In later testing with individual stimuli, normal animals but not those with hippocampal damage, respond weakly to the CS presented only in the second training stage (Rickert et al., 1978; Solomon, 1977). In the overshadowing procedure, animals are trained on a discrimination of compound cues containing a common element. In later testing with individual stimulus elements, normal animals, but not animals with hippocampal damage, respond poorly to the common element (Rickert et al., 1979; Wagner, 1968). In each of these paradigms, animals with hippocampal system damage demonstrated an inability to perceive as irrelevant poorly predictive contextual stimuli.

Winocur's account provides a framework for understanding a variety of data about the influence of context and of contextual manipulations on the pattern of sparing and loss in amnesia, data that have not been accommodated by other major theories of amnesia. Furthermore, the "fusing" together of the discriminative and contextual cues in animals with hippocampal system damage, from Winocur's account, would produce an example of the inflexible memory representation that we have attributed to subjects forced to rely on procedural systems. However, this can only be considered a limited-domain account of amnesia. By emphasizing the representation of a particular type of relationship (in this case, between the discriminative stimuli and the background contextual cues), Winocur's account is mute on the wide range of other relationships whose representation is central to performance on the other paradigms we have considered here, and that are accommodated by our procedural-declarative account. Those other relationships include the spatial relationships among distal cues necessary for performance on the radial-arm maze and water maze tasks, and the temporal relationships among successively presented (or sampled) cues in the radial-arm maze, in DNMS, and in the successive-cue variant of the olfactory discrimination learning task. Furthermore, it cannot offer any generally applicable understanding of the issue of flexible versus inflexible representations we have shown to be so central to the human amnesia findings. As a consequence, it just cannot provide an account of the full pattern of sparing and loss following hippocampal system damage.

Summary

The three hypotheses succeed in capturing an important aspect of hippocampal function, and thus provide an account of some of the amnesia data, by attributing representation of conditional and contextual relationships to the hippocampal system. Clearly, this is an important function of the hippocampal system. By focusing on only some of the relationships that the procedural-declarative account ascribes to hippocampal functioning, however, these proposals constitute limited-domain accounts. As we have indicated above, they fail to provide an account of the full pattern of spared versus impaired performances in amnesia. Furthermore, they offer no explanation of the physiological findings of hippocampal encoding of all sorts of relationships among multiple stimuli and of the functional or behavioral significance of those stimuli. These relationships, too, are part of hippocampal representation, as described in the procedural-declarative account we have offered.

MEMORY OR REPRESENTATIONAL MEMORY VERSUS HABIT OR DISPOSITIONAL MEMORY

The final account to be considered here actually comprises two proposals, one from Mishkin and colleagues (Mishkin & Petri, 1984; Mishkin et al., 1984) and the other from Thomas (1984), that are sufficiently similar to consider them jointly. This account has distinguished between a memory system that permits comparison of available cues to some representation of other cues that were experienced previously but are not actually present during performance, and a system that supports classical and instrumental conditioning of stimulus-stimulus or stimulus-response contingencies and that thereby accomplishes the development of "habits" or "dispositions."

This account has not been explicated in terms of the characteristics and distinguishing features of the two systems in the way the other accounts have; that is, they are not described in representational or processing terms. Mishkin has made the point that this proposal is fundamentally similar to Hirsh's proposal, although he offers no explanation of the ways in which this is and is not so. If the accounts really are to be considered as having the same processing and performance implications, then we need go no further in evaluating this proposal, as we have already considered Hirsh's account, above. However, the nature and extent of the similarity are not clear to us, so we shall proceed to evaluate it on its own terms. Unfortunately, it has not been applied to the paradigms we have considered here; thus, we shall have to evaluate it somewhat differently than we have the other alternative accounts.

What seems to be the case is that the "habit" or "dispositional memory" system is viewed as being equivalent to the kind of learning system proposed by conditioning theorists, whereas the "memory" or "representational memory" system is seen as having whatever features cognitive theorists attribute to memory. Mishkin and Thomas see the habit system or dispositional memory as either not a memory system at all or as a nonrepresentational memory system. But how can a system that guides increasingly skilled or well-adapted performances as a function of experience not be a memory system? How exactly can a system accomplish experience-dependent change in behavioral performance in the absence of some representation of (or caused by) previous experience? We have discussed in chapter 3 several examples of modifications of brain physiology and brain wiring that are illustrative of phenomena we would attribute to our procedural memory system and that this alternative proposal would presumably attribute to their nonmemory or nonrepresentational system. Surely these brain alterations reflect (or constitute the neural substrates of) memory for—and, indeed, are some form of representation of—previous training experiences, every bit as much as are the brain changes that occur in more "cognitive" or "representational" or declarative memory–dependent performances. Yet, this alternative approach would seem to preclude considering such brain alterations as being the same as, or being described with the same vocabulary as, the changes representative of their "memory" or "representational memory" system.

A consequence of this position is that it becomes impossible to ask such crucial questions as: What is it about hippocampal representation or hippocampal-dependent memory that distinguishes it from non-hippocampal-dependent memory representations? And, What is it about the hippocampal system that results in its mediating one but not the other of these types of memory representation? These questions have been at the heart of our entire presentation in this book, and, we think, have been answered in the procedural-declarative theory we have offered here. In contrast, by distinguishing between some kind of cognitive-representational memory system and some noncognitive-nonrepresentational memory (or nonmemory) system, this alternative account would seem to be at something of a dead end, in terms of connecting the proposal to anatomical and physiological data and to the other categories of performance data we have considered at length here. With regard to the latter, in the absence of some statement about the characteristics and properties of their two systems, it is not possible to see how the two systems support various behavioral performances and how the specific pattern of sparing and loss that results from hippocampal system damage can be understood (except by reference to learning and forgetting rate characteristics—Mishkin et al., 1984, pp. 71–74).

Our discomfort about this alternative account is greatest when considering the human amnesia data. It is difficult to see how a stimulus-response conditioning account of word priming or category exemplar priming could be generated, much less an account of cognitive skill learning. That is, it is not clear how facilitation in reading or naming, or a biasing in generating category exemplars, could occur following a single exposure to words or line drawings without some representation (we think a procedural memory representation) of the stimuli presented earlier.

Summary and an Observation

This account has some superficial similarity with the procedural-declarative account we have offered and has been cited in conjunction with the earlier statements of the procedural-declarative distinction on many occasions by a variety of authors. Certainly, declarative memory is the kind of memory that best captures the layperson's use of the term, as we indicated in chapter 3. Hence, the use of the term *memory* for one of the dissociated systems may well be seen to capture the same phenomena as we ascribe to declarative memory. Moreover, the repetition priming effects and skill learning phenomena that we claim to be mediated by procedural memory have something of the feel of "dispositions" or "habits." Thus, at a purely descriptive level, the terms used in this account map fairly comfortably onto the procedural-declarative account. Yet, this surface similarity does not extend to the content of the accounts.

12 Comparing the Theory to Other Accounts: Human Amnesia

We turn now to a comparison of the procedural-declarative theory with alternative proposals from the human amnesia literature. The nature of the proposals we will consider, and consequently the way in which we will consider them, differs significantly from our treatment of the animal model literature in chapter 11. Most of the competing proposals that we considered in that treatment were alternative dichotomizations of memory, each concerned primarily with a limited subset of the data on spared versus impaired learning performances after hippocampal system damage. For each of the proposals, we systematically evaluated its ability to extend to the data from each of the major paradigms, from both the human and animal model literatures, as well as to handle the anatomical and physiological findings. The competing proposals from the human amnesia literature, however, differ from those in chapter 11 in ways that make it difficult to evaluate them in the same way. They all attempt to address the basic behavioral dissociation between sparing and loss, rather than being limited to individual paradigms; they almost universally ignore the animal models (it is, after all, human amnesia—not rat or monkey amnesia—that they wish to understand) and make no contact with the anatomical or physiological data; and are explicated largely without discussion of the representational or processing characteristics entailed. Also, many of the proposals are related intimately to various aspects of the procedural-declarative theory articulated here.

Accordingly, after discussing the semantic-episodic memory distinction, which will be treated much like the accounts in chapter 11, we will spend most of our time indicating the ways in which the alternative accounts differ from the procedural-declarative theory, and the implications of those differences in terms of the data for which they cannot provide coverage.

SEMANTIC VERSUS EPISODIC MEMORY

Tulving (1972) proposed a distinction between *episodic* memory, containing autobiographical records of personally experienced events occurring in specifiable temporal and spatial contexts, and *semantic* memory, consisting of world knowledge stored in a context-free fashion. This account of normal human memory (and further elaborations of it: Tulving, 1983, 1985, 1987) has been applied by a number of different investigators to the pattern of impairment and sparing in amnesic patients, with the claim that amnesia represents a selective impairment of episodic memory (e.g., Cermak, 1982; Kinsbourne, 1987; Kinsbourne & Wood, 1975; Parkin, 1987; Schacter & Tulving, 1982, 1983; Tulving, 1983, 1984, 1985; Wood, Ebert & Kinsbourne, 1982). This view of amnesia followed first from the characterization of amnesic patients as demonstrating intact knowledge about the world, including preserved language, perceptual, and social skills, and spared general intelligence, while suffering from profoundly impaired memory for their day-to-day events, their recent history, and even their current whereabouts. It followed secondly from the observation that the tests of new learning on which amnesic patients fail so badly in the laboratory almost invariably probe episodic memory, for example, in requiring recall or recognition of the items presented during some previous learning *episode;* whereas the examples of preserved learning, such as skill learning and repetition priming, all involve the expression of memory in a manner that does *not* require recollection of previous episodes.

Although attractive in many ways, this account cannot accommodate the full range of impaired versus spared performances considered in this book. This is particularly true for the paradigms in the animal model literature, where the critical variables determining sparing versus loss are just not accommodated within the semantic-episode framework. In the water maze task, the critical variable discussed earlier was whether the start location was held constant or was variable across trials; in the radial-arm maze task, the critical variable was whether performance was assessed for once-baited or never-baited arms; in our olfactory discrimination learning work, performance was spared or impaired depending on whether the very same odor stimuli were presented successively or simultaneously; and in other discrimination learning work, profound impairments were seen on many conditional discrimination tasks but not *un*conditional discrimination tasks. There is no account of any of these variables within the semantic-episodic proposal.

Turning to the human amnesia data, the semantic-episodic account fails to capture the basic features of spared versus impaired memory abilities, as we have discussed elsewhere (Cohen, 1984; Gabrieli, Cohen, & Corkin, 1988; Squire & Cohen, 1984; Zola-Morgan, Cohen, & Squire, 1983). Consider the first claim of support for the semantic-episodic account cited above, namely that amnesic patients show intact world knowledge but impaired memory for the events of daily life. The problem with this is that it confounds semantic and episodic memory with premorbid and postmorbid memory. Semantic memory here refers to the information that supports performance on intelligence tests, or on tests of naming, language, or perceptual skills; these are all memories that are acquired premorbidly—before the onset of amnesia. Indeed, such memories are acquired rather early in life, long before amnesia onset. By contrast, episodic memory here refers to memory for recent daily events, information that is exclusively postmorbid (after the onset of amnesia) and thus susceptible to anterograde amnesia. When semantic and episodic memory are both assessed within *either* the anterograde (postmorbid) *or* the retrograde (premorbid) domain, the claimed pattern of sparing and loss seems to break down. Amnesic patients have frequently been reported to exhibit retrograde loss of memory for personal events *and* for world knowledge, the latter in the form of memory for public events or the identity of famous persons (see discussion in Butters & Albert, 1982; Kopelman, 1989; MacKinnon & Squire, 1989; Ostergaard, 1987; Zola-Morgan et al., 1983). Likewise, H.M.'s anterograde amnesia was shown to cause impairment in learning not only about his daily activities but also about such prototypically semantic information as new vocabulary[1] (Gabrieli et al., 1988; see chapter 11 of this book for details).

The second claim offered in support of the semantic-episodic account was that the difference between preserved and impaired memory performances revolved around whether they required recollection of previous learning episodes. That is, examples of preserved memory performances, such as skill learning and repetition priming effects, were said to reflect performance facilitation without requiring explicit access to memory for particular episodes; and this in turn was taken as reflecting the influence of a preserved semantic memory. This claim is also problematic. Skill learning and repetition priming in amnesic patients do indeed reflect performance facilitations that occur in the absence of memory for the learning experiences. But attributing such phenomena to the operation of a preserved semantic memory and damaged episodic memory does not conform with the evidence. Amnesic patients are profoundly impaired on other tasks that fit this definition of semantic memory, in which performance need not depend on getting access to previous learning episodes. The deficit shown by H.M. in learning new vocabulary (Gabrieli et al., 1988), is particularly illuminating here. In that study, as we discussed in chapter 11, vocabulary-learning performance was measured indirectly or implicitly: On repeated trials he was asked to indicate which definitions or common synonyms "went best with" one or another of the new vocabulary words, or to indicate which of the new vocabulary words "went best with" sentence frames. At no time was he required to recollect the previous training experiences with the words or in any other way gain access to any previous learning episode. Rather, learning was taken to be any increase in matching or completion success. Yet his performance was profoundly impaired (see figure 11.3). Indeed, it was concluded that he "could not learn, in a laboratory setting, the meaning of any word that he did not already know" (Gabrieli et al., 1988, p. 161).

Accordingly, either impairment or sparing can occur on tests of semantic memory; the variables determining whether impairment or sparing will be observed across these different tasks are outside the scope of the semantic-episodic account. It is noteworthy that in more recent work by Tulving together with Schacter (e.g., Schacter, 1990a; Schacter et al., 1990; Tulving & Schacter, 1990) the (perceptually based) repetition priming phenomena preserved in amnesia has been attributed to the *perceptual representation system* (PRS), a system that is neither semantic nor episodic. We shall return to their PRS proposal later in this chapter.

The criticism leveled at the semantic-episodic distinction concerns only its potential applicability to sparing and impairment of memory in amnesia. Stepping aside from consideration of the phenomenology of amnesia, the distinction between semantic and episodic memory may well be useful in articulating a full taxonomy of memory systems, an agenda expressed most clearly by Tulving (1983, 1985, 1987). Thus, we and others (Cermak et al., 1985; Cohen, 1984; Schacter & Tulving, 1983; Squire, 1986, 1987; Squire & Zola-Morgan, 1991) have suggested that semantic and episodic memory may be considered as components of the declarative memory system, and thus both distinguishable from procedural memory. Tulving (1987) and Kinsbourne (1987) have each offered different formulations of the relationship between semantic, episodic, and procedural memory. More work and debate on these issues should be expected.

EXPLICIT VERSUS IMPLICIT MEMORY

The distinction between explicit and implicit memory offered by Schacter and Graf (Graf & Schacter, 1985; Schacter, 1987b; Schacter & Graf, 1986) revolves around whether or not conscious recollection of a "prior study episode" is necessary for memory performance. Tests of explicit memory depend on conscious recollection of the learning event, and refer the subject to some particular study episode or learning event (e.g., in the query: What did you have for breakfast yesterday?, or in the instructions for a multiple-choice recognition memory test: Which of the following items did you see on the previous list?). Tests of implicit memory refer subjects to some processing task (e.g., What is the first word that comes to mind that completes the stem *mot____*?, or Generate the first several exemplars that come to mind of the category *vehicles*), and then measure the extent to which previous exposure to the to-be-tested stimulus materials changes the speed or accuracy of performance on the processing task; no conscious recollection of the learning event is required. As applied to amnesia, the claim is that amnesia is a selective deficit of explicit memory, leaving implicit memory fully intact.

As a description, the above captures the essence of the dissociation between impaired and spared memory abilities. Indeed, from our earliest statements of the procedural-declarative account (Cohen, 1981, 1984; Cohen et al., 1985), we have characterized procedural memory as being represented implicitly in the various processors, and declarative memory as being based on explicit representations and entailing explicit remembering. However, we have then gone on to outline a theory of the nature of the procedural and declarative representations that support spared and impaired memory performances, respectively, and of how the hippocampal system supports (and gives rise to the critical features of) declarative memory.

Unfortunately, the explicit-implicit memory distinction, as proposed, offers no theory about or characterization of multiple memory systems. It is less a proposal about memory systems than it is a statement of the conditions necessary, or the tests best suited, for eliciting the dissociable memory performances. It speaks about different kinds of memory only in the sense of saying that there exists one kind of memory that is elicited with explicit tests, namely, when directed toward conscious recollection of the learning event, and another kind of memory that is elicited with implicit tests, that is, when directed away from conscious recollection. This observation that the explicit-implicit memory distinction is really about memory *measures* and not about memory systems has been made by a number of authors; it was made particularly persuasively by Richardson-Klavehn and Bjork (1988), who suggested that it would be more useful to distinguish between direct tests of memory and indirect tests of memory.

Accordingly, the explicit-implicit distinction cannot really be evaluated with respect to all of the data with which we have challenged the procedural-declarative theory and the other alternative accounts. With the criterial difference in explicit versus implicit memory tasks being whether or not the subject is directed toward using and depends on conscious recollection, there is no obvious way to apply it to the animal model data. For the procedural-declarative theory, by contrast, we intentionally articulated the representational characteristics of the two memory systems in such a way as to permit the theory to be extended to animal model data. Similarly, the explicit memory–implicit memory proposal, other than to ascribe, without explanation, explicit memory functions to the hippocampal system, makes absolutely no contact with the anatomical and physiological data we have considered.

Finally, even as a description of the dissociable memory phenomena in human amnesia, the explicit-implicit memory distinction is problematic. The criterion of whether or not the subject is directed toward using and depends on conscious recollection is not adequate to correctly categorize all of the behavioral data we have considered. Let us give two examples. The first is the Gabrieli et al. (1988) vocabulary-learning study that we discussed in the preceding section and in chapter 11. Subjects were given implicit memory test instructions conforming perfectly with the explicit-implicit memory framework. They were directed away from conscious recollection of the previous learning events, and memory was assessed in terms of any improvement in performance across multiple trials. Yet H.M.'s performance was profoundly impaired. The second is the studies of priming for word pairs, in which the performance of amnesic patients does not measure up to the performance of normal controls. The key feature of both of these tasks, according to the procedural-declarative theory, is that relationships between (nonderivable pairings of) perceptually distinct items must be learned—between the vocabulary words and their meanings or synonyms, in the first case, and between the arbitrarily paired words, in the second case. The ability to learn such relationships depends uniquely on hippocampal-mediated declarative memory, and thus would be expected to be impaired in amnesic patients *no matter whether direct or indirect tests of memory are employed.* The finding that there is indeed impairment, even with indirect tests of memory, supports the procedural-declarative theory, but it is in conflict with the explicit-implicit memory distinction. There is an interesting irony here in thinking about declarative memory as being the kind of memory assessed directly and procedural memory as the kind of memory assessed indirectly. From the perspective of how we interact with our environment—process information, comprehend objects and events in the world, and act on the world—the mapping of procedural-declarative memory onto indirect-direct is exactly reversed. Procedural memory has a direct influence on our processing and action systems, and is elicited directly by a given processing task. By contrast, declarative memory has only an indirect effect on our processing and actions, mediated by the representations stored in declarative memory and by the various processes (and processors) that act upon them.

COGNITIVE MEDIATIONAL OR EVALUATIVE MEMORY HYPOTHESIS

Warrington and Weiskrantz (1982) and Baddeley (1982) have suggested that impairments are observed on those tasks for which it is *not* sufficient to have an incremental facilitation of performance, but rather requires what Weiskrantz (1978) called "conscious remembering" or what Baddeley (1982) (and, earlier, William James, 1890; see Cohen et al., 1985) called "recollection." It is exactly this type of memory phenomenon that we mean by "explicit remembering" (Cohen, 1984; Cohen et al., 1985), which we see as following from the fundamental nature of declarative memory, and that Schacter (Graf & Schacter, 1985; Schacter, 1987b; Schacter & Graf, 1986) means by "explicit memory" (see above). On Warrington and Weiskrantz's (1982) view, this type or quality of memory results from the operation of a *cognitive mediational system* which permits information to be "manipulated, interrelated, and stored in a continually changing record of events" (p. 242). The disconnection of this system from other—particularly semantic memory—systems is what causes amnesic deficits. Baddeley's (1982) very similar view is that amnesic deficits reflect an impairment in *evaluative memory*, which ordinarily provides the means for accessing, evaluating, and effortfully manipulating stored information.

These views are quite similar to our notion of the declarative memory system. More than anything else, what distinguishes our account from theirs is that whereas they attribute the ability to manipulate and interrelate memories to the operation of a special frontal-lobe "cognitive mediational system" on input from various neocortical knowledge systems, we attribute it to the representational characteristics of declarative memory. We have emphasized the *input* to the declarative system, consisting of the *outcomes* of the various processing modules, the *features* of declarative representation, namely *flexibility and promiscuity*, and the *relational organization* of declarative memory. The ability to flexibly manipulate and interrelate stored information is a property of declarative representation; together with the ability of this information to be promiscuously accessed by all manner of processes, it gives rise to the ability to consciously or explicitly remember previous learning episodes and their processing outcomes. While systems in the frontal lobe are certainly involved in cognitively mediated behaviors, on our account it is only one of the systems to which declarative memory is promiscuously accessible, and only one of the systems that can partake of the relational character of hippocampal-mediated declarative memory.

The notion we have advanced is that the anatomical and physiological properties of the hippocampal system and the resulting characteristics of declarative memory are what tie all of the behavioral work to all of the neuroscientific data. The alternative proposals by Warrington and Weiskrantz and by Baddeley make no contact with these other data about the hippocampal system.

Our account also offers some idea about the properties of memory that are spared in amnesia—procedural memory. The procedural-declarative theory offers a representational description of this other form of memory that can explain why it survives amnesia. It describes the *in*flexibility and dedicatedness of procedural representations, that are dedicated to the particular processing modules whose tuning and modification provide its substrate. In the absence of representational flexibility, procedural representations cannot be expressed in novel testing situations but rather only in repetitions of the original learning situation, providing an account of the dissociation between impaired explicit remembering and spared acquisition and expression of skilled performance. This level of explanation is not part of the cognitive mediational account.

DECLARATIVE VERSUS NONDECLARATIVE MEMORY

In Squire's recent writings (Squire, 1987, 1992; Squire & Zola-Morgan, 1991), there has been a movement away from the original procedural-declarative formulation toward a view in which declarative memory is distinguished from a collection of capacities collectively labeled *nondeclarative*. This move was prompted by findings that some of the various types of memory performances spared in amnesia can be dissociated in the memory disturbances seen in other patient populations, such as in Alzheimer's or Huntington's disease (Gabrieli, 1991; Heindel et al., 1988, 1989). To the extent that this serves to remind us that dichotomizing memory into procedural and declarative systems is just a step in the process of articulating a more complete multiple memory systems view— a point we stressed at the end of chapter 1—it is to be applauded.

However, to the extent that memory performances that are spared following hippocampal system damage share certain fundamental properties, it would be a mistake to ignore their commonalities. On our view, these performances share a common representational basis. They all depend on a dedicated, inflexible, nonrelational form of representation. They are all manifestations of experience that can be expressed only inflexibly, in repetitions of the original learning experience. They are each tied to modifications of specific processing networks. Therefore, we think it appropriate to consider them all examples of the operation of procedural memory.

That is *not* to say that the dissociations among different examples of preserved learning are to be ignored, or that procedural memory is a monolithic entity. On the contrary, we believe that procedural memory and declarative memory each consist of a set of component systems (see the section, below, on *perceptual representation system*), and that the properties of these component systems should by all means be investigated and characterized carefully. But just as evidence supporting the distinction between semantic and episodic memory would *not* convince us to abandon the notion of declarative memory, so too would evidence of dissociations among different examples of performances preserved in amnesia *not* convince us to abandon the category of procedural memory. With regard to semantic and episodic memory, notwithstanding their differences, they both share what we take to be the defining properties of declarative memory. We consider them as distinct components or examples of declarative memory. Likewise, the different categories of performances preserved in amnesia share what we take to be the defining properties of procedural memory, and hence we consider them to be distinguishable components or examples of procedural memory.

This is more than just an issue of semantics. The real problem we see in regarding the various kinds of memory performances spared in amnesia as a collection of different *nondeclarative* memory capacities is that doing so puts all the emphasis on the level of behavioral phenomenology and too little on the level of underlying representational basis. It is by addressing the representational differences between hippocampal-dependent and hippocampal-independent memory performances, and by considering the representational and processing implications of the anatomy and physiology of the hippocampal system, that we have been able to formulate a comprehensive theory of memory, amnesia, and the hippocampal system, bringing together the various lines of converging evidence. Theoretical accounts in this area must be informed and constrained by more than behavioral associations and dissociations.

One final point is that the procedural-declarative framework *predicts* certain dissociations along the lines that have been found. Because procedural memory reflects and is manifested by dedicated changes in one or another of the neocortical processors, cases in which one or another processor itself is compromised will produce domain-specific procedural deficits. This is exactly what is seen in patients with early-stage Alzheimer's disease, in whom the visual cortical areas in which basic visual processing is accomplished remain unaffected by the disease at a time when language areas are compromised. As a result, they show intact "perceptual priming," which is based on the perceptual features of the stimuli, and impaired "conceptual priming," which is based on the linguistic properties of the stimuli (Gabrieli, 1991; Keane et al., 1991).

PERCEPTUAL REPRESENTATIONAL SYSTEM

Schacter and Tulving (Schacter, 1990a; Schacter et al., 1990; Tulving & Schacter, 1990) have proposed that repetition priming effects are mediated by the *perceptual representation system* (PRS), a memory system that is distinct from both semantic and episodic memory systems. According to this proposal, PRS stores information about the visual forms of words and objects, that is, *structural descriptions* of the items encountered through the visual modality. It is unconnected to other (e.g., semantic) information about those items or to information about the specific episodes in which they are encountered. Perceptual identification of words and objects depends critically on PRS, and also results in the storage of additional memories in that system. Facilitation of performance in accomplishing the perceptual identification of words or objects that have been recently repeated (i.e., perceptually based repetition priming) reflects the representations of visual form information stored in the PRS about the stimuli during their prior presentations.

This proposal was offered to account for the dissociation between perceptually based priming phenomena and explicit remembering of the stimulus materials or recollection of the training experiences. Because the representations in PRS of experience with visual objects and words support basic perceptual processing without calling on any (declarative) memories of the learning episodes or of their semantic contents, perceptual processing and perceptually based priming would be expected to proceed independently of explicit remembering. Schacter and Tulving have also argued that the representations in PRS are "hyperspecific," accounting for sensitivity of priming effects to the match between the testing context and the original processing context. As far as it goes, it conforms nicely to the data.

However, the PRS proposal offers no account of conceptually based priming, such as in the category exemplar priming task discussed in chapter 8, in which prior exposure to words from particular categories biases subjects to include those words disproportionately when later asked to generate whatever exemplars come to mind of that category (Graf et al., 1985). In addition, there is no account at all of skill learning, even though it too is preserved in amnesia and shows the same dissociation between skilled performance and explicit remembering. Hence, this is clearly a limited-domain account. Perhaps the best way to think of this account is as an *example of procedural memory*, supporting experience-induced tuning and modifications of a particular subset of processing networks, namely those involved in early visual perceptual processing. On the procedural-declarative view, PRS is one of the various neocortical processing networks we claim show procedural memory–based modifications as a result of experience.

UNITARY SYSTEM OR "PROCESSING" ACCOUNTS

An alternative view, which has been offered by a number of investigators concerned primarily or exclusively with normal memory performances, is that the observed performance dissociations come from differences in the processing demands (and retrieval requirements) that various tasks place on a unitary memory system (e.g., Jacoby, 1988, 1991; Roediger, 1990; Roediger & Blaxton, 1987b: Roediger et al., 1989). On this view, there is a unitary memory system that represents all learning events. The ability to retrieve or gain access to memory representations is said to be a function of the match or overlap between processing operations performed during the learning event and those performed at test time, based on the principles of transfer-appropriate processing (Morris, Bransford, & Franks, 1977) or encoding specificity (Tulving & Thomson, 1973). The way in which this idea is applied to the dissociation between explicit remembering and the acquisition and expression of skilled performance (in these cases, repetition priming in particular) is that the tests used to assess these different performances require different retrieval-time processes, which in turn makes them sensitive to different types of encoding-time processes. More specifically, tests of priming tend to require *data-driven processing*, relying heavily on *automatic* processing of the perceptual matches between stimuli presented during the learning event and at test time; whereas tests of explicit remembering tend to require *conceptually driven processing*, relying heavily on controlled, *conscious* processing of the meaningful contents of the learning event and the testing event.

Applying this idea to the data against which we have challenged the procedural-declarative theory and the other alternative accounts suggests serious shortcomings; it clearly provides only a limited-domain account. Although it does provide an interpretation of the dissociation between priming and explicit remembering in normal subjects, it does *not* provide a compelling account of why explicit remembering is selectively impaired in amnesic patients. That is, as noted in our discussion in chapter 2 of unitary system accounts, it is necessary for proponents of such views to postulate some kind of processing deficit in amnesic patients that would explain the selectivity of their memory impairment. Jacoby (1984) has suggested that amnesic patients have a deficit in attributional or intentional retrieval processes that prevent them from making intentional use of the (fully intact) representations they have stored of their learning experiences; only when tested with indirect memory tests, resulting in *incidental* retrieval, is it possible for the representations to be revealed. Another possibility, based on the above descriptions of automatic data-driven versus conscious conceptually driven processing, is that amnesic patients might have a selective deficit in conscious conceptually driven processing. Unfortunately, there is no evidence that amnesic patients have a special deficit in any of these processes. Their normal on-line processing of language and their intact reasoning abilities argues against any general deficit in conceptually driven processing. Furthermore, they *do* show normal conceptually driven priming, as noted above' and in chapter 8, contrary to the expectations of this account. And they *can* show normal learning of cognitive skills that require conceptually driven processing (see chapter 8), contrary to the expectations of this account.

Moreover, the automatic versus controlled or conscious processing idea is problematic in this context. We have already provided evidence that engaging in processing not only causes automatic procedural memory–based changes in the neocortical processors engaged by the learning event, but that there is also the automatic and obligatory declarative memory–based storage of the outcomes of processing. A further problem with invoking a deficit in consciously mediated processing in amnesic patients as a means of explaining the behavioral dissociations is that it prevents this account from making any contact with the animal model data, in which the same behavioral dissociations are seen, or with the anatomical and physiological data that we have considered. By contrast, as we discussed above, the procedural-declarative theory is able to make contact with the animal data and neuroscientific considerations by explaining the dissociations in terms of fundamental differences between the representational properties of procedural versus declarative memory and by accounting for those representational properties in terms of the brain substrates of procedural and, particularly, declarative memory.

This alternative to multiple memory system approaches has raised some important and interesting questions about normal memory processing, and has forced the literature on normal memory to confront difficult issues about representation and processing. However, it does not offer us a way to understand amnesia and the hippocampal system. One possibly unexpected observation needs to be made here, which is that the transfer-appropriate processing idea is an important aspect of our view of procedural memory. That is, although transfer-appropriate processing and encoding specificity were first raised in the 1970s to account for certain declarative memory phenomena, it is clear now that procedural memory is disproportionately sensitive to the match in processing performed during the learning event versus at test time, emphasizing the inflexibility of procedural memory–based performances.

13 On the Functional Role of the Hippocampal System in Memory

In any instance of interacting with the environment, various processing systems of the brain become engaged in identifying, appreciating, and responding appropriately to the objects and persons we encounter and to the events in which we participate. These processors depend critically on memory systems in the brain that provide the knowledge derived from previous experiences, serving to inform and guide our processing. The major thesis of the present book has been that memory serves this function in two different ways.

One way is by directly tuning and modifying the processors, shaping them in conformance with—and optimizing them for—the regularities of the stimuli with which they are actually confronted. This is the province of procedural memory, mediated by the plasticities inherent in each of the brain's processors. Current views of learning algorithms capable of modifying neural networks in accordance with experience provide us with at least one way of understanding this type of memory mechanism: Incremental changes occur in the strengths or weights of connections among the network elements, tuning and shaping the networks to gradually transform the way in which they operate.

The other way in which memory serves to inform and guide our processing is by storing and relating all of the outcomes of processing during learning events, maintaining and providing access to a database that can be drawn on by any processor when circumstances warrant. This is the province of declarative memory, critically dependent on the hippocampal system. We turn now, in this final chapter, to a description of the engagement of the hippocampal system by a single learning event, in an attempt to illustrate the nature of the functional role played by the hippocampal system in memory.

The hippocampal system, as we have seen, is anatomically placed to receive the convergence of input from the highest-order unimodal, multimodal, and supramodal processors of the brain. During a learning event, the brain's reaction to relevant stimuli capturing one's attention includes generation of the hippocampal theta rhythm (at least in nonhuman species). The cellular mechanisms reflected in this rhythm effectively time-lock the contemporaneous arrival of the multiple channels of exteroceptive sensory input with behaviorally generated events and purely internal stimuli whose various functional representations in associational cortices converge on the hippocampal network. These various channels or streams of inputs are projected onto hippocampal neurons in the form of overlapping gradients, serving to distribute the co-activations across the hippocampal network.

Primed by the synchronization reflected in the theta rhythm, hippocampal cells maximally co-activated by the converging inputs that reflect the learning event can take advantage of a particularly robust mechanism of synaptic plasticity called long-term potentiation. This hippocampal synaptic mechanism has at least two properties crucial to understanding the way in which the hippocampal system plays its role in declarative memory. First, its physiology makes it a type of convergence detector: Converging inputs arriving in close temporal contiguity cause a stable increase in synaptic efficacy lasting for hours to weeks. Second, these cellular changes are induced very rapidly to support a fully formed representation of the pattern of co-activations on a single trial. However, this representation is *not* the permanent record of the entire event or scene— the fact that hippocampal system damage does *not* cause loss of all stored memories (i.e., the fact that retrograde amnesia is temporally limited) rules this out. More about this in a moment.

In so doing, the hippocampal network serves to "chunk" or "bind" together the converging processing outcomes reflecting the learning event. Wickelgren (1979) spoke about the hippocampal system as performing a chunking function, thereby permitting the creation of what he called "vertical associations." We think of it, alternatively, as "solving the *binding problem* for memory" (Cohen, 1986) in a way that parallels current views of the binding problem in perception.

To explain, many investigators working in the area of (visual) perception hold that there are multiple, functionally distinct streams of processing, each dedicated to particular features or properties of (visual) objects, such as color, contour, orientation, and so forth (e.g., Cowey, 1985; Kaas, 1992; Zeki, 1990). On this view, processing a given stimulus results in concurrent activation in several distinct cortical maps, separately representing the different features of that object in parallel. If there are multiple objects in a given scene, each activating the appropriate feature values of the different maps, the problem emerges of how the overall system can keep track of which activations across the maps belong to the same object. That is, if the scene contains several cars, people, trees, and buildings of varying types, then there will be multiple feature values activated in each of the (color, contour, orientation, etc.) maps; that being the case, how can the overall system tell which color and which contour went with (should be bound to) which orientation in the scene? This is the binding problem in perception. Treisman (1969, 1988) and others have argued that the solution to this problem comes from the serial application of selective attention to different locations in space, serving to bind together the particular values across disparate maps that share the same spatial location.

A related issue emerges for declarative memory of scenes or events. The declarative system, as we have indicated, represents the outcomes of processing of the various processors engaged by a given learning event, with each processor projecting its separate output onto the hippocampal system. Thus, the hippocampal system will receive information from the visual system about the visual objects present during the learning event, information from the auditory system about the sounds emitted during the learning event, information from the olfactory system about the odors present during the learning event, and so forth. These various objects will be remembered by virtue of the participation of the hippocampal system in the declarative memory circuit. But what about the event (or scene) itself? There is no single processing system that "detects" or recognizes events and scenes along the lines of the visual object recognition system; and, hence, there is no single input to the hippocampal system to trigger declarative memory for the learning event as a whole. How, then, is an event actually remembered other than as the sum of its constituent parts?

The temporal and spatial convergence of projections from the neocortical processors onto the hippocampal network, and the ability of hippocampal plasticity to permit the rapid inducing of cellular changes capable of supporting a fully formed representation of the pattern of co-activations across hippocampal elements on a single trial, provides the means for declarative long-term memory of the event. Storage of patterns of activation across the hippocampal network for each learning event, representing the conjunction of co-activations of various neocortical networks, may permit the hippocampal system to "maintain the coherence" of the neocortical co-activations that constitute the original event, as proposed by Squire, Cohen, and Nadel (1984). Teyler and DiScenna (1985) have suggested that the hippocampus stores the "addresses" of the various neocortical sites activated by the original learning event, thus serving an "indexing" function. Whenever, on subsequent occasions, a portion or aspect of the original event is re-presented, activating a subset of the cortical networks originally activated, the connections between neocortical processors and the hippocampal system permits the original pattern of co-activations to be completed or recovered.

Damasio (1989a,b) has written at some length about the issue of binding co-occurrences of activity patterns from different neural networks in "convergence zones" of the brain, including the hippocampus. His ideas about memory in the brain are also tied strongly to the issues of perception and attention discussed by Treisman, as considered above. Others have also noted the possibility of hippocampus playing some kind of chunking or binding function (e.g., Squire et al., 1990).

Thus the hippocampal system, rather than generating a representation that serves as the permanent record of the event or scene, apparently stores—for a time after learning—a representation from which declarative memory of the event or scene can be *reconstructed* from the permanent representations of the various attributes or features of the event or scene stored within the various neocortical processors. This idea of an intermediary role of the hippocampal system in permitting access to memories actually stored in various neocortical processing networks, together with the view of hippocampal system as solving the binding problem for memory, makes contact with two important features or properties of declarative memory that we proposed in chapter 3. First is the property of compositionality that is demonstrated by declarative memory. That is, representations exist of both the learning event or scene as a whole and of the individual objects that are its constituents. Thus, the hippocampal-mediated representation must be able to permit access not only to the full pattern of co-activations reflective of the event as a whole, but also the activations within individual processors reflective of their separate processing outcomes. Accordingly, our view that the hippocampal system does not actually store the long-term memory for the learning event, or in some other way bring together the convergent inputs into a single combined representation, but rather provides the means for gaining access to the various neocortical representations that collectively define the learning event, is crucial. It permits simultaneous access to representations of the constituent elements *and* their conjunctions.

Second is the representational flexibility of declarative memory and its relational properties. The storage of multiple patterns of co-activations across the same hippocampal network elements ensures that when new events share features with items stored previously, the already stored representations will share in the activation of network elements caused by new events. Activation of representations of prior events will interact with the representation and storage of current events. Out of the interactions of current and stored representations in the hippocampal network emerges a "memory space" encoding and updating of representations of significant relations among new items and all other related items still excitable by hippocampal activity. Such reinstantiations occur repetitively over time, re-exciting and possibly modifying long-term neocortical representations, enabling memory consolidation.

Furthermore, this relational processing, and the ability of partial patterns to re-activate the entire hippocampal network, permits representations to be activated across vastly different (including entirely novel) contexts. The resulting representational flexibility also permits the ability to "manipulate" stored representations— that is, to activate and operate on the representations in the course of processing by other brain systems, particularly in the frontal lobes, that provide for deliberative, problem-solving, and introspective behaviors. Accordingly, it would seem that the representational flexibility of declarative representation is crucial for conscious recollection and for integrative cognitive processing, with declarative memory serving as the database on which such processing operates.

Notes

CHAPTER 1

1. In more recent years, however, the effects of normal aging (H.M. was born in 1926) and of 50 years of administration of anticonvulsant medication have begun to take a toll, resulting in some decreases in performance abilities, particularly in the motor domain, and also in certain language and perhaps other cognitive performances.

2. Note, however, that many of these researchers are also interested in and contribute work to the issues that are central to the theme of this book. Consequently, that aspect of these researchers' work will be represented here.

CHAPTER 2

1. This assertion must, of course, be tempered by an appreciation of the difficulty of detecting systematic differences in behavioral impairments following damage to different hippocampal system structures in *human patients*. Detection of such systematic differences would require conducting and accumulating behavioral studies of a sufficient number of patients whose accidentally occurring brain injuries were restricted to one or another of the different structures within the hippocampal system, and obtaining reliable radiological and/or neuropathological identification of the different injury sites. It may be that further work will reveal some differences that will prove significant. Based on the currently available evidence, however, no such differences are apparent.

2. This is *not* to imply that they are a homogeneous group with respect to either the details of their behavioral performances or the precise nature of their impairment. While it would be important to study such differences, as long as the differences do *not* extend to the domain of memory for which impairment is observed we can consider all such patients in the discussion here of the sparing and loss of memory following hippocampal system damage.

3. Quite apart from the current amnesia data, this statement draws from analogy with other areas of neuropsychological inquiry. The neuropsy-

chological analysis of such cognitive capacities as reading, writing, calculation, and visual perception has taught us that brain damage can cause selective disruption of different component cognitive processes within a domain. Despite similarities at a gross performance level, more precise assessment reveals performances that are impaired in different ways, reflecting the damage to different component processes. Given that amnesic deficits can result from damage to different—if nonetheless anatomically interconnected—brain structures, the possibility that amnesia too is actually a collection of different kinds of impairment (i.e., *amnesias*) seems eminently reasonable, if still unproven. This is, in the end, an empirical question that will be resolved with more data.

CHAPTER 3

1. We refer here to anatomically distinct brain areas or brain systems that provide the substrate for functionally distinct processing systems or modules.

2. We thank Gary Dell for pointing out the relevance of these ideas for our view of hippocampally mediated declarative memory.

3. Current interest in the issue of *situated cognition* also reminds us (thanks to a discussion with Dedre Gentner) that even declarative memories, e.g., of some specific single event, may be much more readily accessible when cued by a highly related context than by any other (see discussion of encoding specificity [Tulving & Thomson, 1973] and transfer appropriate processing [Morris, Bransford, & Franks, 1977] in chapter 12). However, such memories, once cued, have all the representational flexibility and promiscuity that we have been discussing as characteristic of declarative representations.

4. Some connectionist models have a more "localist" flavor, in which stored representations at a given level in the system are *not* distributed across all of the processing elements. These models share with more fully distributed connectionist models, however, the critical feature of having the connection weights be modifiable by experience in a manner that permits the incremental tuning and biasing of the system so as to support the acquisition and expression of skilled performance. As discussed in the text, it is the way in which such systems are modified by experience that captures the essence of our view of procedural learning.

5. N.J.C. is grateful to Don Norman and Dave Rumelhart for directing him to that work in the latter 1970s and for suggesting that he incorporate those ideas into his conceptualization of the dissociation he was seeing in amnesic performance.

CHAPTER 4

1. Neurons with large, overlapping receptive fields have much *greater* resolution ability than neurons with small, nonoverlapping receptive fields. In a network of neurons with large, overlapping receptive fields, each individual neuron would be able to code information only coarsely, but the network would have very great specificity.

CHAPTER 7

1. At least one study comparing DNMS and DMS in human amnesic patients (Freed & Corkin, 1988) found the opposite effect for the patient H.M. He performed *better* in the DNMS task than he did in the DMS task. However, it should be noted that the performance of control subjects was also superior for DNMS than for DMS, contrary to the findings with monkeys. Moreover, this study involved assessing H.M.'s performance after providing him with 20 times as much exposure to the stimulus materials as was provided to control subjects, making it impossible to compare with the animal model studies.

CHAPTER 8

1. Morton (e.g., 1979) has argued that we possess memory representations of linguistic objects (i.e., words) and of visual objects, called logogens and pictogens, respectively, that support our ability to identify such objects. Recent exposure to such objects may cause a lingering activation of the relevant representations, resulting in a state of affairs in which subsequent repetition of the objects would more easily or more rapidly lead to activation of the corresponding representation.

CHAPTER 12

1. It has been argued that in the absence of intact episodic memory, new learning of semantic memory would be expected to be impaired, because of an obligatory seriality of episodic and semantic memory processing (see Tulving, 1987). This view of the relationship between episodic and semantic memory does not seem to be amenable to empirical test (i.e., it seems unfalsifiable).

References

Aggleton, J. P. (1985). One trial object recognition by rats. *Quarterly Journal of Experimental Psychology, 37B,* 279–294.

Aggleton, J. P., Blindt, H. S., Rawlins, J. N. P. (1989). Effects of amygdaloid and amygdaloid-hippocampal lesions on object recognition and spatial working memory in rats. *Behavioral Neuroscience, 5,* 962–974.

Aggleton, J. P., Hunt, P. R., & Rawlins, J. N. P. (1986). The effects of hippocampal lesions upon spatial and non-spatial tests of working memory. *Behavioral Brain Research, 19,* 133–146.

Aggleton, J. P., Nicol, R. M., Huston, A. E., & Fairbairn, A. F. (1988). The performance of amnesic subjects on tests of experimental amnesia in animals: Delayed matching-to-sample and concurrent learning. *Neuropsychologia, 26,* 265–272.

Allard, T. T., Clark, S. A., Jenkins, W. M., & Merzenich, M. M. (1991). Reorganization of somatosensory area 3b representation in adult owl monkeys following digital syndactyly. *Journal of Neurophysiology, 66,* 1048–1058.

Amaral, D. G. (1987). Memory: Anatomical organization of candidate brain regions. In J. M. Brookhart & V. B. Montcastle (Eds.), *Handbook of physiology: The nervous system V. Higher functions of the nervous system* (Vol. Ed. F. Plum, pp. 211–294). Bethesda, MD: American Physiological Society.

Amaral, D. G., Insausti, R., & Cowan, W. M. (1987). The entorhinal cortex of the monkey: I. Cytoarchitectonic organization. *Journal of Comparative Neurology, 264,* 326–355.

Amaral, D. G., & Witter, M. P. (1989). The three-dimensional organization of the hippocampal formation: A review of anatomical data. *Neuroscience, 31,* 571–591.

Anderson, J. R. (1983). *The architecture of cognition.* Cambridge, MA: Harvard University Press.

Bachevalier, J., Parkinson, J. K., & Mishkin, M. (1985). Visual recognition in monkeys: Effects of separate versus combined transection of fornix and amydalofugal pathways. *Experimental Brain Research, 57,* 554–561.

Baddeley, A. D. (1982). Implications of neuropsychological evidence for theories of normal memory. In D. E. Broadbent & L. Weiskrantz (Eds.), *Philosophical Transactions of the Royal Society of London, Vol. 298* (pp. 59–72). London: The Royal Society.

Barnes, C. A. (1979). Memory deficits associated with senescence: A neurophysiological and behavioral study in the rat. *Journal of Comparative Physiology and Psychology, 93,* 74–104.

Barnes, C. A. (1988). Spatial learning and memory processes: The search for their neurobiological mechanisms in the rat. *Trends in Neurosciences, 11,* 163–169.

Barr, A. & Feigenbaum, E. A. (1982). *The handbook of artificial intelligence. Volume II.* Los Altos, CA: William Kaufman.

Baylis. G. C., & Rolls, E. T. (1987). Responses of neurons in the inferior temporal cortex in short term and serial recognition memory tasks. *Experimental Brain Research, 65,* 614–622.

Baylis, G. C., Rolls, E. T., & Leonard, C. M. (1987). Functional subdivisions of the temporal lobe neocortex. *Journal of Neuroscience, 7,* 330–342.

Benson, D. F., Marsden, C. D., & Meadows, J. C. (1974). The amnesic syndrome of posterior cerebral artery occlusion. *Acta Neurologica Scandinavica, 50,* 133–145.

Benzing, W. C., & Squire, L. R. (1989). Preserved learning and memory in amnesia: Intact adaptation-level effects and learning of stereoscopic depth. *Behavioral Neuroscience, 103,* 538–547.

Berger, T. W., & Orr, W. B. (1983). Hippocampectomy selectively disrupts discrimination reversal learning of the rabbit nictitating membrane response. *Behavioral Brain Research, 8,* 49–68.

Berger, T. W., Rinaldi, P. C., Weisz, D. J., & Thompson, R. F. (1983). Single-unit analysis of different hippocampal cell types during classical conditioning of rabbit nictitating membrane response. *Journal of Neurophysiology, 50,* 1197–1219.

Berry, D. C., & Broadbent, D. E. (1984). On the relationship between task performance and associated verbalizable knowledge. *Quarterly Journal of Experimental Psychology, 36A,* 209–231.

Blakemore, C. (1974). Developmental factors in the formation of feature extracting neurons. In F. O. Schmitt & F. G. Worden (Eds.), *The neurosciences: Third study program* (pp. 105–113). Cambridge, MA: MIT Press.

Bliss, T. V. P., & Lomo, T. (1973). Long-lasting potentiation of synaptic transmission in the dentate area of the anaesthetized rabbit following stimulation of the perforant path. *Journal of Physiology, 232,* 331–365.

Blue, J. H. (1983). Hippocampal lesions syndrome: Switching to and from a place hypothesis. *Quarterly Journal of Experimental Psychology, 35B,* 299–314.

Boeijinga, P. H., & Van Groen, T. (1984). Inputs from the olfactory bulb and olfactory cortex to the entorhinal cortex in the cat. II. Physiological studies. *Experimental Brain Research, 57*, 40–48.

Bostock, E., Muller, R. U., & Kubie, J. L. (1986). Firing fields of hippocampal neurons: A stimulus manipulation that alters place cell mapping of the environment. *Society for Neuroscience Abstracts, 12*, 522.

Broadbent, D. E. FitzGerald, P., & Broadbent, M. H. P. (1986). Implicit and explicit knowledge in the control of complex systems. *British Journal of Psychology, 77*, 33–50.

Brooks, D. N., & Baddeley, A. (1976). What can amnesic patients learn? *Neuropsychologia, 14*, 111–122.

Brown, M. W. (1982). Effect of context on the response of single units recorded from the hippocampal region of behaviourally trained monkeys. In C. A. Marsan & H. Matthies (Eds.), *Neuronal plasticity and memory formation* (pp. 557–573). New York: Raven Press.

Bruner, J. S. (1969). Modalities of memory. In G. A. Talland, & N. C. Waugh (Eds.), *The pathology of memory* (pp. 253–259). New York: Academic Press.

Butters, N., & Albert, M. S. (1982). Processes underlying failures to recall remote events. In L. S. Cermak (Ed.), *Human memory and amnesia*. Hillsdale, NJ: Erlbaum.

Butters, N., & Cermak, L. S. (1980). *Alcoholic Korsakoff's syndrome: An information-processing approach to amnesia*. New York: Academic Press.

Butters, N., & Miliotis, P. (1985). Amnesic disorders. In K. M. Heilman & E. Valenstein (Eds.), *Clinical neuropsychology*, 2nd edition (pp. 403–452). Oxford: Oxford University Press.

Butters, N., Wolfe, J., Martone, M., Granholm, E., & Cermak, L. (1985). Memory disorders associated with Huntington's disease: Verbal recall, verbal recognition, and procedural memory. *Neuropsychologia, 23*, 729–743.

Cahusac, P. M. B., & Miyashita, Y. (1988). Hippocampal activity related to processing of single sensory-motor associations. *Neuroscience Letters, 9*, 265–272.

Cahusac, P. M. B., Miyashita, Y., & Rolls, E. T. (1989). Responses of hippocampal formation neurons in the monkey related to delayed spatial response and object-place memory tasks. *Behavioral Brain Research, 33*, 229–240.

Caramazza, A. (1986). On drawing inferences about the structure of normal cognitive systems from the analysis of patterns of impaired performance: The case for single-patient studies. *Brain and Cognition, 5*, 41–66.

Cermak, L. S. (Ed.) (1982). *Human memory and amnesia*. Hillsdale, NJ: Erlbaum.

Cermak, L. S., Blackford, S. P., O'Connor, M., & Bleich, R. P. (1988). The implicit memory ability of a patient with amnesia due to encephalitis. *Brain and Cognition, 7*, 145–156.

Cermak, L. S., Lewis, R., Butters, N., & Goodglass, H. (1973). Role of verbal mediation in performance of motor tasks by Korsakoff patients. *Perceptual and Motor Skills, 37*, 259–262.

Cermak, L. S., Talbot, N., Chandler, K., & Wolbarst, L. R. (1985). The perceptual priming phenomenon in amnesia. *Neuropsychologia, 23(5)*, 615–622.

Charness, N., Milberg, W., & Alexander, M. P. (1988). Teaching an amnesic a complex cognitive skill. *Brain and Cognition, 8*, 253–272.

Cohen, N. J. (1981). *Neuropsychological evidence for a distinction between procedural and declarative knowledge in human memory and amnesia*. Unpublished doctoral dissertation, University of California, San Diego.

Cohen, N. J. (1984). Preserved learning capacity in amnesia: Evidence for multiple memory systems. In L. R. Squire & N. Butters (Eds.), *Neuropsychology of memory* (pp. 83–103). New York: Guilford Press.

Cohen, N. J. (1985). Levels of analysis in memory research: The neuropsychological approach. In N. M. Weinberger, J. L. McGaugh, & G. Lynch (Eds.), *Memory systems of the brain* (pp. 419–432). New York: Guilford Press.

Cohen, N. J. (1986). Hippocampal function as solving the "binding problem" for memory. Unpublished *Memory Working Group* Report.

Cohen, N. J., Abrams, I., Harley, W. A., Tabor, L., & Sejnowski, T. (1986). Skill learning and repetition priming in symmetry detection: Parallel studies of human subjects and connectionist models. *Proceedings of the Eighth Annual Conference of the Cognitive Science Society* (pp. 23–44). Hillsdale, NJ: Erlbaum.

Cohen, N. J., & Corkin, S. (1981). The amnesic patient H.M.: Learning and retention of cognitive skill. *Society for Neuroscience Abstracts, 7*, 517–518.

Cohen, N. J., & Eichenbaum, H. (1991). The theory that wouldn't die: A critical look at the spatial mapping theory of hippocampal function. *Hippocampus, 1*, 265–268.

Cohen, N. J., Eichenbaum, H., Deacedo, B. S., & Corkin, S. (1985). Different memory systems underlying acquisition of procedural and declarative knowledge. In D. S. Olton, E. Gamzu, & S. Corkin (Eds.), *Memory dysfunctions: An integration of animal and human research from preclinical and clinical perspectives* (pp. 54–71). New York: New York Academy of Sciences.

Cohen, N. J., & Shapiro, M. (1985). Minding the general memory store: Further considerations of the role of the hippocampus in memory. *Behavioral and Brain Sciences, 8*, 498.

Cohen, N. J., & Squire, L. R. (1980). Preserved learning and retention of pattern-analyzing skill in amnesia: Dissociation of knowing how and knowing that. *Science, 210*, 207–209.

Coltheart, M. (1985). Cognitive neuropsychology and the study of reading. In M. L. Posner & O. S. M. Marin (Eds.), *Attention and performance, Vol. 11* (pp. 3–37). Hillsdale, NJ: Erlbaum.

Corkin, S. (1965). Tactually guided maze-learning in man: Effects of unilateral cortical excisions and bilateral hippocampal lesions. *Neuropsychologia, 3*, 339–351.

Corkin, S. (1968). Acquisition of motor skill after bilateral medial temporal lobe excision. *Neuropsychologia, 6*, 255–265.

Corkin, S. (1982). Some relationships between global amnesias and the memory impairments in Alzheimer's disease. In S. Corkin, K. L. Davis, J. H. Growdon & E. Usdin (Eds.), *Alzheimer's disease: A report of progress in research* (pp. 149–164). New York: Raven Press.

Corkin, S. (1984). Lasting consequences of bilateral medial temporal lobectomy: Clinical course and experimental findings in H. M. *Seminars in Neurology, 4*, 249–259.

Correll, R. E., & Scoville, W. B. (1965a). Effects of medial temporal lesions on visual discrimination performance. *Journal of Comparative Physiology and Psychology, 60*, 175–181.

Correll, R. E., & Scoville, W. B. (1965b). Performance on delayed match following lesions of medial temporal lube structures. *Journal of Comparative and Physiological Psychology, 60*, 360–367.

Correll, R. E., & Scoville, W. B. (1967). Significance of delay in the performance of monkeys with medial temporal lobe resections. *Experimental Brain Research, 4*, 85–96.

Correll, R. E., & Scoville, W. B. (1970). Relationship of ITI to acquisition of serial visual discriminations following temporal rhinencephalic resection in monkeys. *Journal of Comparative and Physiological Psychology, 70*, 464–469.

Corsi, P. M. (1972). *Human memory and the medial temporal regions of the brain.* Ph.D. thesis, McGill University, Montreal.

Cowey, A. (1985). Aspects of cortical organization related to selective attention and selective impairments of visual perception: A tutorial review. In M. I. Posner & O. S. M. Marin (Eds.), *Attention and performance. XI.* Hillsdale, NJ: Erlbaum.

Crovitz, H. F., Harvey, M. T., & McClanahan, S. (1981). Hidden memory: A rapid method for the study of amnesia using perceptual learning. *Cortex, 17*, 273–278.

Crowne, D. P., & Radcliffe, D. D. (1975). Some characteristics and functional relations of the electrical activity of the primate hippocampus and a hypothesis of hippocampal function. In R. L. Isaacson & K. H. Pribram (Eds.), *The hippocampus. Volume 2: Neurophysiology and behavior*. New York: Plenum Press.

Damasio, A. R. (1989a). The brain binds entities and events by multiregional activation from convergence zones. *Neural Computation, 1*, 123–132.

Damasio, A. R. (1989b). Multiregional co-attended retroactivation: A new model of the neural substrates of cognition. *Cognition, 33*, 25–62.

Damasio, A. R., Eslinger, P. J., Damasio, H., Van Hoesen, G. W., & Cornell, S. (1985). Multimodal amnesic syndrome following bilateral temporal and basal forebrain damage. *Archives of Neurology, 42*, 252–259.

Daum, I., Channon, S. & Canvan, A. G. M. (1989). Classical conditioning in patients with severe memory problems. *Journal of Neurology, Neurosurgery and Psychiatry, 52*, 47–51.

Davidson, T. L., & Jarrard, L. E. (1989). Retention of concurrent conditional discriminations in rats with ibotenate lesions of the hippocampus. *Psychobiology, 17*, 49–60.

Deacon, T. W., Eichenbaum, H., Rosenberg, P., Eckman, K. W. (1983). Afferent connections of the perirhinal cortex in the rat. *Journal of Comparative Neurology, 200*, 168–190.

Dennett, D. C. (1984). Cognitive wheels: The frame problem in AI. In C. Hookaway, (Ed.), *Minds, machines, and evolution*. Cambridge: Cambridge University Press.

Desimone, R., Albright, T. D., Gross, C. G., & Bruce, C. (1984). Stimulus-selective properties of inferior temporal neurons in the macaque. *Journal of Neuroscience, 4*, 2051–2062.

Devenport, L. D., Hale, R. L., & Stidham, J. A. (1988). Sampling behavior in the radial maze and operant chamber: Role of the hippocampus and prefrontal area. *Behavioral Neuroscience, 102*, 489–498.

Diamond, D. M., Dunwiddie, T. V., Rose, G. M. (1988). Characteristics of hippocampal primed burst potentiation *in vitro* and in the awake rat. *Journal of Neuroscience, 8*, 4079–4088.

Diamond, D. M., & Weinberger, N. M. (1986). Classical conditioning rapidly induces specific changes in frequency receptive fields of single neurons in secondary and ventral ectosylvian cortical fields. *Brain Research, 372*, 357–360.

Diamond, R., & Rozin, P. (1984). Activation of existing memories in the amnesic syndrome. *Journal of Abnormal Psychology, 93*, 98–105.

DiMattia, B. D., & Kesner, R. P. (1988). Spatial cognitive maps: Differential role of parietal cortex and hippocampal formation. *Behavioral Neuroscience, 102*, 471–480.

Douglas, R. J. (1967). The hippocampus and behavior. *Psychological Bulletin, 67,* 416–442.

Drachman, D. A., & Adams, R. D. (1962). Acute herpes simplex and inclusion body encephalitis. *Archives of Neurology, 7,* 45–63.

Drachman, D. A., & Arbit, J. (1966). Memory and hippocampal complex. II. Is memory a multiple process? *Archives of Neurology, 15,* 52–61.

Dulany, D. E., Carlson, R. A., & Dewey, G. I. (1984). A case of syntactical learning and judgment: How conscious and how abstract? *Journal of Experimental Psychology: General, 114,* 25–32.

Eichenbaum, H., & Buckingham, J. (1991). Studies on hippocampal processing: Experiment, theory, and model. In M. Gabriel & J. Moore (Eds.), *Learning and computational neuroscience: Foundations of adaptive networks* (pp. 171–231). Cambridge, MA: MIT Press.

Eichenbaum, H., & Cohen, N. J. (1988). Representation in the hippocampus: What do the neurons code? *Trends in Neurosciences, 11,* 244–248.

Eichenbaum, H., Cohen, N. J., Otto, T., & Wible, C. G. (1991). Memory representation in the hippocampus: Functional domain and functional organization. In L. R. Squire, G. Lynch, N. M. Weinberger, & J. L. McGaugh (Eds.), *Memory: Organization and locus of change* (in press). Oxford University Press.

Eichenbaum, H., Fagan, A., & Cohen, N. J. (1986). Normal olfactory discrimination learning set and facilitation of reversal learning after combined and separate lesions of the fornix and amygdala in rats: Implications for preserved learning in amnesia. *Journal of Neuroscience, 6,* 1876–1884.

Eichenbaum, H., Fagan, A., Mathews, P., & Cohen, N. J. (1988). Hippocampal system dysfunction and odor discrimination learning in rats: Impairment or facilitation depending on representational demands. *Behavioral Neuroscience, 102,* 3531–3542.

Eichenbaum, H., Kuperstein, M., Fagan, A., & Nagode, J. (1987). Cue-sampling and goal-approach correlates of hippocampal unit activity in rats performing an odor discrimination task. *Journal of Neuroscience, 7,* 716–732.

Eichenbaum, H., Mathews, P., & Cohen, N. J. (1989). Further studies of hippocampal representation during odor discrimination learning. *Behavioral Neuroscience, 103,* 1207–1216.

Eichenbaum, H., Otto, T., & Cohen, N. J. (1992). The hippocampus—What does it do? *Behavioral and Neural Biology, 57,* 2–36.

Eichenbaum, H., Stewart, C., & Morris, R. G. M. (1990). Hippocampal representation in spatial learning. *Journal of Neuroscience, 10,* 331–339.

Eichenbaum, H., Wiener, S. I., Shapiro, M., & Cohen, N. J. (1989). The organization of spatial coding in the hippocampus: A study of neural ensemble activity. *Journal of Neuroscience, 9,* 2764–2775.

Ellis, A. W., & Young, A. W. (1988). *Human cognitive neuropsychology.* Hove, London: Erlbaum.

Farah, M. J. (1990). *Visual agnosia.* Cambridge, MA: MIT Press.

Feldon, J., Rawlins, J. N. P., & Gry, J. A. (1985). Fornix-fimbria section and the partial reinforcement extinction effect. *Experimental Brain Research, 58,* 435–439.

Fodor, J. A., & Pylyshyn, Z. W. (1988). Connectionism and cognitive architecture: A critical analysis. *Cognition, 28,* 3–71.

Foster, T. C., Castro, C. A., & McNaughton, B. L. (1990). Spatial selectivity of rat hippocampal neurons: Dependence on preparedness for movement. *Science, 244,* 1580–1582.

Foster, T. C., Christian, E. P., Hampson, R. E., Campbell, K. A., & Deadwyler, S. A. (1987). Sequential dependencies regulate sensory evoked responses of single units in the rat hippocampus. *Brain Research, 40,* 86–96.

Freed, D. M., & Corkin, S. (1988). Rate of forgetting in H.M.: 6-month recognition. *Behavioral Neuroscience, 102,* 823–827.

Freed, D. M., Corkin, S., & Cohen, N. J. (1987). Forgetting in H.M.: A second look. *Neuropsychologia, 25,* 461–471.

Fuster, J. M., & Jervey, J. P. (1981). Inferotemporal neurons distinguish and retain behaviourally relevant features of visual stimuli. *Science, 212,* 952–955.

Fuster, J. M., & Jervey, J. P. (1982). Neuronal firing in the inferotemporal cortex of the monkey in a visual memory task. *Journal of Neuroscience, 2,* 361–375.

Gabrieli, J. D. E. (1991). Differential effects of aging and age-related neurological diseases on memory subsystems of the brain. In F. Boller & J. Grafman (Eds.), *The handbook of neuropsychology.* New York: Elsevier.

Gabrieli, J. D. E., Cohen, N. J., & Corkin, S. (1988). The impaired learning of semantic knowledge following bilateral medial temporal-lobe resection. *Brain and Cognition, 7,* 157–177.

Gabrieli, J. D. E., Milberg, W., Keane, M. M., & Corkin. (1990). Intact priming of patterns despite impaired memory. *Neuropsychologia, 28,* 417–427.

Gaffan, D. (1972). Loss of recognition memory in rats with lesions of the fornix. *Neuropsychologia, 10,* 327–341.

Gaffan, D. (1974). Recognition impaired and association intact in the memory of monkeys after transection of the fornix. *Journal of Comparative Physiological Psychology, 86,* 1100–1109.

Gaffan, D. (1977). Monkey's recognition memory for complex pictures and the effects of fornix transection. *Quarterly Journal of Experimental Psychology, 29,* 505–514.

Gaffan, D., & Harrison, S. (1989a). A comparison on the effects of fornix transection and sulcus principalis ablation upon spatial learning by monkeys. *Behavioral Brain Research, 31,* 207–220.

Gaffan, D., & Harrison, S. (1989b). Place memory and scene memory: Effects of fornix transection in the monkey. *Experimental Brain Research, 74,* 202–212.

Gaffan, D., & Saunders, R. C. (1985). Running recognition of configural stimuli by fornix transected monkeys. *Quarterly Journal of Experimental Psychology, 37B,* 61–71.

Gaffan, D., Saunders, R. C., Gaffan, E. A., Harrison, S., C. Shields, & Owen, M. J. (1984). Effects of fornix transection upon associative memory in monkeys: Role of the hippocampus in learned action. *Quarterly Journal of Experimental Psychology, 36B,* 173–221.

Garrud, P., Rawlins, J. N. P., Mackintosh, N. J., Goodall, G., Cotton, M. M., & Feldon, J. (1984). Successful overshadowing and blocking in hippocampectomized rats. *Behavioral Brain Research, 12,* 39–53.

Glisky, E. L., & Schacter, D. L. (1987). Acquisition of domain-specific knowledge in organic amnesia: Training for computer-related work. *Neuropsychologia, 25,* 893–906.

Glisky, E. L., & Schacter, D. L. (1989). Extending the limits of complex learning in organic amnesia: Computer training in a vocational domain. *Neuropsychologia, 27,* 107–120.

Glisky, E. L., Schacter, D. L., & Tulving, E. (1986). Computer learning by memory impaired patients: Acquisition and retention of complex knowledge. *Neuropsychologia, 24,* 313–328.

Goldman-Rakic, P. S., Selemon, L. D., & Schwartz, M. L. (1984). Dual pathways connecting the dorsolateral prefrontal cortex with the hippocampal formation and parahippocampal cortex in the rhesis monkey. *Neuroscience, 12,* 719–743.

Good, M., & Honey, R. C. (1991). Conditioning and contextual retrieval in hippocampal rats. *Behavioral Neuroscience, 105,* 499–509.

Gordon, B. (1988). Preserved learning of novel information in amnesia: Evidence for multiple memory systems. *Brain and Cognition, 7,* 257–282.

Gould, S. J. (1984). Review of "A feeling for the organism: The life and work of Barbara McClintock." *The New York Review of Books, 31,* 3–4.

Graf, P., & Mandler, G. (1984). Activation makes words more accessible, but not necessarily more retrievable. *Journal of Verbal Learning and Verbal Behavior, 23,* 553–568.

Graf, P., & Schacter, D. L. (1985). Implicit and explicit memory for new associations in normal and amnesic subjects. *Journal of Experimental Psychology: Learning, Memory and Cognition, 11,* 501–518.

Graf, P., & Schacter, D. L. (1987). Selective effects of interference on implicit and explicit memory for new associations. *Journal of Experimental Psychology: Learning, Memory, and Cognition, 13*, 45–53.

Graf, P., Shimamura, A. P., & Squire, L. R. (1985). Priming across modalities and priming across category levels: Extending the domain of preserved function in amnesia. *Journal of Experimental Psychology: Learning, Memory, and Cognition, 11*, 386–396.

Graf, P., Squire, L. R., & Mandler, G. (1984). The information that amnesic patients do not forget. *Journal of Experimental Psychology: Learning, Memory, and Cognition, 10*, 164–178.

Gray, J. A. (1982). *The neuropsychology of anxiety: An investigation into the functions of the septo-hippocampal system.* Oxford: Oxford University Press.

Gray, J. A., & McNaughton, N. (1983). Comparison of the behavioral effects of septal and hippocampal lesions: A review. *Neuroscience and Biobehavioral Reviews, 7*, 119–188.

Gray, J. A., & Rawlins, J. N. P. (1986). Comparator and buffer memory: An attempt to integrate two models of hippocampal functions. In R. L. Isaacson and K. H. Pribram (Eds.), *The hippocampus, Vol. 4* (pp. 159–202). New York: Plenum Press.

Gross, C. G., Bender, B., & Gerstein, G. L. (1979). Visual properties of neurons in the inferotemporal cortex of the macaque. *Journal of Neuroscience, 17*, 215–229.

Gross, C. G., Roche-Miranda, C. E., & Bender, D. B. (1972). Visual properties of neurons in the inferotemporal cortex of the macaque. *Journal of Neurophysiology, 35*, 96–111.

Habets, A. M. M. C., Lopes da Silva, F. H., & de Quartel, F. W. (1980). Autoradiography of the olfactory-hippocampal pathway in the cat with special reference to the perforant path. *Experimental Brain Research, 38*, 257–265.

Haist, F., Musen, G., & Squire, L. R. (1991). Intact priming of words and nonwords in amnesia. *Psychobiology, 19*, 275–285.

Halgren, E. (1984). Human hippocampal and amygdala recording and stimulation: Evidence for a neural model of recent memory. In L. R. Squire & N. Butters (Eds.), *The neuropsychology of memory* (pp. 165–182). New York: Guilford Press.

Halgren, E., Babb, T. L., & Crandal, P. H. (1978). Activity of human hippocampal formation and amygdala neurons during memory testing. *EEG and Clinical Neurophysiology, 45*, 585–601.

Hayes, J. R., & Simon, H. A. (1977). Psychological differences among problem isomorphs. In J. Castellan, D. B. Pisoni, & G. Potts (Eds.), *Cognitive theory, Vol. 2*, Hillsdale, NJ: Erlbaum.

Hebb, D. O. (1961). Distinctive features of learning in the higher animal. In J. F. Delafresnaye (Ed.), *Brain mechanisms in learning.* Oxford: Blackwell.

Heindel, W. C., Butters, N., & Salmon, D. P. (1988). Impaired learning of a motor skill in patients with Huntington's disease. *Behavioral Neuroscience, 102,* 141–147.

Heindel, W. C., Salmon, D. P., Shults, C. W., Walicke, P. A., & Butters, N. (1989). Neuropsychological evidence for multiple implicit memory systems: A comparison of Alzheimer's, Huntington's, and Parkinson's disease patients. *Journal of Neuroscience, 9,* 582–587.

Heit, G., Smith, M. E., & Halgren, E. (1988). Neural encoding of individual words and faces by the human hippocampus and amygdala. *Nature, 333,* 773–775.

Hill, A. J., & Best, P. J. (1981). Effects of deafness and blindness on the spatial correlates of hippocampal unit activity in the rat. *Experimental Neurology, 74,* 204–217.

Hinton, G. E., McClelland, J. L., & Rumelhart, D. E. (1986). Distributed representations. In D. E. Rumelhart, & J. L. McClelland (Eds.), *Parallel distributed processing: Explorations in the microstructure of cognition.* Cambridge, MA: MIT Press.

Hintzman, D. L. (1990). Human learning and memory: Connections and dissociations. *Annual Review of Psychology, 41,* 109–139.

Hirsh, R. (1970). Lack of variability or perseveration: Describing the effect of hippocampal ablation. *Physiology and Behavior, 5,* 1249–1254.

Hirsh, R. (1974). The hippocampus and contextual retrieval of information from memory: A theory. *Behavioral Biology, 12,* 421–444.

Hirsh, R. (1980). The hippocampus, conditional operations, and cognition. *Physiological Psychology, 8,* 175–182.

Hirsh, R., Davis, R., & Holt, L. (1979). Fornico-thalamus fibers, motivational states, and contextual retrieval. *Experimental Neurology, 65,* 373–390.

Hirsh, R., Holt, L., & Mosseri, A. (1978). Hippocampal mossy fibers, motivational states, and contextural retrieval. *Experimental Neurology, 62,* 68–79.

Hirst, W., Johnson, M. K., Phelps, E. A., Risse, G., & Volpe, B. T. (1986). Recognition and recall in amnesics. *Journal of Experimental Psychology: Learning, Memory and Cognition, 12,* 445–451.

Hirst, W., Phelps, E. A., Johnson, M. K., & Volpe, B. T. (1988). Amnesia and second language learning. *Brain and Cognition, 8,* 105–116.

Honig, W. K. (1978). Studies of working memory in the pigeon. In S. H. Hulse, H. Fowler & W. K. Honig (Eds.), *Cognitive processes in animal behavior* (pp. 211–248). Hillsdale, NJ: Erlbaum.

Horel, J. A., & Pytko, D. E. (1982). Behavioral effects of local cooling in temporal lobe of monkeys. *Journal of Neurophysiology, 47,* 11–22.

Hsiao, S., & Isaacson, R. L. (1971). Learning of food and water positions by hippocampus damaged rats. *Physiological Behavior, 6,* 81–83.

Hubel, D. H., & Wiesel, T. N. (1979). Brain mechanisms of vision. *Scientific American, 241,* 150–162.

Hubel, D. H., Wiesel, T. N., & LeVay, S. (1977). Plasticity of ocular dominance columns in the monkey striate cortex. *Philosophical Transactions Royal Society of London: Biology, 278,* 377–409.

Humphreys, G. W., & Riddoch, M. J. (1987a). *To see but not to see: A case study of visual agnosia.* London: Erlbaum.

Humphreys, G. W., & Riddoch, M. J. (1987b). The fractionation of visual agnosia. In G. W. Humphreys & M. J. Riddoch (Eds.), *Visual object processing* (pp. 281–306). London: Erlbaum

Humphreys, M. S., Bain, J. D., & Pike, R. (1989). Different ways to cue a coherent memory system: A theory for episodic, semantic, and procedural tasks, *Psychological Review, 96,* 208–233.

Insausti, R., Amaral, D. G., & Cowan, W. M. (1987a). The entorhinal cortex of the monkey: II. Cortical afferents. *Journal of Comparative Neurology, 264,* 356–395.

Insausti, R., Amaral, D. G., & Cowan, W. M. (1987b). The entorhinal cortex of the monkey: III. Subcortical afferents. *Journal of Comparative Neurology, 264,* 396–408.

Isaacson, R. L., & Kimble, D. P. (1972). Lesions of the limbic system: Their effects upon hypotheses and frustration. *Behavioral Biology, 7,* 767–793.

Iversen, S. D. (1976). Do hippocampal lesions produce amnesia in animals? *International Review of Neurobiology, 19,* 1–49.

Iversen, S. D. (1977). Temporal lobe amnesia. In C. W. M. Whitty & O. L. Zangwill (Eds.), *Amnesia* (pp. 136–182). London: Butterworth.

Jacoby, L. L. (1983). Perceptual enhancement: Persistent effects of an experience. *Journal of Experimental Psychology: Learning, Memory and Cognition, 9,* 21–38.

Jacoby, L. L. (1984). Incidental versus intentional retrieval: Remembering and awareness as separate issues. In L. R. Squire and N. Butters (Eds.), *Neuropsychology of memory* (pp. 145–156). New York: Guilford Press.

Jacoby, L. L. (1988). Memory observed and memory unobserved. In U. Neisser, & E. Winograd (Eds.), *Remembering reconsidered: Ecological and traditional approaches to the study of memory* (pp. 145–177). New York: Cambridge University Press.

Jacoby, L. L. (1991). A process dissociation framework: Separating automatic from intentional uses of memory. *Journal of Memory and Language, 30,* 513–541.

Jacoby, L. L., & Witherspoon, D. (1982). Remembering without awareness. *Canadian Journal of Psychology, 36,* 300–324.

James, W. (1890). *Principles of psychology.* New York: Holt.

Jarrard, L. E. (1986). Selective hippocampal lesions and behavior: Implications for current research and theorizing. In R. L. Isaacson & K. H. Pribram (Eds.), *The Hippocampus: Vol. 4.* New York: Plenum Press.

Jarrard, L. E., & Davidson, T. L. (1990). Acquisition of concurrent conditional discriminations in rats with ibotenate lesions of hippocampus and of subiculum. *Psychobiology, 18,* 68–73.

Jarrard, L. E., & Davidson, T. L. (1991). On the hippocampus and learned conditional responding: Effects of aspiration versus ibotenate lesions. *Hippocampus, 1,* 107–117.

Jarrard, L. E., Okaichi, H., Steward, O. & Goldschmidt, R. (1984). On the importance of the dentate gyrus and hippocampal connections in the performance of a complex place and cue task. *Behavioral Neuroscience, 98,* 946–954.

Johnson, M. K., Kim, J. K., & Risse, G. (1985). Do alcoholic Korsakoff's syndrome patients acquire affective reactions? *Journal of Experiment Psychology: Learning, Memory and Cognition,* 1–47.

Kaas, J. H. (1992). Processing areas and modules in the sensory-perceptual cortex. In G. M. Edelman, W. E. Gall, & W. M. Cowan (Eds.), *Signal and sense: Local and global order in perceptual maps.* New York: Wiley.

Karat, J. A. (1982). A model of problem solving with incomplete constraint knowledge. *Cognitive Psychology, 14,* 538–559.

Keane, M. M., Gabrieli, J. D. E., Kjelgaard, M. M., Growdon, J. J., & Corkin, S. (1988). Dissociation between two kinds of priming in global amnesia and Alzheimer's disease. *Society for Neuroscience Abstracts, 14,* 1290.

Keane, M. M., Gabrieli, J. D. E., Fennema, A. C., Growdon, J. H., & Corkin, S. (1991). Evidence for a dissociation between perceptual and conceptual priming in Alzheimer's disease. *Behavioral Neuroscience, 105,* 326–342.

Kesner, R. P. (1991). Neurobiological views of memory. In J. L. Martinez, Jr., & R. P. Kesner (Eds.), *Learning and memory: A biological view.* San Diego: Academic Press.

Kesner, R. P., & Novak, J. (1982). Serial position curve: Role of the dorsal hippocampus. *Science, 218,* 173–174.

Kimble, D. P. (1963). The effects of bilateral hippocampal lesions in rats. *Journal of Comparative and Physiological Psychology, 56,* 273–283.

Kimble, D. P. (1968). Hippocampus and internal inhibition. *Psychological Bulletin, 70,* 285–295.

Kimble, D. P., & Kimble, R. J. (1970). The effect of hippocampal lesions on extinction and "hypothesis" behavior in rats. *Physiology and Behavior, 5,* 735–738.

Kinsbourne, M. (1987). Brain mechanisms and memory. *Human Neurobiology, 6*, 81–92.

Kinsbourne, M., & Wood, F. (1975). Short-term memory processes and the amnesic syndrome. In D. Deutsch & J. A. Deutsch (Eds.), *Short-term memory* (pp. 258–291). New York: Academic Press.

Kolers, P. A. (1979). A pattern-analyzing basis of recognition. In L. S. Cermak & F. I. M. Craik (Eds.), *Levels of processing in human memory* (pp. 363–387). Hillsdale, NJ: Erlbaum.

Kopelman, M. D. (1989). Remote and autobiographical memory, temporal context memory and frontal atrophy in Korsakoff and Alzheimer patients. *Neuropsychologia, 27*, 437–460.

Kosel, K. C., Van Hoesen, G. W., & West, J. R. (1981). Olfactory bulb projections to the parahippocampal area of the rat. *Journal of Comparative Neurology, 198*, 467–487.

Kruschke, J. K. (1992). ALCOVE: An exemplar-based connectionist model of category learning. *Psychological Review, 99*, 22–44.

Kubie, J. L., & Ranck, J. B. Jr. (1984). Hippocampal neuronal firing, context, and learning. In L. R. Squire & N. Butters (Eds.), *Neuropsychology of memory*. New York: Guilford Press.

Larson, J., & Lynch, G. (1986). Induction of synaptic potentiation in hippocampus by patterned stimulation involves two events. *Science, 232*, 985–988.

Larson, J., Wong, D., & Lynch, G. (1986). Patterned stimulation at the theta frequency is optimal for the induction of hippocampal long-term potentiation. *Brain Research, 368*, 347–350.

Leaton, R. N., & Borszcz, G. S. (1990). Hippocampal lesions and temporally chained conditioned stimuli in a conditioned suppression paradigm. *Psychobiology, 18*, 81–88.

LeDoux, J. E. (1991). Systems and synapses of emotional memory. In L. R. Squire, N. M. Weinberger, G. Lynch, & J. L. McGaugh (Eds.), *Memory: Organization and locus of change*. New York: Oxford University Press.

Leis, T. L., Pallage, V., Toniolo, G., & Will, B. (1984). Working memory theory of hippocampal function needs qualification. *Behavioral Neurology and Biology, 42*, 140–157.

Levin, H. S., Papanicolaou, A. & Eisenberg, H. M. (1984). Observations on amnesia after non-missile head injury. In L. R. Squire & N. Butters (Eds.), *Neuropsychology of memory* (pp. 247–257). New York: Guilford Press.

Lewicki, P. (1986). *Nonconscious social information processing*. New York: Academic Press.

Lewicki, P., Hill, T., & Bizot, E. (1988). Acquisition of procedural knowledge about a pattern of stimuli that cannot be articulated. *Cognitive Psychology, 20*, 24–37.

Loechner, K. J., & Weisz, D. J. (1987). Hippocampectomy and feature-positive discrimination. *Behavioral Brain Research, 26,* 63–73.

Logan, G. (1988). Toward an instance theory of automatization. *Psychological Review, 85,* 492–527.

Lynch, G. (1986). *Synapses, circuits, and the beginnings of memory.* Cambridge, MA: MIT Press.

MacKinnon, D., & Squire, L. R. (1989). Autobiographical memory in amnesia. *Psychobiology, 17,* 247–256.

Mahut, H., & Moss, M. (1984). Consolidation of memory: The hippocampus revisited. In L. R. Squire & N. Butters (Eds.), *Neuropsychology of memory* (pp. 297–315). New York: Guilford Press.

Mahut, H., Zola-Morgan, S., & Moss, M. (1982). Hippocampal resections impair associative learning and recognition memory in the monkey. *Journal of Neuroscience, 1,* 227–240.

Malamut, B. L., Saunders, R. C., & Mishkin, M. (1984). Monkeys with combined amygdala-hippocampal lesions succeed in object discrimination learning despite 24-hour intertrial intervals. *Behavioral Neuroscience, 98,* 759–769.

Markowska, A. L., Olton, D. S., Murray, E. A., & Gaffan, D. (1989). A comparative analysis of the role of fornix and cingulate cortex in memory: Rats. *Behavioral Brain Research, 74,* 255–269.

Martone, M., Butters, N., Payne, M., Becker, J., & Sax, D. S. (1984). Dissociations between skill learning and verbal recognition in amnesia and dementia. *Archives of Neurology, 41,* 965–970.

Masson, M. E. J. (1986). Identification of typographically transformed words: Instance-based skill acquisition. *Journal of Experimental Psychology: Learning, Memory, and Cognition, 12,* 479–488.

Mayes, A. R., & Goodling, P. (1989). Enhancement of word completion priming in amnesics by cuing with previously novel associates. *Neuropsychologia, 27,* 1057–1072.

McAndrews, M. P., Glisky, E. L., & Schacter, D. L. (1987). When priming persists: Long-lasting implicit memory for a single episode in amnesic patients. *Neuropsychologia, 25,* 497–506.

McCarthy, R. A., & Warrington, E. K. (1990). *Cognitive neuropsychology.* San Diego: Academic Press.

McClelland, J. L., & Rumelhart, D. E. (1981). An interactive activation model of context effects in letter perception. Part 1: An account of basic findings. *Psychological Review, 88,* 375–407.

McClelland, J. L., & Rumelhart, D. E. (1986). Amnesia and distributed memory. In J. L. McClelland & D. E. Rumelhart (Eds.), *Parallel distributed processing: Explorations in the microstructure of cognition* (pp. 503–527). Cambridge, MA: MIT Press.

McNaughton, B. L., Barnes, C. A., & O'Keefe, J. (1983). The contributions of position, direction, and velocity to single unit activity in the hippocampus. *Experimental Brain Research, 52,* 41–49.

McNaughton, B. L., Douglas, R. M., & Goddard, G. V. (1978). Synaptic enhancement in fascia dentata: Cooperativity among coactive afferents. *Brain Research, 157,* 277–293.

McNaughton, B. L., & Morris, R. G. M. (1987). Hippocampal synaptic enhancement and information storage within a distributed memory system. *Trends in Neurosciences, 10,* 408–415.

Meck, W. H., Church, R. M., & Olton, D. S. (1984). Hippocampus, time, and memory. *Behavioral Neuroscience, 98,* 3–22.

Merzenich, M. M., Recanzone, G. H., Jenkins, W. M., & Grajski, K. A. (1990). Adaptive mechanisms in cortical networks underlying cortical contributions to learning and nondeclarative memory. In *Cold Spring Harbor symposia on quantitative biology. Vol. 55: The brain.* New York: Cold Spring Harbor Laboratory.

Meudell, P. R., & Mayes, A. R. (1981). The Claparède phenomenon: A further example in amnesics, a demonstration of a similar effect in normal people with attenuated memory, and a reinterpretation. *Current Psychological Research, 1,* 75–88.

Mikami, A., & Kubota, A. (1980). Inferotemporal neuron activities and color discrimination with delay. *Brain Research, 182,* 65–78.

Milberg, W., Alexander, M. P., Charness, N., McGlinchey-Berrot, R., & Barrett, A. (1988). Learning of a complex arithmetic skill in amnesia: Evidence for a dissociation between compilation and production. *Brain and Cognition, 8,* 91–104.

Milner, B. (1962). Les troubles de la mémoire accompagnant des lésions hippocampiques bilatérales. In P. Passouant (Ed.), *Physiologie de l'hippocampe.* Paris: Centre de la Recherche Scientifique.

Milner, B. (1965). Memory disturbance after bilateral hippocampal lesions. In P. M. Milner & S. E. Glickman (Eds.), *Cognitive processes and the brain.* Princeton, NJ: Van Nostrand.

Milner, B. (1966). Amnesia following operation on the temporal lobe. In C. W. M. Whitty & O. L. Zangwill (Eds.), *Amnesia* (pp. 109–133). London: Butterworth.

Milner, B., Corkin, S., & Teuber, H. L. (1968). Further analysis of the hippocampal amnesic syndrome: 14-year followup study of H.M. *Neuropsychologia, 6,* 215–234.

Milner, B., & Teuber, H. L. (1968). Alteration of perception and memory in man: Reflections on methods. In L. Weiskrantz (Ed.), *Analysis of behavioral change* (pp. 268–375). New York: Harper & Row.

Mishkin, M. (1978). Memory in monkeys severely impaired by combined but not separate removal of the amygdala and hippocampus. *Nature, 273,* 297–298.

Mishkin, M. (1982). A memory system in the monkey. *Philosophical Transactions of the Royal Society, B298,* 85–95.

Mishkin, M., & Delacour, J. (1975). An analysis of short-term visual memory in the monkey. *Journal of Experimental Psychology* [Animal Behavior], *1,* 326–334.

Mishkin, M., Malamut, B., & Bachevalier, J. (1984). Memories and habits: Two neural systems. In J. L. McGaugh, G. Lynch & N. M. Weinberger (Eds.), *The neurobiology of learning and memory* (pp. 65–77). New York: Guilford Press.

Mishkin, M., & Petri, H. L. (1984). Memories and habits: Some implications for the analysis of learning and retention. In N. Butters & L. R. Squire (Eds.), *Neuropsychology of memory.* New York: Guilford Press.

Miyashita, Y., & Chang, H. S. (1988). Neuronal correlate of pictoral short-term memory in the primate temporal cortex. *Nature, 331,* 68–70.

Morris, C. D., Bransford, J. D., & Franks, J. J. (1977). Levels of processing versus transfer appropriate processing. *Journal of Verbal Learning and Verbal Behavior 16,* 519–533.

Morris, R. G. M. (1981). Spatial localization does not require the presence of local cues. *Learning and Motivation, 12,* 239–260.

Morris, R. G. M. (1984). Developments of a water-maze procedure for studying spatial learning in the rat. *Journal of Neuroscience Methods, 11,* 47–60.

Morris, R. G. M. (1991). Is the hippocampus disportionately involved in spatial learning? Address given at the Society of Neuroscience Meeting, New Orleans.

Moscovitch, M. (1984). The sufficient conditions for demonstrating preserved memory in amnesia: A task analysis. In L. R. Squire & N. Butters (Eds.), *Neuropsychology of memory* (pp. 104–114). New York: Guilford Press.

Moscovitch, M., Winocur, G., & McLachlan, D. (1986). Memory as assessed by recognition and reading time in normal and memory impaired people with Alzheimer's disease and other neurological disorders. *Journal of Experimental Psychology: General, 115,* 331–347.

Moss, M., Mahut, H., & Zola-Morgan, S. (1981). Concurrent discrimination learning of monkeys after hippocampal, entorhinal, or fornix lesions. *Journal of Neuroscience. 1,* 227–240.

Moyer, J. R., Deyo, R. A., & Disterhoft, J. F. (1990). Hippocampectomy disrupts trace eyeblink conditioning in rabbits. *Behavioral Neuroscience, 104,* 243–252.

Muller, R. U., & Kubie, J. L. (1987). The effects of changes in the environment on the spatial firing of hippocampal complex-spike cells. *Journal of Neuroscience, 7*, 1951–1968.

Muller, R. U., & Kubie, J. L. (1989). The firing of hippocampal place predicts the future position of moving rats. *Journal of Neuroscience, 9*, 4101–4110.

Muller, R. R., Kubie, J. L., & Ranck, J. B., Jr. (1987). Spatial firing patterns of hippocampal complex spike cells in a fixed environment. *Journal of Neuroscience, 7*, 1935–1950.

Mumby, D. G., Pinel, J. P. J., & Wood, E. R. (1990). A new paradigm for testing nonspatial working memory in rats: Nonrecurring items delayed nonmatching to sample. *Psychobiology, 18*, 321–326.

Munro, P. W. (1984). A model for generalization and specification by single neurons. *Biological Cybernetics, 51*, 169–179.

Murray, E. A., Davidson, M., Gaffan, D., Olton, D. S., & Suomi, S. (1989). Effects of fornix transection and cingulate cortical ablation on spatial memory in rhesis monkeys. *Experimental Brain Research, 74*, 173–186.

Murray, E. A., & Mishkin, M. (1986). Visual recognition in monkeys following rhinal cortical ablations combined with either amygdalectomy or hippocampectomy. *Journal of Neuroscience, 6*, 1991–2003.

Musen, G., & Squire, L. R. (1990). Implicit memory: No evidence for rapid acquisition of new associations in amnesic patients or normal subjects. *Society for Neuroscience Abstracts, 16*, 287.

Musen, G., & Squire, L. R. (1991). Normal acquisition of novel verbal information in amnesia. *Journal of Experimental Psychology: Learning, Memory and Cognition, 17*, 1095–1104.

Musen, G., Shimamura, A. P., & Squire, L. L. (1990). Intact text-specific reading skill in amnesia. *Journal of Experimental Psychology: Learning, Memory and Cognition, 16*, 1068–1076.

Musen, G., & Triesmann, A. (1990). Implicit memory and explicit memory for visual patterns. *Journal of Experimental Psychology: Learning, Memory and Cognition, 16*, 127–137.

Nadel, L. (1991). The hippocampus and space revisited. *Hippocampus, 1*, 221–229.

Newell, A. (1973). Productions systems: Models of control structures. In W. G. Chase, (Ed.), *Visual information processing*. New York: Academic Press.

Nissen, M. J., & Bullemer, P. (1987). Attentional requirements of learning: Evidence from performance measures. *Cognitive Psychology, 19*, 1–32.

Nissen, M. J., Cohen, N. J., & Corkin, S. (1981). The amnesic patient H.M.: Learning and retention of perceptual skills. *Society for Neuroscience Abstracts, 7*, 517.

Nissen, M. J., Willingham, D., & Hartman, M. (1989). Explicit and implicit remembering: When is learning preserved in amnesia? *Neuropsychologia, 27,* 341–352.

Norman, D. A., & Rumelhart, D. E. (1975). In D. A. Norman, D. E. Rumelhart, & the LNR Research Group, *Explorations in cognition.* San Francisco: Freeman.

Okaichi, H. (1987). Performance and dominant strategies on place and cue tasks following hippocampal lesions in rats. *Psychobiology, 15,* 58–63.

O'Keefe, J. A. (1976). Place units in the hippocampus of the freely moving rat. *Experimental Neurology, 51,* 78–109.

O'Keefe, J. A. (1979). A review of hippocampal place cells. *Progress in Neurobiology, 13,* 419–439.

O'Keefe, J. A. (1989). Computations the hippocampus might perform. In L. Nadel, L. A. Cooper, P. Culicover, & R. M. Harnish (Eds.), *Neural connections, mental computation.* Cambridge, MA: MIT Press.

O'Keefe, J. A., & Conway, D. H. (1978). Hippocampal place units in the freely moving rat: Why they fire when they fire. *Experimental Brain Research, 31,* 573–590.

O'Keefe, J. A., & Conway, D. H. (1980). On the trail of the hippocampal engram. *Physiology and Psychology, 2,* 229–238.

O'Keefe, J. A., & Nadel, L. (1978). *The hippocampus as a cognitive map.* London: Oxford University Press.

O'Keefe, J. A., & Speakman, A. (1987). Single unit activity in the rat hippocampus during a spatial memory task. *Experimental Brain Research, 68,* 1–27.

Olton, D. S., Becker, J. T., & Handelmann, G. E. (1979). Hippocampus, space, and memory. *Behavioral and Brain Sciences, 2,* 313–365.

Olton, D. S., Branch, M., & Best, P. (1978). Spatial correlates of hippocampus unit activity. *Experimental Neurology, 58,* 387–409.

Olton, D. S., Meck, W. H., & Church, R. M. (1987). Separation of hippocampal and amygdaloid involvement in temporal memory dysfunctions. *Brain Research, 404,* 180–188.

Olton, D. S., & Papas, B. C. (1979). Spatial memory and hippocampal function. *Neuropsychologia, 17,* 669–682.

Olton, D. S., & Samuelson, R. J. (1976). Remembrance of places passed: Spatial memory in rats. *Journal of Experimental Psychology* [Animal Behavior], *2,* 97–116.

Ono, T., Nakamura, K., Fukuda, M., & Tamura, R. (1991). Place recognition responses of neurons in monkey hippocampus. *Neuroscience Letters, 121,* 194–198.

Orbach, J., Milner, B., & Rasmussen, T. (1960). Learning and retention in monkeys after amygdala-hippocampus resection. *Archives of Neurology, 3*, 230–251.

Osborne, B., & Black, A. H. (1978). A detailed analysis of behavior during the transition from acquisition to extinction in rats with fornix lesions. *Behavioral Biology, 23*, 271–290.

Ostergaard, A. L. (1987). Episodic, semantic, and procedural memory in a case of amnesia at an early age. *Neuropsychologia, 25*, 341–357.

Otto, T., & Eichenbaum, H. (1992). Dissociable roles of the hippocampus and orbitofrontal cortex in an odor-guided delayed nonmatch to sample task. *Behavioral Neuroscience, 105*, 111–119.

Otto, T., Schottler, F., Staubli, U., Eichenbaum, H., & Lynch, G. (1991). The hippocampus and olfactory discrimination learning: Effects of entorhinal cortex lesions on learning-set acquisition and on odor memory in a successive-cue, go/no-go task. *Behavioral Neuroscience, 105*, 111–119.

Packard, M. G., Hirsh, R., & White, N. M. (1989). Differential effects of fornix and caudate lesions on two radial arm maze tasks: Evidence for multiple memory systems. *Journal of Neuroscience, 9*, 1465–1472.

Parkin, A. J. (1987). *Memory and amnesia.* Oxford: Basil Blackwell.

Pavlides, C., Greenstein, Y. J., Grudman, M., & Winson, J. (1988). Long-term potentiation in the dentate gyrus is induced preferentially on the positive phase of theta rhythm. *Brain Research, 439*, 383–387.

Perrett, D. I., Rolls, E. T., & Caan, E. (1982). Visual neurons responsive to faces in the monkey temporal cortex. *Experimental Brain Research, 47*, 329–342.

Perruchet, P., & Pacteau, C. (1990). Synthetic grammar learning: Implicit rule abstraction or explicit fragmentary knowledge? *Journal of Experimental Psychology: General, 119(3)*, 264–275.

Petersen, S. E., Fox, P. T., Posner, M. I., Mintun, M. A., & Raichle, M. E. (1989). Positron emission tomographic studies of the processing of single words. *Journal of Cognitive Neuroscience, 1*, 153–170.

Petersen, S. E., Fox, P. T., Snyder, A. Z., & Raichle, M. E. (1990). Activation of extrastriate and frontal cortical areas by visual words and word-like stimuli. *Science, 249*, 1041–1044.

Port, R. L., Beggs, A. L., & Patterson, M. M. (1987). Hippocampal substrate of sensory associations. *Physiology and Behavior, 39*, 643–647.

Port, R. L., Mikail, A. A., & Patterson, M. M. (1985). Differential effect of hippocampectomy on classically conditioned rabbit nictitating membrane response related to interstimulus interval. *Behavioral Neuroscience, 99*, 200–208.

Posner, M. I. (1973). *Cognition: An introduction.* Glenview, IL: Scott, Foresman.

Posner, M. I., Inhoff, A. W., Friedrich, F. J., & Cohen, A. (1987). Isolating attentional systems: A cognitive-anatomical analysis. *Psychobiology, 15,* 107–121.

Purves, D., & Lichtman, J. W. (1985). *Principles of neural development.* Sunderland, MA: Sinauer.

Quirk, G. J., Muller, R. U., & Kubie, J. L. (1990). The firing of hippocampal place cells in the dark depends on the rat's recent experience. *Journal of Neuroscience, 10,* 2008–2017.

Raffaele, K. C., & Olton, D. S. (1988). Hippocampal and amygdaloid involvement in working memory for nonspatial stimuli. *Behavioral Neuroscience, 102,* 349–355.

Rawlins, J. N. P. (1985). Associations across time: The hippocampus as a temporary memory store. *Brain and Behavioral Science, 8,* 479–496.

Rawlins, J. N. P., Feldon, J., & Butt, S. (1985). The effects of delaying reward on choice preference in rats with hippocampal or selective sepatial lesions. *Behavioral Brain Research, 15,* 191–203.

Rawlins, J. N. P., Maxwell, T. J., & Sinden, J. D. (1988). The effects of fornix section on win-stay/lose-shift and win-shift/lose-stay performance in the rat. *Behavioral Brain Research, 31,* 17–28.

Rawlins, J. N. P., Winocur, G., & Gray, J. A. (1983). The hippocampus, collateral behavior and timing. *Behavioral Neuroscience, 97,* 857–872.

Reber, A. S. (1967). Implicit learning of artificial grammars. *Journal of Verbal Learning and Verbal Behavior, 77,* 317–327.

Reber, A. S. (1976). Implicit learning of synthetic languages: The role of instructional set. *Journal of Experimental Psychology: Human Learning and Memory, 2,* 88–94.

Reber, A. S. (1989). Implicit learning and tacit knowledge. *Journal of Experimental Psychology: General, 118,* 219–235.

Recanzone, G. H., Merzenich, M. M., Jenkins, W. M., Grajski, K. A., & Dinse, H. R. (1992). Topographic reorganization of the hand representation in cortical area 3b of owl monkeys trained in a frequency-discrimination task. *Journal of Neurophysiology, 67,* 1031–1056.

Rescorla, R. A. (1973). Effect of US habituation following conditioning. *Journal of Comparative and Physiological Psychology, 82,* 137–143.

Richardson-Klavehn, A., & Bjork, R. A. (1988). Measures of memory. *Annual Review of Psychology, 39,* 475–543.

Rickert, E. J., Bennett, T. L., Lane, P., & French, J. (1978). Hippocampectomy and the attenuation of blocking. *Behavioral Biology, 22,* 147–160.

Rickert, E. J., Lorden, J. F., Dawson, R., Smyly, E., & Callahan, M. F. (1979). Stimulus processing and stimulus selection in rats with hippocampal lesions. *Behavioral and Neural Biology, 27,* 454–465.

Roediger, H. L. (1990). Implicit memory: Retention without remembering. *American Psychologist, 45,* 1043–1056.

Roediger, H. L., & Blaxton, T. A. (1987a). Effects of varying modality, surface features, and retention interval on priming in word-fragment completion. *Memory and Cognition, 15,* 379–388.

Roediger, H. L., & Blaxton, T. A. (1987b). Retrieval modes produce dissociations in memory for surface information. In D. S. Gorfein & R. R. Hoffman (Eds.), *Memory and learning: The Ebbinghaus centennial conference* (pp. 349–379). Hillsdale, NJ: Erlbaum.

Roediger, H. L., Weldon, M. S., & Challis, B. H. (1989). Explaining dissociations between implicit and explicit measures of retention: A processing account. In H. L. Roediger & F. I. M. Craik (Eds.), *Varieties of memory and consciousness: Essays in honor of Endel Tulving* (pp. 3–41). Hillsdale, NJ: Erlbaum.

Rolls, E. T. (1987). Information representation, processing and storage in the brain: Analysis at the single neuron level. In J.-P. Changeux and M. Konishi (Eds.), *The scientific basis of clinical neurology* (pp. 503–540). Chichester: Wiley.

Rolls, E. T. (1989). Functions of neuronal networks in the hippocampus and neocortex in memory. In J. H. Byrne & W. O. Berry (Eds.), *Neural models of plasticity: Theoretical and empirical approaches.* New York: Academic Press.

Rolls, E. T., Miyashita, Y., Cahusac, P., Kesner, R. P., Niki, H. D., Feigenbaum, J. D., & Bach, L. (1989). Hippocampal neurons in the monkey with activity related to the place where a stimulus is shown. *Journal of Neuroscience, 9,* 1835–1846.

Rolls, E. T., & O'Mara, S. M. (1991). Are there place cells in the primate hippocampus? *Society for Neuroscience Abstracts, 17,* 1101.

Room, P., & Groenewegen, H. J. (1986). Connections of the parahippocampal cortex in the cat. I. Cortical afferents. *Journal of Comparative Neurology, 251,* 415–450.

Room, P., Groenewegen, H. J., & Lohman, A. H. M. (1984). Inputs from the olfactory bulb and olfactory cortex to the entorhinal cortex in the cat. I. Anatomical observations. *Experimental Brain Research, 56,* 488–496.

Rose, F. C., & Symonds, C. P. (1960). Persistent memory defect following encephalitis. *Brain, 83,* 195–212.

Rose, G. M., & Dunwiddie, T. V. (1986). Induction of hippocampal long-term potentiation using physiologically patterned stimulation. *Neuroscience Letters, 69,* 244–248.

Rosene, D. L., & Van Hoesen, G. W. (1987). The hippocampal formation of the primate brain. A review of some comparative aspects of cytoarchitecture and connections. In E. G. Jones and A. Peters (Eds.), *Cerebral cortex, Vol. 6: Further aspects of cortical function, including hippocampus.* New York: Plenum Press.

Ross, B. H. (1984). Remindings and their effects in learning a cognitive skill. *Cognitive Psychology, 16,* 371–416.

Ross, B. H. (1987). This is like that: The use of earlier problems and the separation of similarity effects. *Journal of Experimental Psychology: Learning, Memory, and Cognition, 13,* 629–639.

Ross, R. T., Orr, W. B., Holland, P. C., & Berger, T. W. (1984). Hippocampectomy disrupts acquisition and retention of learned conditioning and responding. *Behavioral Neuroscience, 2,* 211–225.

Rothblatt, L. A., & Kromer, L. F. (1991). Object recognition memory in the rat: The role of the hippocampus. *Behavioral Brain Research, 42,* 25–32.

Rueckl, J. (1990). Similarity effects in word and pseudoword repetition priming. *Journal of Experimental Psychology: Learning, Memory and Cognition, 16,* 374–391.

Rumelhart, D. E., Hinton, G. E., & Williams, R. J. (1986). Learning internal representations by error propagation. In D. E. Rumelhart & J. L. McClelland (Eds.), *Parallel distributed processing: Explorations in the microstructure of cognition. Vol. 1.* Cambridge, MA: MIT Press.

Rumelhart, D. E., & McClelland, J. (1982). An interactive activation model of context effects in letter perception: Part 2. The contextual enhancement effect and some tests and extensions of the model. *Psychological Review, 89,* 60–94.

Rumelhart, D. E., & McClelland, J. (Eds.) (1986). *Parallel distributed processing.* Cambridge, MA: MIT Press.

Russell, W. R., & Nathan, P. W. (1946). Traumatic amnesia. *Brain, 68,* 280–300.

Sagar, H. H., Cohen, N. J., Corkin, S., & Growdon, J. M. (1985). Dissociations among processes in remote memory. In D. S. Olton, E. Gamzu, & S. Corkin (Eds.), *Memory dysfunctions, Vol. 444* (pp. 533–535). New York: *Annals of the New York Academy of Sciences.*

Saint-Cyr, J. A., Taylor, A. E., & Lang, A. E. (1988). Procedural learning and neostriatal dysfunction in man. *Brain, 111,* 941–959.

Sakurai, Y. (1990). Hippocampal cells have behavioral correlates during performance of an auditory working memory task in the rat. *Behavioral Neuroscience, 104,* 253–263.

Sanderson, P. M. (1989). Verbalizable knowledge and skilled task performance: Association, dissociation, and mental models. *Journal of Experimental Psychology: Learning, Memory and Cognition, 15(4),* 729–747.

Sato, T. (1988). Effects of attention and stimulus interaction on visual responses of inferior temporal neurons in macaque. *Journal of Neurophysiology, 60*, 344–364.

Saunders, R. C., & Weiskrantz, L. (1989). The effects of fornix transection and combined fornix transection, mammillary body lesions and hippocampal ablations on object pair association memory in the rhesus monkey. *Behavioral Brain Research, 35*, 85–94.

Savoy, R. L., & Gabrieli, J. E. E. (1988). Normal McCollough effect in Alzheimer's disease and global amnesia. *Society for Neuroscience Abstracts. 14*, 217.

Schacter, D. L. (1987). Implicit memory: History and current status. *Journal of Experimental Psychology: Learning, Memory, and Cognition, 13*, 501–508.

Schacter, D. L. (1990a). Perceptual representation systems and implicit memory: Toward a resolution of the multiple memory systems debate. In A. Diamond (Ed.), *Development and neural bases of higher cognitive functions* (pp. 543–571). Annals of the New York Academy of Science. New York: New York Academy of Sciences and MIT/Bradford Press.

Schacter, D. L. (1990b) Toward a cognitive neuropsychology of awareness: Implicit knowledge and anosognosia. *Journal of Clinical and Experimental Neuropsychology, 12*, 155–178.

Schacter, D. L., & Crovitz, H. F. (1977). Memory function after closed head injury: A review of the quantitative research. *Cortex, 13*, 150–176.

Schacter, D. L., & Glisky, E. (1986). Memory remediation. In B. Uzzel (Ed.), *Clinical neuropsychology of intervention* (pp. 257–282). Holland: Nijhoff.

Schacter, D. L., & Graf, P. (1986). Effects of elaborative processing on implicit and explicit memory for new associations. *Journal of Experimental Psychology: Learning, Memory, and Cognition, 12*, 432–444.

Schacter, D. L., & Tulving, E. (1982). Amnesia and memory research. In L. S. Cermak (Ed.), *Human memory and amnesia.* Hillsdale, NJ: Erlbaum.

Schacter, D. L., & Tulving, E. (1983). Memory, amnesia, and the episodic/semantic distinction. In R. L. Isaacson & N. E. Spear (Eds.), *Expression of knowledge.* New York: Plenum Press.

Schacter, D. L., Cooper, L. A., & Delaney, S. M. (1990). Implicit memory for unfamiliar objects depends on access to structural descriptions. *Journal of Experimental Psychology: General, 119*, 5–24.

Schenck, F., & Morris, R. G. M. (1985). Dissociation between components of spatial memory in rats after recovery from the effects of retrohippocampal lesions. *Experimental Brain Research, 58*, 11–28.

Schmajuk, N. A. (1989). The hippocampus and the control of information storage in the brain. In M. Arbib & S. I. Amari (Eds.), *Dynamic interactions in neural networks: Models and data.* New York: Springer-Verlag.

Schmajuk, N. A., & Isaacson, R. L. (1984). Classical contingencies in rats with hippocampal lesions. *Physiology and Behavior, 33,* 889–893.

Schmajuk, N. A., & Moore, J. W. (1988). The hippocampus and the classically conditioned nictitating membrane response: A real-time attentional-associative model. *Psychobiology, 16,* 20–35.

Schmaltz, L. W., & Theios J. (1972). Acquisition and extinction of a classically conditioned response in hippocampectomized rabbits (*Oryctolagus cuniculus*). *Journal of Comparative Physiology and Psychology, 79,* 328–333.

Schwartz, E. L., Desimone, R., Albright, T. D., & Gross, C. G. (1983). Shape recognition and inferior temporal neurons. *Proceedings of the National Academy of Science, 80,* 5776–5778.

Scoville, W. B., & Milner, B. (1957). Loss of recent memory after bilateral hippocampal lesions. *Journal of Neurological and Neurosurgical Psychiatry, 20,* 11–12.

Segal, M., Disterholt, J. F., & Olds, J. (1972). Hippocampal unit activity during classical aversive and appetitive conditioning. *Science, 175,* 792–794.

Shallice, T. (1982). Specific impairments of planning. *Philosophical Transactions of the Royal Society of London B, 298,* 199–209.

Shallice, T. (1988). *From neuropsychology to mental structure.* Cambridge: Cambridge University Press.

Shapiro, M. L., Hetherington, P. A., Eichenbaum, H. B., & Fortin, W. B. (1990). A simple PDP model simulates spatial correlates of hippocampal neuronal activity. *Society of Neuroscience Abstracts, 16,* 473.

Sharp, P. E. (1991). Computer simulation of hippocampal place cells. *Psychobiology, 19,* 103–115.

Shimamura, A. P. (1986). Priming effects in amnesia: Evidence for a dissociable memory function. *Quarterly Journal of Experimental Psychology, 38A,* 618–644.

Shimamura, A. P., & Squire, L. R. (1989). Impaired priming of new associations in amnesia. *Journal of Experimental Psychology: Learning, Memory and Cognition, 15,* 721–728.

Simon, H. A. (1975). The functional equivalence of problem solving skills. *Cognitive Psychology, 7,* 268–288.

Simon, H. A., & Hayes, J. R. (1976). The understanding process: Problem isomorphs. *Cognitive Psychology, 8,* 165–190.

Sinden, J. D., Rawlins, J. N. P., Gray, J. A., & Jarrard, L. E. (1986). Selective cytotoxic lesions of the hippocampal formation and DRL performance in rats. *Behavioral Neuroscience, 100,* 320–329.

Sloman, S. A., Hayman, C. A. G., Ohta, N., & Tulving, E. (1988). Forgetting and interference in fragment completion. *Journal of Experimental Psychology: Learning, Memory and Cognition, 14,* 223–239.

Sloman, S. A., & Rumelhart, D. E. (1991). Reducing interference in distributed memory through episodic gating. In A. F. Healey, S. M. Kosslyn, & R. M. Shiffrin (Eds.), *From learning theory to cognitive processes: Essays in honor of William E. Estes*, NJ: Erlbaum.

Snodgrass, J. G. (1989). How many memory systems are there really?: Some evidence from the picture fragment completion task. In C. Izawa (Ed.), *Current issues in cognitive processes: The Tulane Floweree symposium on cognition* (pp. 135–173). Hillsdale, NJ: Erlbaum.

Snodgrass, J. G., & Feenan, K. (1990). Priming effects in picture fragment completion: Support for the perceptual closure hypothesis. *Journal of Experimental Psychology: General, 119*, 276–296.

Solomon, P. R. (1977). Role of the hippocampus in blocking and conditioned inhibition of the rabbit's nictitating membrane response. *Journal of Comparative and Physiological Psychology, 91*, 407–417.

Solomon, P. R., & Moore, J. W. (1975). Latent inhibition and stimulus generalization of the classically conditioned nictitating membrane response in rabbits. (*Oryctolagus cuniculus*) following dorsal hippocampal ablation. *Journal of Comparative Physiology and Psychology, 89*, 1192–1203.

Solomon, P. R., Vander Schaff, E. R., Norbe, A. C., Weisz, D. J., & Thompson, R. F. (1986). Hippocampus and trace conditioning of the rabbit's nictitating response. *Behavioral Neuroscience, 100*, 729–744.

Squire, L. R. (1982a). The neuropsychology of human memory. *Annual Review of Neuroscience, 5*, 241–273.

Squire, L. R. (1982b). Comparisons between forms of amnesia: Some deficits are unique to Korsakoff's syndrome. *Journal of Experimental Psychology: Learning, Memory and Cognition, 8*, 560–571.

Squire, L. R. (1986). Mechanisms of memory. *Science, 232*, 1612–1619.

Squire, L. R. (1987). *Memory and brain*. New York: Oxford University Press.

Squire, L. R. (1992). Memory and the hippocampus: A synthesis from findings with rats, monkeys, and humans. *Psychological Review, 99*, 195–231.

Squire, L. R., & Cohen, N. J. (1984). Human memory and amnesia. In G. Lynch, J. L. McGaugh, & N. M. Weinberger (Eds.), *Neurobiology of learning and memory* (pp. 3–64). New York: Guilford Press.

Squire, L. R., & Frambach, M. (1990). Cognitive skill learning in amnesia. *Psychobiology, 18*, 109–117.

Squire, L. R., Cohen, N. J., & Nadel, L. (1984). The medial temporal region and memory consolidation: A new hypothesis. In H. Eingartner & E. Parker (Eds.), *Memory consolidation* (pp. 185–210). Hillsdale, NJ: Erlbaum.

Squire, L. R., Mishkin, M., & Shimamura, A. (1990). Is the hippocampus disproportionately involved in spatial aspects of representational memory? *Discussions in neuroscience: Learning and memory, Vol. VI* (pp. 39–55). Amsterdam: Elsevier.

Squire, L. R., Shimamura, A. P., & Amaral, D. G. (1989). Memory and the hippocampus. In J. Byrne & W. O. Berry (Eds.), *Neural models of plasticity* (pp. 208–239). New York: Academic Press.

Squire, L. R., Shimamura, A. P., & Graf, P. (1987). Strength and duration of priming effects in normal subjects and amnesic patients. *Neuropsychologia, 25*, 195–210.

Squire, L. R., Ojemann, J. G., Miezin, F. M., Petersen, S. E., Videeen, T., & Raichle, M. (1992). Activation of the hippocampus in normal humans: A functional anatomical study of memory. *Proceedings of the National Academy of Sciences, 89*, 1837–1941.

Squire, L. R., & Zola-Morgan, S. (1983). The neurology of memory: The case for correspondence between the findings for human and nonhuman primate. In J. A. Deutsch (Ed.), *The physiological basis of memory*, 2nd edition. New York: Academic Press.

Squire, L. R., & Zola-Morgan, S. (1988). Memory: Brain systems and behavior. *Trends in Neurosciences, 11*, 170–175.

Squire, L. R., & Zola-Morgan, S. (1991). The medial temporal lobe memory system. *Science, 253*, 1380–1386.

Staubli, U., Ivy, G., & Lynch, G. (1984). Hippocampal denervation causes rapid forgetting of olfactory information in rats. *Proceedings of the National Academy of Sciences, 81*, 5885–5887.

Stewart, M., Fox, S. E. (1990). Do septal neurons pace the hippocampal theta rhythm? *Trends in Neurosciences, 13*, 163–168.

Suess, W. M., & Berlyne, D. E. (1978). Exploratory behavior as a function of hippocampal damage, stimulus complexity, and stimulus novelty in the hooded rat. *Behavioral Biology, 23*, 487–499.

Sutherland, R. J., & Rudy, J. W. (1989). Configural association theory: The role of the hippocampal formation in learning, memory, and amnesia. *Psychobiology, 17*, 129–144.

Sutherland, R. J., Wishaw, I. Q., & Kolb, B. (1983). A behavioral analysis of spatial localization following electrolytic, kainate- or colchicine-induced damage to the hippocampal formation in the rat. *Behavioral Brain Research, 7*, 133–153.

Sutherland, R. J., Macdonald, R. J., Hill, C. R., & Rudy, J. W. (1989). Damage to the hippocampal formation in rats selectively impairs the ability to learn cue relationships. *Behavioral and Neurological Biology, 52*, 331–356.

Talland, G. A. (1965). *Deranged memory*. New York: Academic Press.

Teyer, T. J., & DiScenna, P. (1985). The role of hippocampus in memory: A hypothesis. *Neuroscience and Biobehavioral Reviews, 9,* 377–389.

Thomas, G. J. (1984). Memory: Time binding in organisms. In L. R. Squire & N. Butters (Eds.), *Neuropsychology of memory* (pp. 374–384). New York: Guilford Press.

Thomas, G. J., & Gash, D. M. (1988). Differential effects of hippocampal ablations on dispositional and representational memory in the rat. *Behavioral Neuroscience, 102,* 635–642.

Treisman, A. M. (1969). Strategies and models of selective attention. *Psychological Review, 76,* 282–299.

Treisman, A. (1988). Features and objects: The Fourteenth Bartlett Memorial Lecture. *Quarterly Journal of Experimental Psychology, 40(A).*

Tulving, E. (1972). Episodic and semantic memory. In E. Tulving & W. Donaldson (Eds.), *Organization of memory* (pp. 382–403). New York: Academic Press.

Tulving, E. (1983). *Elements of episodic memory.* New York: Oxford University Press.

Tulving, E. (1984). Precis of *Elements of episodic memory. Behavioral and Brain Sciences, 7,* 223–268.

Tulving, E. (1985). Multiple learning and memory systems. In K. Lagerspetz & P. Niemi, (Eds.), *Psychology in the 1990's.* Amsterdam: North-Holland.

Tulving, E. (1987). Multiple memory systems and consciousness. *Human Neurobiology, 6,* 67–80.

Tulving, E., & Schacter, D. L. (1990). Priming and human memory systems. *Science, 247,* 301–306.

Tulving, E., Schacter, D. L., & Stark, H. A. (1982). Priming effects in word-fragment completion are independent of recognition memory. *Journal of Experimental Psychology: Learning, Memory, and Cognition, 8,* 336–342.

Tulving, E., & Thomson, D. M. (1973). Encoding specificity and retrieval processes in episodic memory. *Psychological Review, 80,* 352–373.

Turner, N., Cupta, K. C., & Mishkin, M. (1979). The locus and cytoarchitecture of the projection areas of the olfactory bulb in macaca muiatta. *Journal of Comparative Neurology, 177,* 381–396.

Vallar, G., & Shallice, T. (Eds.) (1990) *Neuropsychological impairments to short-term memory.* New York: Cambridge University Press.

Van Groen, T., van Harren, F. J., Witter, M. P., & Groenewegen, H. J. (1986). The organization of the reciprocal connections between subiculum and the entorhinal cortex in the cat: I. A neuroanatomical tracing study. *Journal of Comparative Neurology, 250,* 485–497.

Van Hoesen, G. W. (1982). The primate parahippocampal gyrus: New insights regarding its cortical connections. *Trends in Neurosciences, 5,* 345–350.

Van Hoesen, G. W., Pandya, D. N. (1975). Some connections of the entorhinal (area 28) and perirhinal (area 35) cortices of the rhesis monkey. III. Efferent connections. *Brain Research, 95,* 39–59.

Van Hoesen, G. W., Pandya, D. N., & Butters, N. (1972). Cortical afferents to the entorhinal cortex of the rhesis monkey. *Science, 175,* 1471–1473.

Van Hoesen, G. W., Pandya, D. N., & Butters, N. (1975). Some connections of the entorhinal (area 28) and perirhnal (area 35) cortices of the rhesis monkey. II. Frontal lobe afferents. *Brain, 95,* 25–38.

Victor, M., & Agamanolis, D. (1990). Amnesia due to lesions confined to the hippocampus: A clinical-pathologic study. *Journal of Cognitive Neuroscience, 2,* 246–257.

Victor, M., Adams, R. D., & Collins, G. H. (1971). *The Wernicke-Korsakoff syndrome.* Philadelphia: Davis.

Volpe, B. T., & Hirst, W. (1983). The characterization of an amnesic syndrome following hypoxic ischemic injury. *Archives of Neurology, 40,* 436–445.

Warrington, E. K., & Weiskrantz, L. (1968). A new method of testing long-term retention with special reference to amnesic patients. *Nature, 217,* 972–974.

Warrington, E. K., & Weiskrantz, L. (1970). The amnesic syndrome: Consolidation or retrieval? *Nature, 228,* 628–630.

Warrington, E. K., & Weiskrantz, L. (1973). An analysis of short-term and long-term memory deficits in man. In. J. A. Deutsch (Ed.), *The physiological basis of memory.* New York: Academic Press.

Warrington, E. K., & Weiskrantz, L. (1974). The effect of prior learning on subsequent retention in amnesic patients. *Neuropsychologia, 12,* 419–428.

Warrington, E. K., & Weiskrantz, L. (1978). Further analysis of the prior learning effect in amnesic patients. *Neuropsychologia, 16,* 169–177.

Warrington, E. K., & Weiskrantz, L. (1982). Amnesia: A disconnection syndrome? *Neuropsychologia, 20,* 233–248.

Watanabe, T., & Niki, H. (1985). Hippocampal unit activity and delayed response in the monkey. *Brain Research, 325,* 241–254.

Weiskrantz, L. (1978). A comparison of hippocampal pathology in man and other animals. In *Functions of the septo-hippocampal system, Ciba Foundation Symposium 58.* Oxford: Elsevier.

Weiskrantz, L. (1985). On issues and theories of the human amnesic syndrome. In N. Weinberger, J. L. McGaugh, & G. Lynch (Eds.), *Memory systems of the brain.* New York: Guilford Press.

Weiskrantz, L., & Warrington, E. K. (1979). Conditioning in amnesic patients. *Neuropsychologia, 17,* 187–194.

Wible, C. G., & Olton, D. S. (1988). Effect of fimbria-fornix, hippocampal, and hippocampal-amygdala lesions on performance of 8-pair concurrent object discrimination, object reversal, and T-maze alternation in rats. *Society for Neuroscience Abstracts, 14,* 232.

Wible, C. G., Findling, R. L., Shapiro, M., Lang, E. J., Crane, S., & Olton, D. S. (1986). Mnemonic correlates of unit activity in the hippocampus. *Brain Research, 399,* 97–110.

Wickelgren, W. A. (1979). Chunking and consolidation: A theoretical synthesis of semantic networks, configuring in conditioning, S-R versus cognitive learning, normal forgetting, the amnesic syndrome and the hippocampus arousal system. *Psychological Review, 86,* 44–60.

Wiener, S. I., Paul, C. A., & Eichenbaum, H. (1989). Spatial and behavioral correlates of hippocampal neuronal activity. *Journal of Neuroscience, 9,* 2737–2763.

Wiesel, T. N., & Hubel, D. H. (1963). Single cell response in striate cortex of kittens deprived of vision in one eye. *Journal of Neurophysiology, 26,* 1003–1017.

Wiesel, T. N., & Hubel, D. H. (1965). Comparison of the effects of unilateral and bilateral eye closure on cortical unit responses in kittens. *Journal of Neurophysiology, 28,* 1029–1040.

Wigstrom, H., & Gustafsson, B. (1985). On long-lasting potentiation in the hippocampus: A proposed mechanism for its dependence on coincident pre- and postsynaptic activity. *Acta Psychologica Scandinavica, 123,* 519–522.

Williams, M., & Pennybacker, J. (1954). Memory disturbances in third ventricle tumors. *Journal of Neurology, Neurosurgery and Psychiatry, 17,* 115.

Willingham, D. B., Nissen, M. J., & Bullemer, P. (1989). On the development of procedural knowledge. *Journal of Experimental Psychology: Learning, Memory and Cognition, 15,* 1047–1060.

Wilson, F. A. W., Brown, M. W., & Riches, I. P. (1987). Neuronal activity in the inferomedial temporal cortex compared with that in the hippocampal formation: Implications for amnesia of medial temporal lobe origin. In C. D. Woody (Ed.), *Cellular mechanisms of conditioning and behavioral plasticity.* New York: Plenum Press.

Winocur, G. (1980). The hippocampus and cue utilization. *Physiological Psychology, 8,* 280–288.

Winocur, G. (1990). Anterograde and retrograde amnesia in rats with dorsal hippocampal or dorsomedial thalamic lesions. *Behavioral and Brain Research, 38,* 145–154.

Winocur, G., & Gilbert, M. (1984). The hippocampus, context, and information processing. *Behavioral and Neural Biology, 40,* 27–43.

Winocur, G., & Mills, J. A. (1970). Transfer between related and unrelated problems following hippocampal lesions in rats. *Journal of Comparative Physiology and Psychology, 73,* 162–169.

Winocur, G., & Olds, J. (1978). Effects of context manipulation on memory and reversal learning in rats with hippocampal lesions. *Journal of Comparative and Physiological Psychology, 92,* 312–321.

Winocur, G., Rawlins, J. N. P., & Gray, J. A. (1987). The hippocampus and conditioning to contextual cues. *Behavioral Neuroscience, 101,* 617–625.

Winocur, G., Oxbury, S., Agnetti, V., & Davis, C. (1984). Amnesia in a patient with bilateral lesions to the thalamus. *Neuropsychologia, 22,* 123–144.

Winograd, T. (1972). Understanding language. *Cognitive Psychology, 3,* 1–191.

Winson, J. (1972). Inter-species differences in the occurrence of theta. *Behavioral Biology, 7,* 479–487.

Witter, M. P. (1989). Connectivity of the rat hippocampus. In V. Chan-Palay (Ed.) & C. Koeler (Publisher), *The hippocampus: New vistas.* New York: Wiley.

Wood, F. (1974). The amnesic syndrome as a defect in retrieval from episodic memory. Unpublished Ph.D. thesis, Wake Forest University.

Wood, F., Ebert, V., & Kinsbourne, M. (1982). The episodic-semantic memory distinction in memory and amnesia: Clinical and experimental observations. In L. Cermak (Ed.), *Human memory and amnesia* (pp. 167–194). Hillsdale, NJ: Erlbaum.

Zeki, S. (1990). Functional specialization in the visual cortex: The generation of separate constructs and their multistage integration. In G. M. Edelman, W. E. Gall, & W. M. Cowan (Eds.), *Signal and sense: Local and global order in perceptual maps.* New York: Wiley.

Zola, S. M., & Mahut, H. (1973). Paradoxical facilitation of object reversal learning after transection of the fornix in monkeys. *Neuropsychologia, 11,* 271–284.

Zola-Morgan, S., & Squire, L. R. (1984). Preserved learning in monkeys with medial temporal lesions: Sparing of cognitive skills. *Journal of Neuroscience, 4,* 1072–1085.

Zola-Morgan, S., & Squire, L. R. (1985). Medial temporal lesions in monkeys impair memory on a variety of tasks sensitive to human amnesia. *Behavioral Neuroscience, 99,* 22–34.

Zola-Morgan, S., Cohen, N. J., & Squire, L. (1983). Recall of remote episodic memory in amnesia. *Neuropsychologia, 21,* 487–500.

Zola-Morgan, S., Squire, L. R., & Amaral, D. G. (1989a). Lesions of the hippocampal formation but not lesions of the fornix or mammillary nuclei produce long-lasting memory impairment in the monkey. *Journal of Neuroscience, 9*, 898–913.

Zola-Morgan, S., Squire, L. R., & Amaral, D. G. (1989b). Lesions of the amygdala that spare adjacent cortical regions do not impair memory or exacerbate the impairment following lesions of the hippocampal formation. *Journal of Neuroscience, 9*, 1922–1936.

Zola-Morgan, S., Squire, L. R., Amaral, D. G., & Suzuki, W. A. (1989). Lesions of perirhinal and parahippocampal cortex that spare the amygdala and hippocampal formation produce severe memory impairment. *Journal of Neuroscience, 9*, 4355–4370.

Zola-Morgan, S., Squire, L. R., & Mishkin, M. (1982). The neuroanatomy of amnesia: Amygdala-hippocampus vs. temporal stem. *Science, 218*, 1337–1339.

Index